Atlas of
Primary Eyecare Procedures

Atlas of Primary Eyecare Procedures

Murray Fingeret, OD
Chief, Optometry Section
St. Albans Veterans Administration
Extended Care Center/Brooklyn Veterans Administration Medical Center
Brooklyn, New York
Assistant Clinical Professor of Optometry
College of Optometry
State University of New York
New York, New York
Adjunct Assistant Professor of Optometry
Pennsylvania College of Optometry
Philadelphia, Pennsylvania

Linda Casser, OD
Director, Indianapolis Clinics
Indiana University School of Optometry
Indianapolis, Indiana
Associate Professor of Optometry
Department of Clinical Sciences
Indiana University School of Optometry
Bloomington, Indiana

H. Ted Woodcome, OD
Chief, Eye Service
Genesee Valley Group Health
J. C. Wilson Health Center
Rochester, New York
Adjunct Assistant Clinical Professor of Optometry
College of Optometry
State University of New York
New York, New York

Illustrations by Susan C. Tilberry

With a Foreword by
Louis J. Catania, OD

APPLETON & LANGE
Norwalk, Connecticut/San Mateo, California

Notice: Our knowledge in clinical sciences is constantly changing. As new information becomes available, changes in treatment and in the use of drugs become necessary. The authors and the publisher of this volume have taken care to make certain that the doses of drugs and schedules of treatment are correct and compatible with the standards generally accepted at the time of publication. The reader is advised to consult carefully the instruction and information material included in the package insert of each drug or therapeutic agent before administration. This advice is especially important when using new or infrequently used drugs.

Copyright © 1990 by Appleton & Lange
A Publishing Division of Prentice Hall

All rights reserved. This book, or any parts thereof, may not be used or reproduced in any manner without written permission. For information, address Appleton & Lange, 25 Van Zant Street, East Norwalk, Connecticut 06855.

92 93 94 / 10 9 8 7 6 5 4 3 2

Prentice Hall International (UK) Limited, *London*
Prentice Hall of Australia Pty. Limited, *Sydney*
Prentice Hall Canada, Inc., *Toronto*
Prentice Hall Hispanoamericana, S.A., *Mexico*
Prentice Hall of India Private Limited, *New Delhi*
Prentice Hall of Japan, Inc., *Tokyo*
Simon & Schuster Asia Pte. Ltd., *Singapore*
Editora Prentice Hall do Brasil Ltda., *Rio de Janeiro*
Prentice Hall, *Englewood Cliffs, New Jersey*

Library of Congress Cataloging-in-Publication Data

Fingeret, Murray.
    Atlas of primary eyecare procedures / Murray Fingeret, Linda
Casser, H. Ted Woodcome; illustrations by Susan C. Tilberry.
        p.   cm.
    Includes bibliographical references.
    ISBN 0-8385-0134-6
    1. Optometry—Atlases. I. Casser, Linda. II. Woodcome, H. Ted.
III. Title.
    [DNLM: 1. Eye Diseases—diagnosis—atlases. 2. Eye Diseases—
therapy—atlases.   WW 17 F497a]
RE952.F56   1990
617.7—dc20
DNLM/DLC
for Library of Congress   90-11
                                                           CIP

Editor: R. Craig Percy
Designer: Steve Byrum
Index: Jean Wilson

PRINTED IN THE UNITED STATES OF AMERICA

Dedicated to

our families
Janet and Stuart
Keith Locke
AnnMarie, Jonathan, Jessica

Without their support, understanding, and encouragement
this project would not have been possible

Contents

Section IX   Physical Examination Procedures

Section X   Preoperative and Postoperative Cataract Procedures

Foreword

Good primary eyecare requires three things of a practitioner: caring, commitment, and competency. The absence or weakness of any one of these elements effectively reduces primary care to a support service or a technical skill; no doubt valuable, but not primary care.

The elements of caring and commitment are often written about, talked about, and taught in numerous innovative and provocative methods. Notwithstanding all such efforts, there are fundamental character traits and desires required in practitioners and students to be able to successfully acquire and communicate the qualities of caring and commitment. When these traits and desires are present, the results are usually self-evident and rewarding to teacher, student, and patient.

Meanwhile, the third element of primary care, competency, which encompasses examination, diagnosis, and management, is the element most textbooks address. Most optometric texts concentrate on the area of ocular diagnosis because of its critical importance in disease, and on management because of the emphasis on effective outcomes in all primary health care. However, neither effective management nor proper diagnosis would be possible without a knowledge and understanding of the procedures and techniques used. Indeed, such techniques are the means by which practitioners administer their examination, arrive at their diagnosis, and often the method by which they provide their treatment and management.

Not since Arthur H. Keeney's book, *Ocular Examination: Basis and Technique*, written in the early 1970s, has a comprehensive textbook on ocular procedures and techniques been attempted. Never, in fact, has there been an illustrated "atlas" with straightforward, step-by-step descriptions of common eye procedures used regularly in primary eyecare practice. Thus, *Atlas of Primary Eyecare Procedures* is truly a valuable and unique contribution for eyecare practitioners and optometric students who must master appropriate technique before they can hope to arrive at proper diagnoses and management plans.

Now, what if a valuable, needed, and unique textbook the nature of *Atlas of Primary Eyecare Procedures* were able to capture in its technical descriptions, the qualities of caring and commitment mentioned above as the other two fundamental elements in true primary eyecare? That accomplishment would certainly make this textbook the ideal book for every optometric practitioner and student. It would also require some very special authors with the knowledge and skills to complete such a task and the character traits and desires to turn such technical expertise into primary care. Please allow me to share with you the fact that the authors of this textbook, Murray Fingeret, Linda Casser, and Ted Woodcome, are exactly the people in optometry to have achieved this extraordinary task.

I have had the honor and pleasure over a fourteen-year period of working with each of these individuals as students, residents (all at the J. C. Wilson Health Center in Rochester, New York), and now as clinical practitioners and educators in the optometric profession. From my perspective, when it comes to the qualities and skills of caring, commitment, and competency attendant to primary eyecare, these three people have added new dimensions to each of those elements. Although at one point I may have been the teacher, their depth of human qualities, caring, and commitment has turned me into their devoted student. Their contributions and dedication to the optometric profession, patient care, and education continue to help us all grow, improve, and better serve our patients.

It is with a mixture of personal and professional pride and joy that I humbly present to the optometric profession and, indeed, to the health care literature at large, this unique and valuable textbook for eyecare practitioners and students. And it is with even greater pride and joy, on behalf of my profession and the patients who shall benefit from our efforts and the knowledge gained from this book, that I thank the authors and congratulate their achievement.

Louis J. Catania, OD

Introduction

The scope and practice of optometry has continued to evolve over the past 10 to 15 years, along with the diagnostic and therapeutic procedures that help define the profession. Procedures unfamiliar to us a number of years ago are now incorporated into our daily routines. The purpose of the *Atlas of Primary Eyecare Procedures* is to provide a pictorial guide supported by didactic information that enables the clinician to become familiar with many of these important clinical procedures.

Our goal is for students, residents, and practicing optometrists to refer to this book in the clinical setting as these procedures are performed. The *Atlas* is not intended as an all-inclusive textbook covering comprehensive information on the diagnosis, treatment, and management of clinical conditions associated with each technique. A suggested reading list is included for each section to provide the reader with sources of supplementary information.

There are often several generally accepted methods of performing any of these procedures. We have tried to solicit opinions from different clinicians for each procedure and, when applicable, to present alternative approaches. Even so, a bias is inherent in this book whereby the majority of techniques illustrated are those we have used during our primary care experience. These methods do not constitute the "only" way to do a procedure, but are those with which we are most familiar and wish to share with our readers.

Each procedure section is composed of several parts: Description/Indications, Instrumentation, Technique, Interpretation, and Contraindications/ Complications. Before performing any technique the reader should review the procedure in total, become familiar with the equipment, and visualize how the procedure is done, referring back to the illustrations as needed. When attempting a new, unfamiliar procedure, a colleague more experienced in the technique may be a valuable resource to aid in acquiring the skill. Continuing education courses are also available to acquaint each practitioner with many of these techniques. Of course, patient well-being should always be of paramount importance when performing any of these procedures.

Throughout the *Atlas* certain assumptions are made that are not specified in each section: each clinician will wash his or her hands or use gloves as indicated, and any instruments used are appropriately cleaned and asepticized/sterilized before and after each procedure.

We hope the *Atlas* will help expand the scope and mode of practice of the profession of optometry and will further challenge our colleagues in their pursuit of knowledge in providing the highest quality care for their patients.

Murray Fingeret, OD
Linda Casser, OD
H. Ted Woodcome, OD

Acknowledgments

There were many individuals who directly or indirectly contributed to the development of this book. Most will not recognize they did anything special, but their assistance will always be appreciated. During our residencies at the J. C. Wilson Health Center in Rochester, New York, the Eye Service professional and support staff greatly assisted us throughout our training, often going above and beyond what was expected to aid us in any way possible.

In particular, we are indebted to Dr. Louis J. Catania for nurturing us through our initial days in primary care optometry, for providing on-going guidance and inspiration, and for always challenging us to be the best we can be.

For illustrations on the color plates, the first
number is that of the procedure and the second is
the figure number in the procedure. Illustrations on
the color plates are also reproduced in black and
white with their relevant procedures.

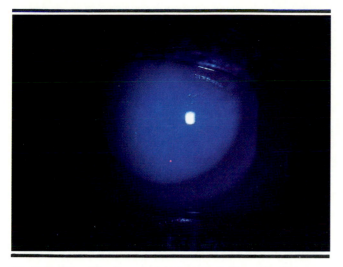

12–1. B. When illuminated with the cobalt filter, the Fleischer ring of keratoconus appears black.

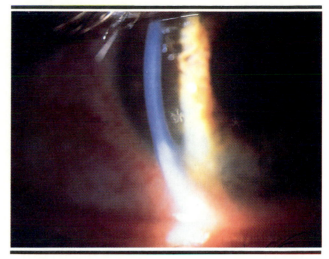

12–3. B. Two small herpes simplex dendritic ulcers are visible in indirect illumination.

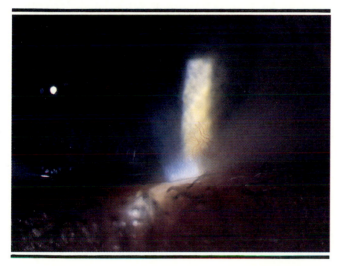

12–4. A. A limbal neovascular tuft is seen in retroillumination.

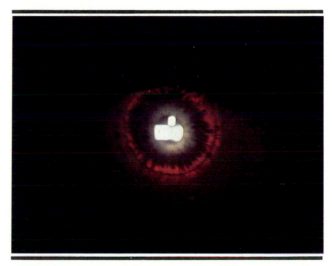

14–2. Extensive peripheral iris transillumination defects are present in this patient with pigment dispersion syndrome. (Courtesy of David W. Sloan, OD.)

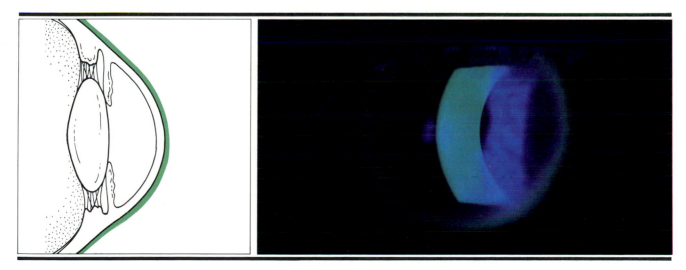

15–3. The intact precorneal tear film (schematic, left) appears uniformly green when stained with fluorescein sodium and illuminated with cobalt filter of the slit lamp (right).

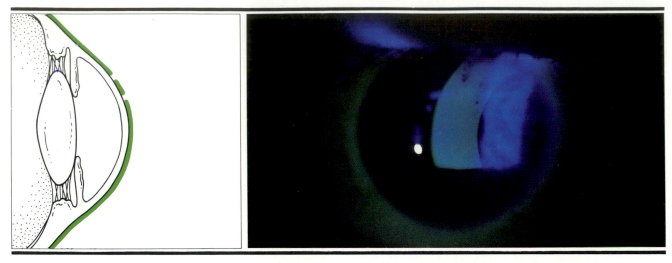

15—4. Dry areas appear as black spots or streaks in the fluorescein-stained precorneal tear film.

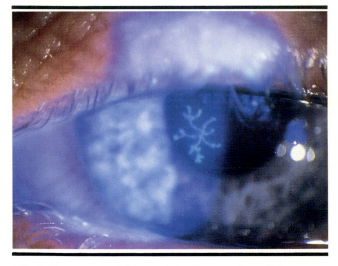

16—4. The cornea exhibits positive fluorescein sodium staining secondary to a herpes simplex dendritic ulcer.

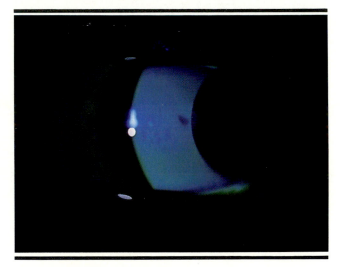

16—5. The cornea exhibits negative fluorescein sodium staining centrally secondary to epithelial bullae resulting from Fuchs' endothelial dystrophy.

16—6. (right) The bulbar conjunctiva and cornea exhibits rose bengal staining secondary to keratitis sicca.

17—4. B. (far right) The corneal reflection of the applanation tonometer probe will appear as two pale blue semicircles, which are used to center the probe.

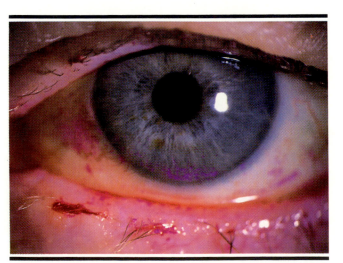

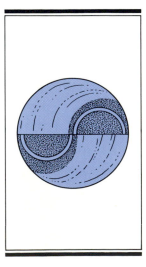

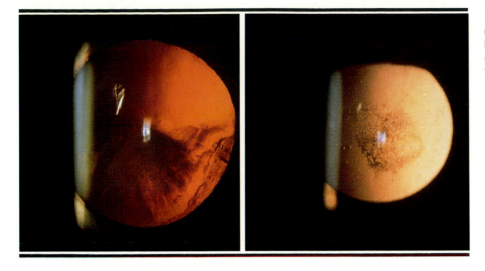

19—6. A. (far left) A cortical cataract as seen using retroillumination. **B.** (left) A posterior subcapsular cataract as seen using retroillumination.

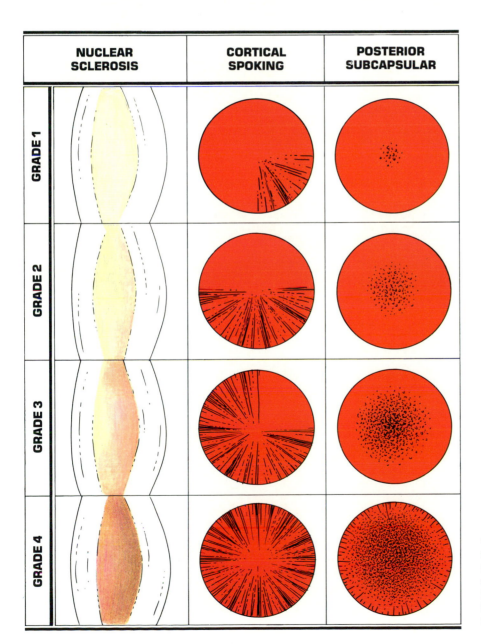

NUCLEAR SCLEROSIS	CORTICAL SPOKING	POSTERIOR SUBCAPSULAR
GRADE 1		
GRADE 2		
GRADE 3		
GRADE 4		

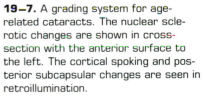

19—7. A grading system for age-related cataracts. The nuclear sclerotic changes are shown in cross-section with the anterior surface to the left. The cortical spoking and posterior subcapsular changes are seen in retroillumination.

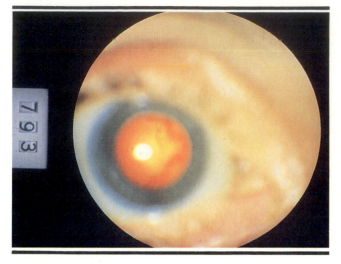

20—5. A. A posterior vitreous detachment may be detected by the large vitreous floater visible with distal direct ophthalmoscopy.

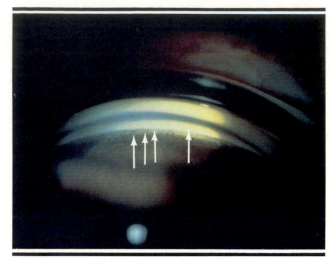

21—4. A wide-open angle as visualized with gonioscopy. The arrows going from left to right indicate the ciliary body band, scleral spur, trabecular meshwork, and Schwalbe's line.

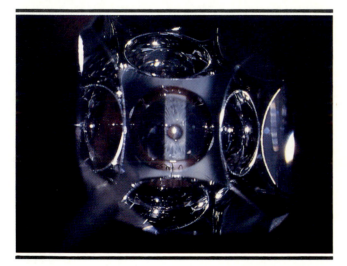

22—4. A. The minified view of the iris and pupil as seen through the center of the 4-mirror goniolens prior to corneal contact.

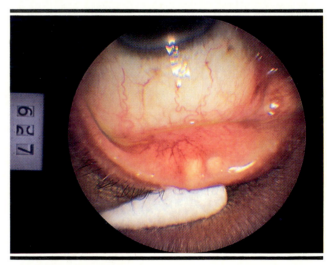

27—2. Occlusive sebaceous distention of the meibomian gland is visible as yellow "streaking" through the overlying palpebral conjunctiva.

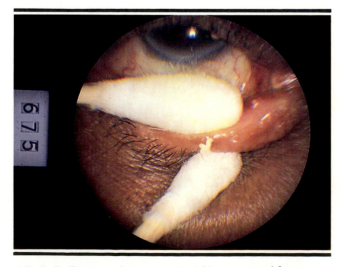

27—4. B. Cheesy sebaceous material is expressed from a meibomian gland in the right lower lid.

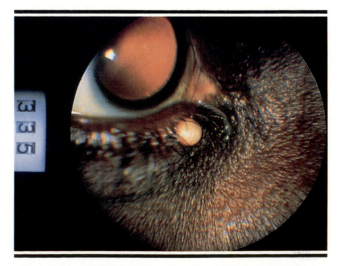

28—1. The superficial sebaceous cyst appears as a well-demarcated, creamy white, smooth, round nodule.

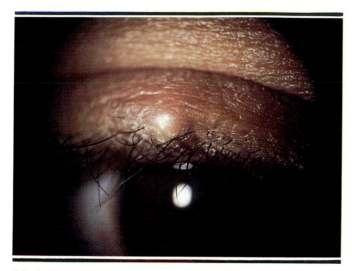

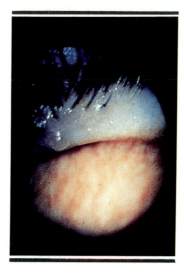

29—1. Sudoriferous cysts appear as one or more small, noninflamed, avascular, clear fluid-filled cysts on the anterior lid margin.

28—2. The deeper sebaceous cyst is more flesh-toned in color and less well demarcated.

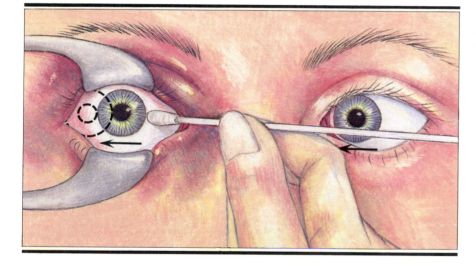

42—4. An ecchymotic right eye is seen with a sixth nerve paresis. With forced duction testing full range of movements is seen.

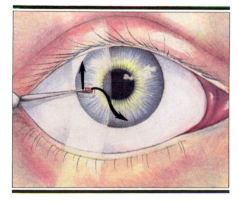

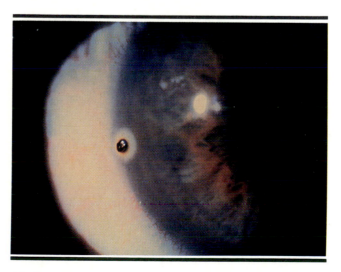

44—7. B. The spud is seen underneath the corneal foreign body. The head is flicked upward to dislodge the foreign body.

45—1. A metallic foreign body on the cornea, surrounded by a ring of rust and edema.

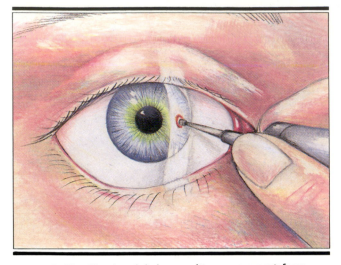

45—4. A. The Algerbrush being used to remove rust from the corneal surface.

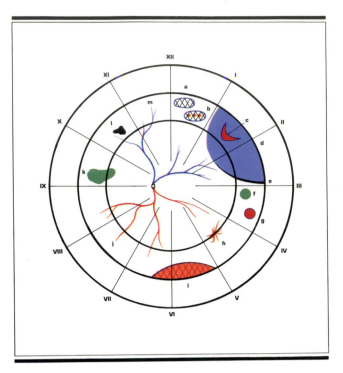

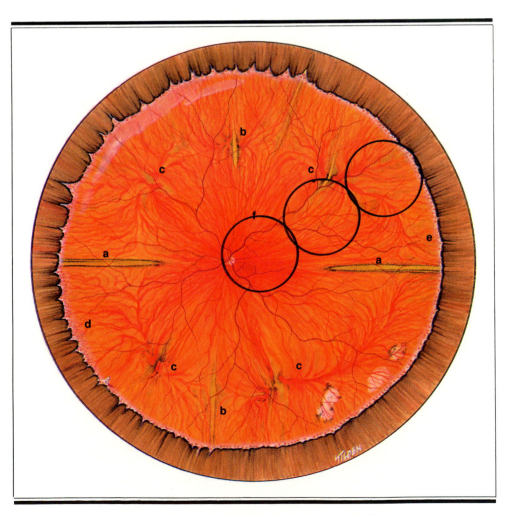

53—6. Ocular fundus with anatomical landmarks. (a) Long posterior ciliary artery and nerve. (b) Short posterior ciliary artery. (c) Vortex vein. (d) Vitreous base (nasal). (e) Vitreous base (temporal). (f) 20 D lens view. (Courtesy of Anthony Cavallerano, OD.)

58—6. (left) The fundus drawing color coding system. (a) Lattice. (b) Lattice with holes. (c) Flap tear. (d) Detached retina. (e) Demarcation line. (f) Operculum. (g) Retinal hole. (h) Vortex vein. (i) Retinal dialysis. (j) Retinal arterioles. (k) Vitreous opacity. (l) Retinal or choroidal nevus. (m) Retinal veins. The universal color code for fundus drawing is given below.

RED

Solid

- Retinal arterioles
- Vortex veins
- Attached retina
- Preretinal and intraretinal hemorrhages
- Normal fovea/red cross
- Retinal neovascularization
- Open areas of retinal breaks (tears/holes)
- Open area of outer layer retinoschisis holes
- Vascular anomalies (collaterals, shunts, etc.)

Crosslined

- Open area of giant tears and retinal dialysis
- Inner area of thinned retina
- Open area of inner layer retinoschisis holes
- Inner area of chorioretinal atrophy

BLACK

- Pigment within detached retina
- Borders of chorioretinal atrophy
- Choroidal nevus
- RPE hypertrophy or choroidal pigment
- Demarcation lines at attached edge of detached retina or within detached retina
- Edge of buckle beneath attached retina
- Sheathed vessels, outlined or solid, depending upon degree
- Pigmented outline of short and long posterior ciliary arteries and nerves
- Posttreatment pigmentation following diathermy, cryotherapy, or photocoagulation

GREEN

Solid

- Cotton wool patches
- Vitreous hemorrhage
- Vitreous membranes
- Intraocular foreign body
- Media opacities (label)
- Ora serrata pearls
- Prepapillary (hyaloid) annular opacity
- Outline of elevated neovascularization
- Retinal operculum

Dotted

- Asteroid hyalosis
- Snowflake deposits on lattice degeneration and retinioschisis

BLUE

Solid

- Retinal veins
- Detached retina
- Detached fovea (blue cross)
- Intraretinal cysts
- Outline of ora serrata
- Outline of lattice degeneration
- Outline of flat neovascularization
- Outline of retinal breaks (holes, tears)
- Outline of thinned retinal areas
- Vitreoretinal traction tufts
- Cystic retinal tufts
- Circumferential, fixed, meridional, or radial folds

Crosslined

- Rolled edges of retinal tear
- White with or without pressure (label)
- Inner layer of retinoschisis
- Detached pars plana epithelium anterior to detached ora serrata
- Outline of change in area or folds of detached retina because of shifting fluid

Stippled

- Peripheral cystoid degeneration

BROWN

- Pigment beneath detached retina
- Choroidal melanoma
- Ciliary processes
- Pars plana cysts
- Uveal tissue
- Striae ciliaris
- Edge of buckle beneath detached retina
- Outline of posterior staphyloma
- Outline of chorioretinal atrophy beneath detached retina
- Choroidal detachment
- Fibrous demarcation lines

YELLOW

Solid

- RPE level deposits
- Serous or hemorrhagic detached fovea drawn as yellow cross
- Long and short ciliary nerves
- Postphotocoagulation retinal edema
- Severe intraretinal and subretinal exudation

Dotted

- Drusen
- Intraretinal and subretinal exudates

58—7. An example of fundus drawing: retinal tear with detachment.

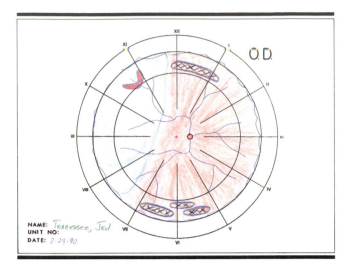

79—1. A. (below left) Protruding suture barbs. **B.** (below right) Same protruding suture barbs seen with fluorescein and the cobalt filter. (Courtesy of David E. Magnus, OD.)

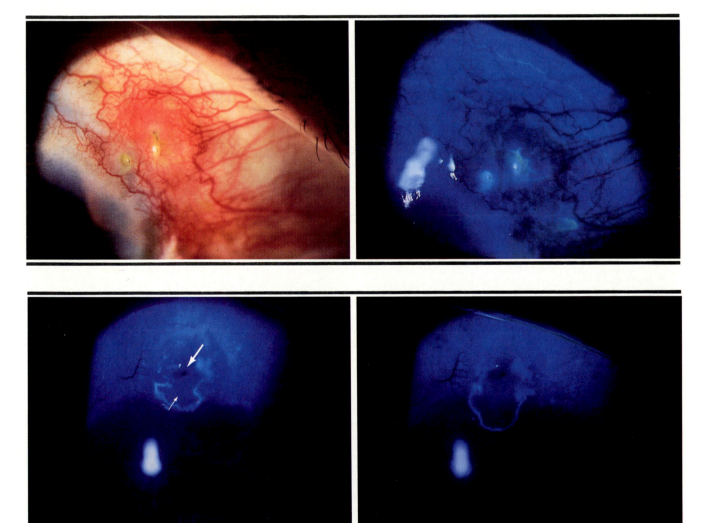

80—1. A. A localized brilliant green fluorescence occurs at the wound site (large arrow), with clear aqueous leaking into the fluorescein (small arrow) demonstrating a positive Seidel test. (Courtesy of David E. Magnus, OD.)

80—1. B. The bright fluorescein is displaced as the aqueous continues to leak. (Courtesy of David E. Magnus, OD.)

Atlas of
Primary Eyecare Procedures

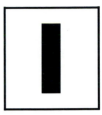

Ophthalmic Pharmaceutical Procedures

1 Drop Instillation and Punctal Occlusion: Adults

Description/Indications. The use of topical ophthalmic pharmaceutical solutions or suspensions is integral to ocular examination, diagnosis, and treatment. The categories of topical ophthalmic drops used diagnostically in-office include anesthetics, mydriatics, miotics, and cycloplegics.

Systemic absorption of topical ophthalmic drops occurs through the nasopharyngeal mucosa via the puncta. Resultant adverse systemic side effects are potentially serious following the use of agents such as topical beta-adrenergic blockers. Systemic absorption of topical ophthalmic drops may be significantly reduced by punctal occlusion to minimize the amount of medication entering the nasolacrimal system. Indications for punctal occlusion following the instillation of ophthalmic drops include the use of 10% phenylephrine to avoid a hypertensive crisis, beta-adrenergic blocking agents to avoid breathing difficulties and bradycardia, and other adrenergic agents to avoid tachycardia and hypertensive crisis.

Instrumentation. Desired ophthalmic solution or suspension, facial tissues.

Technique. Recheck the label of the bottle to ensure that the correct solution or suspension was chosen, and remove the cap. When appropriate, advise the patient that a mild, transient burning sensation may be expected.

Ask the patient to tilt the head back slightly so that the chin is slightly elevated, and to look up and back (Fig. 1). Using the forefinger of one hand, evert the lower lid slightly so that a "trough" is formed by the inferior cul-de-sac. Holding the opened bottle in the opposite hand and stabilizing it by resting the little and/or ring fingers on the patient's cheek or nose as appropriate, squeeze a drop or two as desired into the exposed cul-de-sac (Fig. 2A). Release the lower lid and ask the patient to gently blot away the excess fluid with a tissue, or blot away the excess fluid from the lid area yourself using a tissue. If desired, advise the patient to keep the lids closed for a few seconds, waiting for any associated burning to subside. Alternatively, a one-handed technique may be performed using the little and/or ring fingers to evert the lower lid while the drop is instilled (Fig. 2B).

When indicated, occlude the puncta following drop instillation. Ask the patient to close the eyes and hold your index finger firmly over the nasolacrimal sac, upper and lower canaliculi, and the medial palpebral ligament in the nasal canthus. Use relatively firm pressure to collapse the sac against the nasolacrimal bone for approximately 1 minute (Fig. 3A). Do this for each eye in which drops are instilled. The patient may be advised to bilaterally occlude the puncta himself or herself by straddling the bridge of the nose with thumb and forefinger after closing the eyes (Fig. 3B). Alternatively, instruct the patient to close the eyes for 3 minutes following drop instillation. This will significantly reduce the amount of fluid pumped into the nasolacrimal system through action of the lids and orbicularis oculi muscles.

Contraindications/Complications. The examiner must be familiar with any contraindications that may preclude using a particular drug for a given patient. These contraindications may include drug allergies, drug–drug interactions, certain systemic conditions, and ocular anatomical considerations. Care must be taken to avoid contacting the tip of the dropper to the patient's cilia, lids, conjunctival surface, or tears, as contamination of the bottle's contents may occur.

A patient may exhibit mild to moderate anxiety upon having the eyedrops instilled, so that blepharospasm makes access to the cul-de-sac difficult. Added firmness is then required to open both the upper and lower lids. To instill drops in the right eye using this technique, use your left thumb to hold the lashes of the upper lid against the superior orbital rim. Use the little and/or ring finger of the right hand, which is holding the opened bottle, to simultaneously hold the lower lid (Fig. 4). As the patient looks up and back, squeeze the bottle to instill the drop into the palpebral fissure.

A patient may rarely experience vasovagal syncope following instillation of the drop. Should this occur, basic first-aid measures are taken. These include elevating the feet above the level of the head, passing a broken ammonia inhalant ampule beneath the nostrils, and monitoring the basic vital signs.

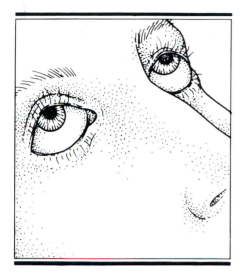

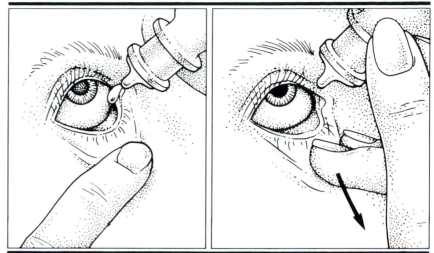

1. Instruct the patient to tilt the head back slightly and to look up and back.

2. A. Evert the lower lid slightly so that a "trough" is formed by the inferior cul-de-sac. Squeeze a drop or two, as desired, into the exposed cul-de-sac.

2. B. Alternatively, use the same hand to evert the lower lid and hold the bottle.

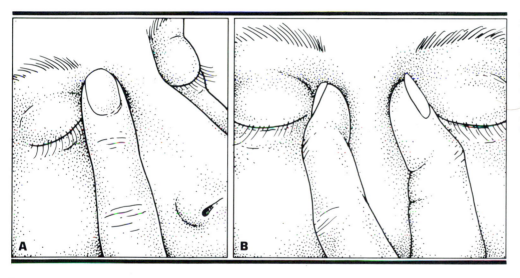

3. A. (far left) Hold your index finger firmly over the medial canthal area to occlude the canaliculi and collapse the lacrimal sac. **B.** (left) Patients themselves may be instructed to occlude the puncta bilaterally following drop instillation.

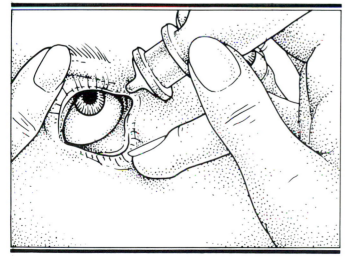

4. If blepharospasm occurs, use the left thumb to hold the upper lid lashes against the superior orbital rim. Use the little finger of the hand holding the dropper bottle to simultaneously hold the lower lid.

2 Drop Instillation and Punctal Occlusion: Young Children

Description/Indications. The use of topical ophthalmic pharmaceutical solutions or suspensions is integral to ocular examination, diagnosis, and treatment even for very young children. The categories of topical ophthalmic drops used diagnostically in-office most frequently include anesthetics, mydriatics, and cycloplegics.

Very young children may be resistant to or apprehensive about drop instillation. When gentle reassurance and persuasion with swift instillation have failed, or if the child becomes slightly combative after successful instillation of one drop in one eye, techniques of mild restraint may be instituted with the help of family members.

Instrumentation. Desired ophthalmic solution or suspension, facial tissues.

Technique. Reassure family members that the child's resistance is usually the result of apprehension rather than discomfort. Recheck the label of the bottle to ensure that the correct solution or suspension was chosen and remove the cap. Recline the young patient halfway in the examination chair. Ask an adult family member of the patient to cross the child's hands in his or her lap and to hold them firmly. Depending upon the size of the child, the family member may be able to use his or her forearms or a free arm to firmly hold the child's legs (Fig. 1).

To overcome the child's blepharospasm, you will need to firmly open the upper and lower lids. Use your left hand to hold the child's forehead steady and your left thumb to hold the upper lid against the superior orbital rim. Use the little and/or ring finger of your right hand, which is holding the opened bottle, to simultaneously hold the lower lid (Fig. 2). Squeeze the bottle and instill the drop into the palpebral fissure. Instill the drop into both eyes as quickly as possible. Blot the excess fluid and tears with tissue.

With extreme resistance of the very young child, it is helpful to have an assistant gently but firmly hold the side of the child's head. Alternatively, the child's arms may be held over his or her head to help hold the sides of the head in place as the drops are instilled (Fig. 3). Further holding of the feet and legs will reduce the child's tendency to kick.

Punctal occlusion may be desirable to reduce systemic absorption in the small child but may not be feasible if the child is restless. To occlude the punc-

tum following drop instillation, hold your index finger or another appropriately sized finger firmly over the nasolacrimal sac, the upper and lower canaliculi, and the medial palpebral ligament in the nasal canthus, while the child's eyes are closed. Use relatively firm pressure to collapse the sac against the nasolacrimal bone for 1 minute (Fig. 4). Do this for each eye in which drops were instilled. Alternatively, instruct a family member, whose hands have been washed, to occlude the puncta.

Contraindications/Complications. The examiner must be familiar with any contraindications of using a particular type of drug for a given patient, including allergies to the drug contents, drug–drug interactions, certain systemic conditions, and ocular anatomical considerations. This is especially important for young children with their smaller body weights. Care must be taken to avoid contacting the tip of the dropper to the patient's cilia, lids, conjunctival surface, or tears, as contamination of the bottle's contents may occur. Discuss with the family member symptoms of central nervous system toxicity of any long-acting anticholinergic agents used such as cyclopentolate or atropine.

Care must be taken to ensure that the child is held firmly but gently. Due to extreme blepharospasm the held upper lid may evert but will not affect instillation of the drop. It may be very difficult to spread the lids apart to instill the drops. In this instance a small pool of drops may be placed in the medial canthal area. Through capillarity some of the fluid will enter the conjunctival sac (reservoir effect). If the child is kicking or moving wildly, the child may injure himself or herself or others, or may damage equipment. Once the drops are instilled, the young child will usually calm down quickly when able to move around freely.

In attempting to instill the drops, the examiner may decide in extreme instances that the risk of physical or emotional trauma outweighs the need for the diagnostic agent. Use of these agents may then be deferred to a time when the child is better able to cooperate. When use of the agent(s) is absolutely necessary, referral may be made or consultation obtained to perform the procedure under mild sedation or even general anesthesia.

It is very unusual for a young child to experience vasovagal syncope following drop instillation. Should this occur, basic first-aid measures are taken.

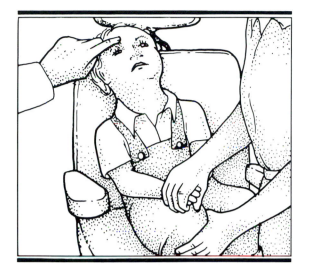

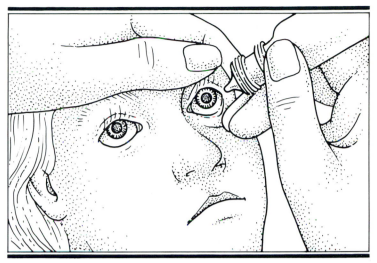

1. Recline the young child in the chair. Instruct a family member to gently restrain the child's hands and legs.

2. Use your left hand to hold the child's forehead and your left thumb to hold the upper lid. Use the little finger of your right hand to hold the lower lid.

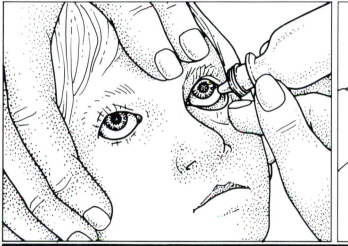

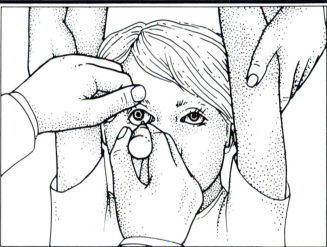

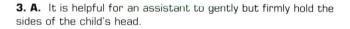

3. A. It is helpful for an assistant to gently but firmly hold the sides of the child's head.

3. B. Alternatively, holding the child's arms over the head will help to hold the head in place.

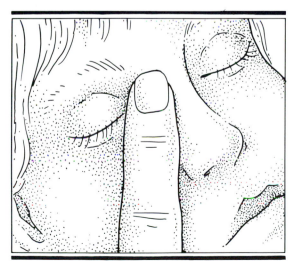

4. Hold a finger over the medial canthal area to minimize systemic absorption of the drops.

3 Pledget Use for Drops

Description/Indications. Small cotton pledgets placed in the conjunctival sac may be utilized as vehicles for the delivery of diagnostic pharmaceutical agents. They are used to maximize pupillary dilation by enhancing ocular contact time.

Maximum pupillary dilation does not always occur despite the use of several potent mydriatic or mydriatic/cycloplegic agents. Optimal dilation can be hampered by conditions such as excessive iris pigmentation, systemic diabetes mellitus, and posterior iris synechiae. The use of a small cotton pledget that has been saturated with the diagnostic agent(s) and placed in the conjunctival sac will increase ocular contact time and enhance the efficacy of the agent(s) in use. This technique is especially helpful in attempting to break posterior iris synechiae.

Instrumentation. Desired ophthalmic mydriatic or mydriatic/cycloplegic solutions, topical ophthalmic anesthetic drop, sterile cotton-tipped applicators, sterile jeweler's forceps, facial tissues.

Technique. Instill 1 to 2 drops of topical ophthalmic anesthetic solution in each eye (see p. 2). Pull off the soft tip of a sterile cotton-tipped applicator, and roll it between your thumb and forefinger to form a tiny ball approximately ⅛ inch in diameter (Fig. 1). Moisten this pledget with a routinely used combination of diagnostic agents such as 1% tropicamide and 2½% phenylephrine. Ask the patient to look up. Holding the pledget in one hand, gently retract the patient's lower lid with the opposite hand. Place the pledget in the inferior cul-de-sac (Fig. 2A). Use a second sterile cotton-tipped applicator to gently push the pledget into the fornix as the patient continues to look upward (Fig. 2B). Alternatively, use a sterile jeweler's forceps to place the pledget in the fornix (Fig. 3).

When necessary and appropriate, use greater concentrations of drugs, different mydriatic agents from those routinely used, or more potent solutions to achieve adequate dilation. Keep the pledget in place for up to 30 to 60 minutes to achieve the desired result. If maximum pupillary dilation is not achieved, instill additional diagnostic agents directly onto the pledget while it is positioned in the conjunctival sac (Fig. 4).

Once in position the pledget will be apparent externally as a small bulge in the lower lid, which the patient may feel as a slight fullness (Fig. 5). Instruct the patient to continue to look up while the pledget is in place or to close the eyes. If the pledget slips or moves, it may be repositioned with the sterile cotton-tipped applicator or jeweler's forceps.

To remove the pledget, ask the patient to look up. While retracting the lower lid with one hand, use the jeweler's forceps to carefully remove the pledget.

Contraindications/Complications. The examiner must be familiar with any contraindications of using a particular type of drug for a given patient, including allergies to the drug contents, drug–drug interactions, certain systemic conditions, and ocular anatomical considerations. Enhanced ocular contact time through the use of a cotton pledget may result in greater ocular and systemic side effects. For this reason some clinicians advise against using 10% phenylephrine on a pledget. Systemic absorption can be minimized if the patient is instructed to keep the eyes closed while the pledget is in place. When adding solution directly onto the pledget, care must be taken to avoid contacting the tip of the dropper to the patient's cilia, lids, conjunctival surface, or tears, as contamination of the bottle's contents may occur.

If the pledget is inadequately placed in the inferior fornix or if the patient moves the eyes excessively following pledget insertion, it may slip out of position, and cause corneal irritation, or it may fall out completely. Any resultant corneal irritation is generally minor and transient, usually requiring treatment only with artificial tears. Care should be taken when manipulating the jeweler's forceps near the globe.

A patient may rarely experience vasovagal syncope following instillation of the pledget. Should this occur, basic first-aid measures are taken. These include elevating the feet above the level of the head, passing a broken ammonia inhalant ampule beneath the nostrils, and monitoring the basic vital signs.

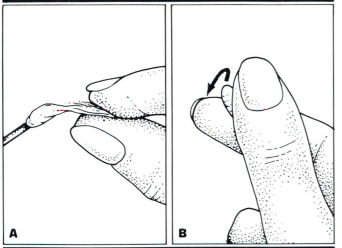

1. A. Pull off the extreme tip of a sterile cotton-tipped applicator. **B.** Roll it between your fingers to form a small ball.

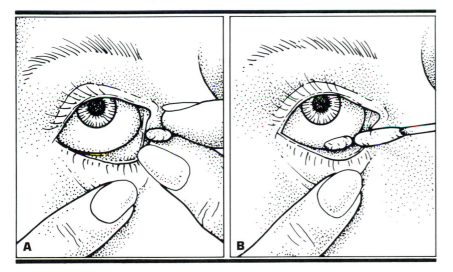

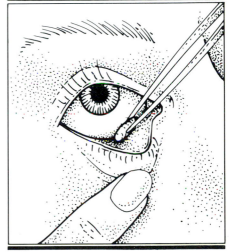

2. A. Place the moistened pledget in the inferior cul-de-sac. **B.** Use a sterile cotton-tipped applicator to position the pledget.

3. A jeweler's forceps may be used to place the pledget into the eye.

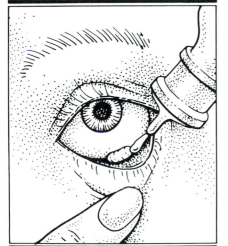

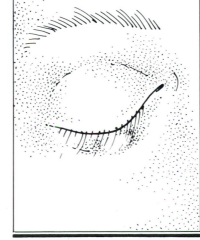

4. (far left) When necessary, resaturate the pledget with the desired pharmaceutical agent(s).

5. (left) The pledget is apparent as a small bulge in the lower lid.

4 Sector Pupil Dilation

Description/Indications. Patients with very narrow anterior chamber angles may require a more detailed evaluation of the media and retina than can be achieved through an undilated pupil, but because of the narrow angles full pupillary dilation is contraindicated. A vertically oval pupil may be produced by focal adrenergic stimulation of the radially oriented iris dilator muscles. This sector pupillary dilation will allow for a more thorough posterior chamber evaluation while minimizing the risk of acute angle closure glaucoma. The use of a sterile cotton-tipped applicator moistened with phenylephrine ophthalmic solution will allow for localized and controlled delivery of the diagnostic agent.

Instrumentation. Phenylephrine in a 2½% ophthalmic solution, topical ophthalmic anesthetic drop, sterile cotton-tipped applicators, facial tissues.

Technique. Instill 1 to 2 drops of topical ophthalmic anesthetic solution in each eye (see p. 2). Moisten the tip of a sterile cotton-tipped applicator with 2 to 3 drops of 2½% phenylephrine (Fig. 1). Ask the patient to look up. While steadying your hand on the patient's cheek, hold the moistened cotton-tipped applicator at the 6 o'clock position of the limbus for 15 to 20 seconds (Fig. 2). Repeat the procedure for the opposite eye if desired using a fresh cotton-tipped applicator. Monitor for sector dilation after approximately 20 to 30 minutes (Fig.

3). If the dilation is inadequate, repeat the technique for another 10 to 15-second interval.

Alternatively, moisten the 5-mm-long tip of a lengthwise portion of a Schirmer tear strip (see p. 108) with either 2½% phenylephrine or 1% epinephrine. Position the strip centrally in the lower lid near the 6 o'clock position of the corneal limbus. When phenylephrine is used for sector dilation, keep the strip in place for approximately 30 seconds; when epinephrine is used keep the strip in place for approximately 1 minute.

Contraindications/Complications. The examiner must be familiar with any contraindications of using a particular type of drug for a given patient, including allergies to the drug contents, drug–drug interactions, certain systemic conditions, and ocular anatomical considerations. Excessive contact time of the moistened cotton-tipped applicator may result in unintentional full pupillary dilation. If the applicator is saturated with too much phenylephrine, contact of the applicator with the globe may "squeeze" excess solution into the sac and will also cause excessive dilation.

If the cotton-tipped applicator slips out of position or if the patient moves the eyes excessively, corneal irritation may result. Any resultant irritation is generally minor and transient, usually requiring treatment only with artificial tears.

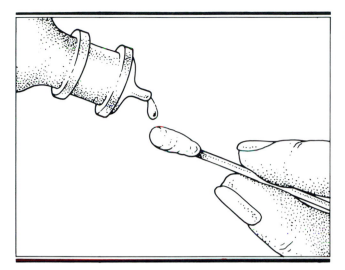

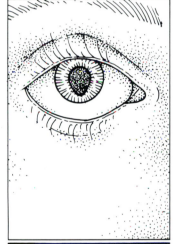

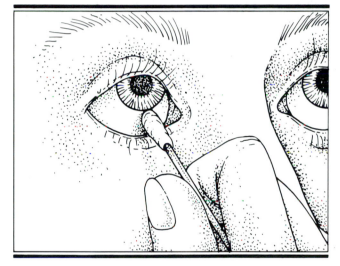

1. Moisten the cotton-tipped applicator with 2–3 drops of 2½% phenylephrine.

2. With the patient looking up, hold the applicator at the 6 o'clock position on the limbus for 15 seconds.

3. Resultant sector dilation of the pupil.

5 Ointment Application: Conjunctival Sac

Description/Indications. The most common indication for in-office ointment application into the conjunctival sac is the use of ophthalmic topical antibiotic ointment in pressure patching for a corneal wound or injury (see p. 156).

Instrumentation. Desired ophthalmic ointment, topical ophthalmic anesthetic solution, facial tissues.

Technique. Recline the patient slightly in the examination chair. As needed following the ocular evaluation, instill another drop of topical ophthalmic anesthetic solution (see p. 2).

Ask the patient to look up over his or her head. Recheck the label of the ointment to ensure that the correct preparation was chosen, and remove the cap of the tube. With the thumb and forefinger of one hand, gently pinch the lower lid away from the globe so that the inferior cul-de-sac forms a small pouch. Simultaneously squeeze a small bolus of ointment into the cul-de-sac while reminding the patient to keep looking upwards (Fig. 1). Twist the tube slightly to interrupt the ointment flow. Release the lower lid.

Release of the lower lid will often cause a small amount of the ointment to exude. To retain this exuded ointment within the conjunctival sac, gently grasp the lashes of the upper lid between the thumb and forefinger of one hand while the patient is looking up (Fig. 2A). Instruct the patient to slowly close the eyes, and while he or she does so, gently lift the upper lid up and over the exuded ointment until the lid margins are apposed (Fig. 2B). Instruct the patient to keep both eyes closed while the pressure patch is applied.

Contraindications/Complications. The examiner must be familiar with any contraindications of using a particular type of ointment for a given patient, including allergies to the drug contents, drug–drug interactions, and so on. Care must be taken to avoid contacting the tip of the tube to the patient's cilia, lids, conjunctival surface, or tears, as contamination of the tube's contents may occur.

If excessive amounts of ointment exude when the patient closes the lids, the examiner may elect to repeat the instillation of ointment before pressure patching. To do so, gently wipe away the excess ointment from the surface of the lids as the patient's eyes are closed. Ointment residue on the lids will make grasping of the slippery lower lid difficult for reinstillation of the medication.

If grasping of the upper lid is used to reduce the amount of ointment exudation when the patient closes the lids, care must be taken not to "overshoot" the lower lid margin with the upper lid. Doing so may result in entrapment of the lower lashes so that they come in contact with the globe under the patch.

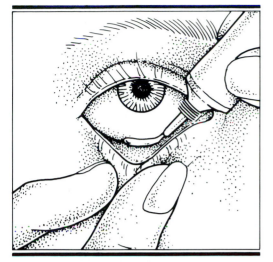

1. Gently pinch the lower lid to form a small pouch as the patient looks up. Apply the ointment into the cul-de-sac.

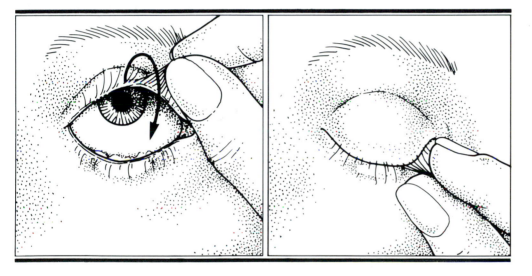

2. A. To minimize ointment exudation, grasp the lashes of the upper lid as the patient looks up.

2. B. Gently lift the upper lid up and over the palpebral aperture as the patient slowly closes the lids.

6 Patient Instructions: Drop Instillation

Description/Indications. For a variety of diagnostic or therapeutic reasons a patient may be instructed to instill drops into his or her own eyes out of the office. In addition to ensuring compliance with medication dosage, it is important that the patient utilize an effective technique to instill the drops. Verbal instructions, written instructions, demonstration, and practice are effective ways of maximizing patient compliance and, therefore, therapeutic effectiveness.

Instrumentation. Desired ophthalmic solution or suspension, facial tissues, wall or stand-mounted mirror.

Technique. Advise the patient to wash the hands, verify that the bottle chosen is correct, and remove the cap of the bottle. Ask the patient to look directly into a mirror. To instill drops into the right eye, have the patient tilt the head slightly to the left and gently pull down the lower lid with the index finger of his or her left hand to form a trough. As the patient holds the dropper bottle in the area of the lateral canthus with right hand, advise him or her to squeeze 1 to 2 drops into the trough formed by the cul-de-sac and then straighten the head (Fig. 1). The procedure is repeated for the left eye by tilting the head to the right, gently retracting the lower lid with the index finger of the right hand, and holding the dropper bottle in the left hand (Fig. 2). Alternatively, if the patient has a strongly dominant hand, the hand holding the bottle may reach across to the lateral canthal area when instilling drops into the contralateral eye.

When indicated, to minimize systemic absorption of the solution or suspension, advise the patient to occlude the puncta bilaterally for 1 minute or to close the eyes for 3 minutes (see p. 2). A tissue may be used to blot away the excess fluid. Advise the patient to wash the hands and recap the bottle.

Contraindications/Complications. The examiner must be familiar with any contraindications of a particular type of drug for a given patient, including allergies to the drug contents, drug–drug interactions, certain systemic conditions, and ocular anatomical considerations. The patient must be advised to avoid contacting the tip of the dropper to the cilia, lids, conjunctival surface, or tears, as contamination of the bottle's contents may occur. If the patient seems to be using an excessive amount of drop refills or if the treated condition is poorly controlled, reassessing the patient's drop instillation technique may be helpful.

When appropriate, it is helpful to advise a patient that certain eyedrops may produce a mild, transient burning sensation. This patient education may prevent poor compliance due to discomfort and can be used as an indicator that the drop was properly instilled. Some preparations may be refrigerated to reduce burning, and the sensation of cold may be used to verify proper instillation. Instruct the patient using steroid suspensions to vigorously shake the bottle 15 to 30 times before instilling the drop.

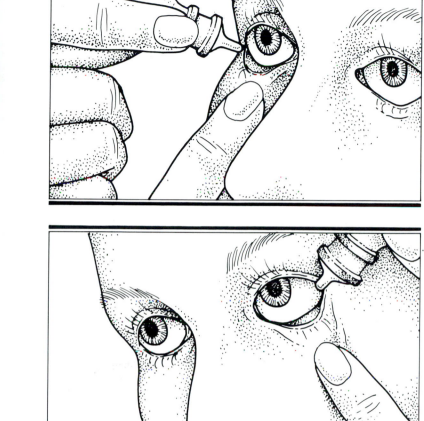

1. The patient looks into a mirror, tilts the head to the left, and retracts the right lower lid. The drop is instilled at the right lateral canthus and the head is straightened.

2. The technique is reversed to instill drops into the left eye.

7 Patient Instructions: Ointment Application to Lid Margins

Description/Indications. Topical ophthalmic ointment is usually the preferred drug vehicle for treating the majority of eyelid conditions. Ointments applied to the lid margins also act as drug reservoirs, providing therapeutic levels of medication to the globe by melting into the conjunctival sac. As a result, ointment applied to the lid may be chosen for the treatment of conjunctival disorders. This technique is especially useful in treating patients for whom manual dexterity is problematic or for treating very young children.

In addition to ensuring compliance with medication dosage, it is important that the patient utilize an effective technique to apply the ointment to his or her lids. Verbal instructions, written instructions, and demonstration are effective ways of maximizing patient compliance.

Instrumentation. Desired ophthalmic ointment, cotton-tipped applicators, facial tissues, wall or stand-mounted mirror.

Technique. Advise the patient to wash the hands, to verify the label on the ointment to be applied, and to remove the cap of the tube. Instruct the patient to apply a ½ to ¾-inch ribbon of ointment onto one index finger (Fig. 1A). Closing the eyes, the ointment is applied along the lid margins, moving from the medial canthus to the lateral canthus (Fig. 1B). Additional reservoir effect is achieved when a small dab of the ointment is placed at the lateral canthus. This technique is repeated for both eyes. If an area of the lid other than the margin is being treated, the ointment is similarly applied in the appropriate area, using a mirror as needed. Instruct the patient to wash the hands and recap the tube.

Alternatively, ointment may be applied to the lid margins using a cotton-tipped applicator. Instruct the patient to apply a ½-inch ribbon of ointment to the applicator tip (Fig. 2A). Advise the patient to look into the mirror and carefully apply the ointment to the upper and lower lid margins (Fig. 2B and C).

When ointment applied to the lid margins is used for its reservoir effect to the conjunctiva, excess lid ointment may be gently wiped away with a tissue after 3 to 5 minutes without reducing the therapeutic effect.

Contraindications/Complications. The examiner must be familiar with any contraindications of using a particular type of drug for a given patient, including allergies to the drug contents and drug–drug interactions. The patient should be advised that transient blurred vision is common following application of ointment to the lid margins. If a cotton-tipped applicator is used to apply ointment to the lid margin, the patient must be instructed to use careful technique while looking in the mirror so that superficial injury to the globe does not occur.

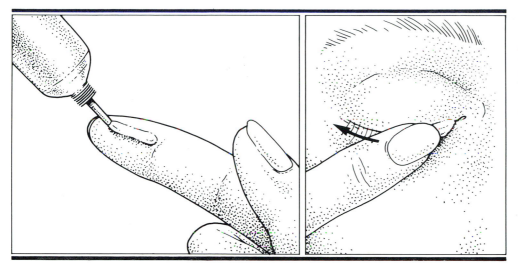

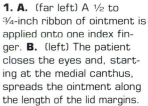

1. A. (far left) A ½ to ¾-inch ribbon of ointment is applied onto one index finger. **B.** (left) The patient closes the eyes and, starting at the medial canthus, spreads the ointment along the length of the lid margins.

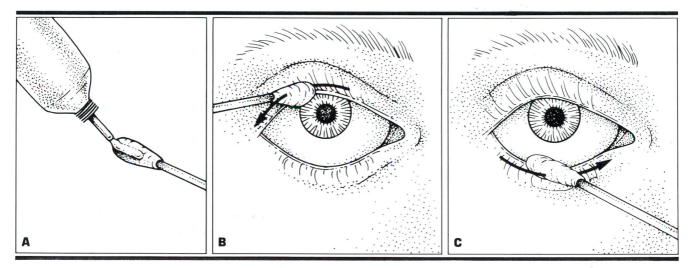

A

B

C

2. A. A ½-inch ribbon of ointment is applied to the cotton-tipped applicator. **B.** While looking in the mirror, ointment is applied with the applicator to the upper lid margin and (**C**) to the lower lid margin.

8 Patient Instructions: Ointment Application to Conjunctival Sac

Description/Indications. Topical ophthalmic ointments applied into the conjunctival sac are prescribed for a number of anterior segment disorders. In addition to ensuring compliance with medication dosage, it is important that the patient utilize an effective technique to apply the ointment into the conjunctival sac. Verbal instructions, written instructions, and demonstration are effective ways of maximizing patient compliance.

Instrumentation. Desired ophthalmic ointment, wall or stand-mounted mirror, facial tissues.

Technique. Advise the patient to wash the hands, verify the label on the ointment to be applied, and remove the cap of the tube. Instruct the patient to look into the mirror and tilt the chin down slightly so that the eyes roll upward. He or she then gently pinches the lower lid away from the globe between the thumb and forefinger of one hand so that the inferior cul-de-sac forms a small pouch (Fig. 1). A ½-inch ribbon of ointment is squeezed into the cul-de-sac and the tube is twisted slightly to interrupt ointment flow. The lower lid is then released (Fig. 1B). The eye may be gently massaged through the closed lid to facilitate spread of the ointment within the sac (Fig. 1C). Excess ointment is gently wiped away with a facial tissue. This procedure is repeated for the opposite eye as indicated. Instruct the patient to wash the hands and recap the tube.

Alternatively, the patient may first apply the ointment to a fingertip and transfer it into the conjunctival sac. Instruct the patient to wash the hands and to apply a ½-inch ribbon of ointment onto the fingertip of one hand (Fig. 2A). While looking into a mirror, the patient pulls down the lower lid with the index or middle finger of the opposite hand to expose the palpebral conjunctival surface (Fig. 2B). He or she then rolls or wipes the ointment onto the palpebral conjunctiva (Fig. 2C). Gently pinching the lower lid away from the globe will help to "pocket" the ointment (Fig. 1B). This technique is especially useful for ointments or gels that are more viscous in nature.

Contraindications/Complications. The examiner must be familiar with any contraindications of using a particular type of ointment for a given patient, including allergies to the drug contents and drug–drug interactions. Some types of ophthalmic ointments or gels have very specific dosage guidelines to determine the amount of medication instilled into the conjunctival sac. The patient must be advised to avoid contacting the tip of the dropper to the cilia, lids, conjunctival surface, or tears, as contamination of the tube's contents may occur. Proper technique must be utilized to prevent inadvertent superficial injury to the globe.

It is important to warn the patient that significant transient blurring of vision will occur following instillation of ointment into the conjunctival sac. Adverse visual effects can be minimized by controlling the amount of ointment applied as well as the timing of dosages.

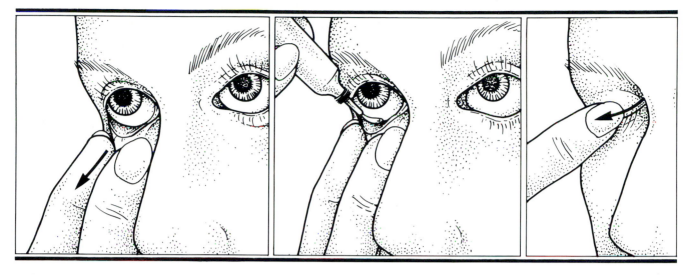

1. A. The patient looks into the mirror and tilts the chin down slightly. The lower lid is gently pinched between the thumb and forefinger of the left hand.

1. B. The ointment is applied into the conjunctival sac and the lid is released.

1. C. The eye may be gently massaged through the closed lid.

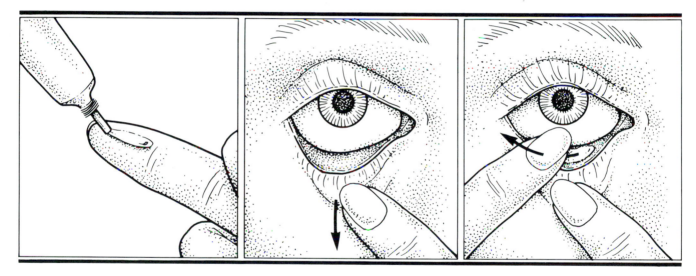

2. A. The patient applies a ½-inch ribbon of ointment onto the fingertip of one hand.

2. B. The patient pulls down the lower lid using the index or middle finger of the opposite hand.

2. C. Patient wipes the ointment onto the exposed palpebral conjunctiva.

I Suggested Readings

Bartlett JD: Dilation of the pupil, in Bartlett JD, Jaanus SD (eds): *Clinical Ocular Pharmacology,* ed 2. Boston, Butterworths, 1989, pp 393–419.

Bartlett JD, Cullen AP: Clinical administration of ocular drugs, in Bartlett JD, Jaanus SD (eds): *Clinical Ocular Pharmacology,* ed 2. Boston, Butterworths, 1989, pp 29–66.

Bienfang BC: Sector pupillary dilatation with an epinephrine strip. *Am J Ophthalmol* 1973;**75**:883–884.

Catania LJ: Management of common eyelid problems. *Practical Hints* series, vol 1, no 1. Dresher, PA, Primary Eyecare, 1982.

Catania LJ: General therapeutic considerations in clinical practice, in *Primary Care of the Anterior Segment.* Norwalk, Appleton & Lange, 1988, pp 1–14.

Chang FW, McCan TA, Hitchcock JR: Sector pupil dilation with phenylephrine and tropicamide. *Am J Optom Physiol Optics* 1985;**62**:482–486.

Samples JR: The use of topical beta adrenergic antagonists for the contemporary therapy of glaucoma. *Contemp Ophthalmic Forum* 1987;**5**:139–147.

Shaffer RN: Problems in the use of autonomic drugs in ophthalmology, in Leopold IH (ed): *Ocular Therapy.* St. Louis, Mosby, 1967, vol 2: *Complications and Management,* pp 18–23.

Terry JE: Diagnostic pharmaceutical agents, clinical uses, in Terry JE (ed): *Ocular Disease: Detection, Diagnosis and Treatment.* Springfield, IL, CC Thomas, 1984, pp 39–41.

Slit Lamp Biomicroscopy and Adjunct Procedures

9 Overview Biomicroscopic Evaluation

Description/Indications. The slit lamp biomicroscopic examination is an integral part of most evaluations performed by the ophthalmic practitioner. It is a noninvasive procedure that poses no risk to the patient. Use of the slit lamp biomicroscope ("slit lamp") is indicated to perform routine ocular health evaluations; to evaluate for ocular trauma, irritation, infection, and inflammation; and to fit and manage contact lens patients. Two of the commonly available attachments for the slit lamp allow the practitioner to perform applanation tonometry (see p. 50) and Hruby lens evaluation (see p. 208). Many slit lamps are adaptable for anterior segment photography. The slit lamp is integral to the use of auxiliary evaluative techniques and procedures described throughout this text.

The scattering of light due to the Tyndall effect will make most of the ocular media visible through biomicroscopy. A variety of slit lamps, including hand-held models, are commercially available, with each having two important components in common: the viewing system and the illumination system. The viewing system consists of a stereoscopic compound microscope adapted to examine the human eye in vivo and mounted on a movable platform. Multiple magnification powers are available. Use of a focusing joystick along with a vertical control knob provides for movement of the microscope in the x, y, and z meridians relative to the patient positioned in the head and chin rest (Fig. 1).

The illumination system is a light source mounted on the microscope that is variable in intensity and orientation and is projected by an optical system upon the eye. Various aperture stops and filters may be introduced to change the configuration and color of the illumination beam. The relative angle between the illumination system and the microscopic viewing system may be varied to achieve the most effective evaluative technique.

It is most clinically effective and efficient to develop a slit lamp examination routine that is identically performed on each patient. In addition, strive to establish a smooth yet dynamic sequencing of examination components resulting from fluid hand movements controlling the joystick and illumination beam settings. If an ocular lesion is detected or if more detailed evaluation of a specific ocular component is desired, additional techniques and illuminations are incorporated as indicated.

This procedure will review a suggested technique for the overview slit lamp evaluation as may be performed during routine patient examination. The two most commonly used illumination techniques for the general slit lamp evaluation are diffuse illumination and direct focal illumination. More structure and purpose-specific techniques are discussed in subsequent procedures.

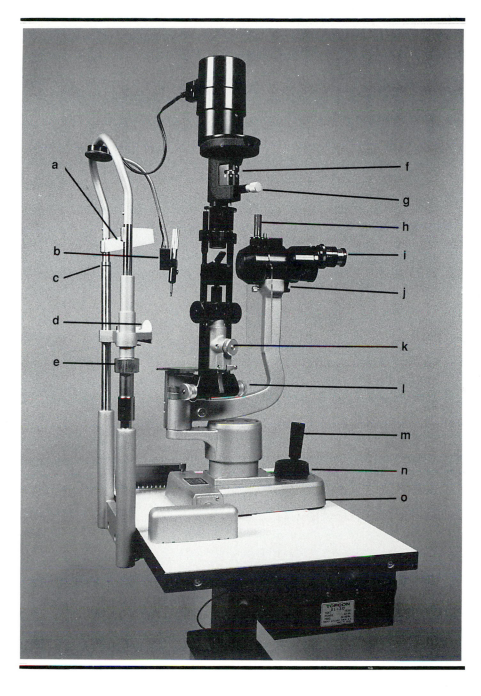

1. The major components of the slit lamp biomicroscope. (a) Forehead rest. (b) Fixation light. (c) Canthus alignment mark. (d) Chin rest. (e) Chin rest height adjustment knob. (f) Beam filters control. (g) Beam height control. (h) Tonometer mount stem. (i) Eyepieces. (j) Magnification lever. (k) Click stop knob. (l) Beam width control. (m) Joystick. (n) Vertical control knob. (o) Slit lamp base.

Diffuse illumination refers to a wide beam that is directed obliquely for general scanning of the anterior segment (Fig. 2). The field of view is maximized by using a low magnification setting. *Direct focal illumination* refers to the focusing of the light beam and the microscope in the same specific area. It does not refer to coaxial placement of the light source with the microscope. Usually medium to high magnification is used depending upon the structure being evaluated. The parallelepiped and optic section are two commonly used types of direct focal illumination, especially important for evaluating the cornea and crystalline lens. The parallelepiped illuminates a three-dimensional tissue area and is effective for detecting tissue lesions (Fig. 3). An optic section illuminates a two-dimensional area of tissue that is viewed obliquely, similar to examining a histological section, and is used to localize the depth of lesions (Fig. 4).

Instrumentation. Slit lamp biomicroscope.

Technique

Basic Slit Lamp Setup: Set the oculars of the microscope to your pupillary distance. Set the power of the ocular eyepieces to zero or to your spherical equivalent refractive error as appropriate. Position the patient comfortably in the slit lamp. Adjust the height of the chin rest so the patient's lateral canthus is aligned with the black line on the upright bar (Fig. 1). Raise or lower the examination chair so the patient can easily rest the forehead against the head strap without straining excessively to reach it (chair too low) or hunching over (chair too high). Advise the patient to grasp the handholds if available. Turn the illumination rheostat to its lowest setting before turning on the slit lamp. Advise the patient that you will be touching the eyelids periodically during the slit lamp examination.

Diffuse Illumination: Position the microscope directly in front of the eye. Adjust the magnification knob to 6X or 10X. Position the light source at approximately 60 degrees from the microscope. Place the microscope and beam in coincident focus with the beam "in click." Adjust the apertures so that the beam is approximately 3 to 4 mm wide and of maximum height. Use the joystick and vertical control knob to focus the microscope on the desired structure illuminated by the diffuse beam (Fig. 2).

Direct Focal Illumination: Position the microscope directly in front of the eye and the light source at approximately 60 degrees from the microscope. Place the microscope and beam in coincident focus with the beam "in click." Adjust the beam to its maximum height and narrow the beam to 1 to 2 mm in width to illuminate a parallelepiped-shaped section of the cornea. Use the joystick to sharply focus the microscope and parallelepiped simultaneously (Fig. 3). To form an optic section, narrow the beam width until it is almost extinguished (Fig. 4).

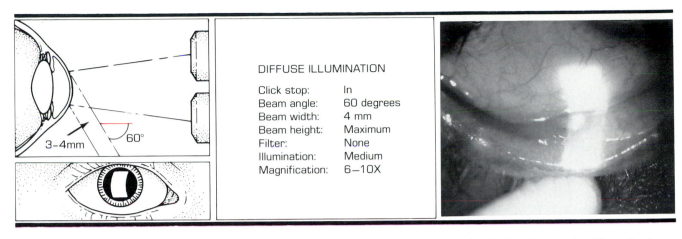

2. Diffuse illumination refers to a wide beam that is directed obliquely for general scanning. In the photograph, diffuse illumination is being used to evaluate the inferior palpebral conjunctiva.

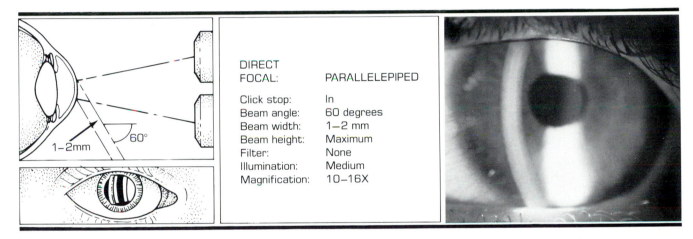

3. A parallelepiped illuminates a three-dimensional tissue area. In the photograph a parallelepiped is illuminating the cornea.

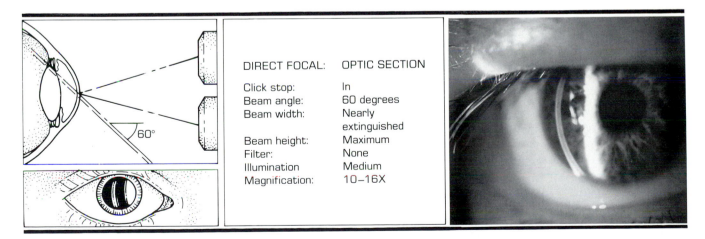

4. An optic section illuminates a two-dimensional tissue area. In the photograph an optic section is focused on the cornea.

Overview Biomicroscopic Evaluation: To evaluate the right eye first, position the beam 60 degrees to the left (temporally) of the axially aligned microscope. Turn on the slit lamp and increase the illumination so that the structures are adequately illuminated but without inducing patient discomfort. Instruct the patient to fixate toward your right ear or over your right shoulder so that the eyes are in primary gaze. Alternatively, the slit lamp fixation light may be placed in front of the left eye, but the patient will have a tendency to converge the eyes to see it. Initially a gross focusing movement of the slit lamp base toward the patient may be made while holding the joystick vertically. Subsequently, use your right hand to control the joystick and vertical positioning knob; use your left hand to control the beam height and width levers. Adjust the magnification knob to 6X to 10X and open the slit beam to create diffuse illumination (Fig. 5).

Beginning at the lateral canthus, scan the inferior lid margin, lash, and lid skin area while moving the microscope nasally. Once the nasal canthus is reached, elevate the beam and scan the upper lid while moving temporally. Once the temporal canthus is reached, ask the patient to look up, retract the lower lid gently with your left thumb or index finger, and scan the inferior palpebral and bulbar conjunctival areas while moving the beam nasally. Once the nasal canthal area is reached, ask the patient to look down, gently retract the upper lid with your left thumb, and scan the superior bulbar conjunctiva while moving the beam temporally (Fig. 5).

With the diffuse beam once again at the temporal canthal area, ask the patient to look to his or her left, and scan the temporal bulbar conjunctiva. Ask the patient to again look straight ahead. Turn the magnification to 10X to 16X. Using your left hand, narrow the beam to an optic section and position it at the temporal limbus for Van Herick angle estimation (see p. 26). Widen the beam to a 1-mm parallelepiped and scan across the cornea. When the nasal third of the cornea is reached, gently swing the beam to the right of the microscope; switch your left hand to the joystick and your right hand to the illumination housing. Complete the parallelepiped scan of the nasal cornea, including a slight overlap of observation at the point of beam rotation. When the nasal limbus is reached, use your right hand to narrow the beam to an optic section for Van Herick angle estimation (Fig. 6). Lower the magnification to 6X to 10X, widen the beam to diffuse illumination, and ask the patient to look to his or her right to scan the nasal bulbar conjunctiva, plica, and caruncle. Ask the patient to look straight ahead, focus the microscope slightly forward with the joystick, and evaluate the iris while scanning temporally (Fig. 7). Near the temporal pupil margin the beam may be repositioned temporally. Repeat the procedure for the left eye and record your findings.

Evaluation of the crystalline lens and anterior vitreous with the slit lamp biomicroscope are best performed following pupillary dilation and are covered elsewhere (see pp. 62 and 68).

Contraindications/Complications. Slit lamp biomicroscopy is a non-invasive procedure that poses no risk to the patient. Challenges in positioning may occur with certain patient types. An assistant or family member may need to gently but firmly hold the head of a very young or elderly patient against the chin and head rests. Very small children may sit on a family member's lap or on a booster seat cushion, or may even stand on the footrest of the examination chair. Occasionally, a patient may have neck or back problems that prevent positioning in a slit lamp. A slit lamp mounted on an adjustable free-standing table may be helpful for use with patients in wheelchairs. Patient comfort will be compromised if the illumination is set too high or the beam too wide.

Novice biomicroscopists tend to commit certain errors in technique that will make initial interpretation difficult. If the source is positioned out of click stop, properly focused direct illumination is impossible. Using a magnification too high for general viewing results in a loss of perspective of relative structures and a tendency to overinterpret normal findings as abnormal. If an optic section rather than a parallelepiped is used to initially evaluate the cornea, most subtle corneal findings will be missed, particularly as a result of small patient eye movements. Switching the slit lamp beam from the temporal to the nasal position at the apex of the cornea will produce a filament reflection that obscures central corneal findings. If the upper and lower lids obscure the superior and inferior portions of the cornea, respectively, the lids must be retracted for complete corneal evaluation. Too small an angle between the microscope and the illumination beam will result in inadequate visualization of the structural layers.

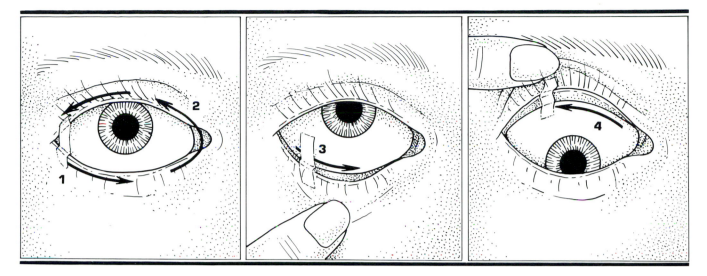

5. Use diffuse illumination to scan the lids, inferior bulbar/palpebral conjunctiva, and superior bulbar conjunctiva in the order shown.

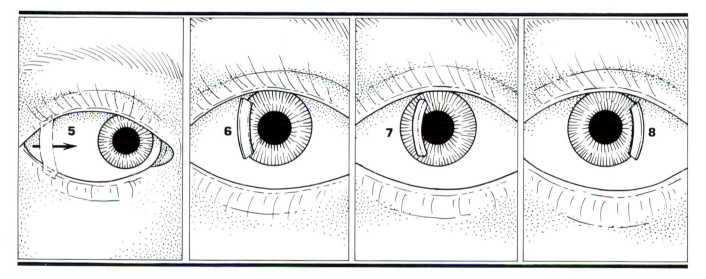

6. Use diffuse illumination to scan the temporal bulbar conjunctiva (5). Increase the magnification and use an optic section for temporal Van Herick angle estimation (6). Use a 1-mm parellelepiped to scan the cornea, switching the beam position for the nasal third of the cornea (7). Use an optic section for nasal Van Herick angle estimation (8).

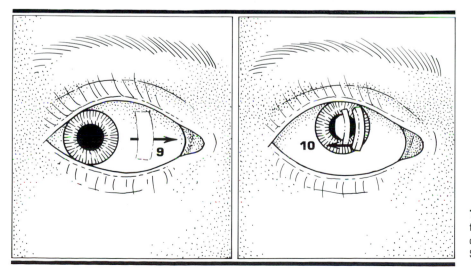

7. Lowering the magnification, use diffuse illumination to scan the nasal bulbar conjunctiva as the patient looks right. Scan temporally to evaluate the iris.

10 Van Herick Angle Estimation

Description/Indications. The depth of the anterior chamber angle must be assessed prior to pupillary dilation. The Van Herick angle estimation technique is an efficient and reliable method to evaluate the depth of the anterior chamber angle using the slit lamp biomicroscope without applying a gonioscopic lens. This technique must be incorporated into the routine slit lamp examination (see p. 24). In addition, this technique may elicit the first clinical sign of narrow-angle or acute-angle closure glaucoma in a symptomatic patient who presents acutely.

When an optic section is focused on the cornea in the limbal region, the cornea will be seen in cross-section with the slit beam reflected off the front surface of the iris. In the presence of an open anterior chamber angle and clear aqueous humor, the anterior chamber is optically empty and appears as a black space between the cornea and iris (see Fig. 2). The width of the space formed by the anterior chamber angle relative to the width of the corneal section is used as a measure for chamber angle width estimation.

Instrumentation. Slit lamp biomicroscope.

Technique. Position the patient comfortably at the slit lamp and adjust the eyepieces of the microscope properly (see p. 22). Make certain that the beam is in the "click" position and that the patient's eyes are in primary gaze. To assess the right eye, ask the patient to fixate toward your right ear or over your right shoulder.

Position the light source 60 degrees to the left (temporally) of the microscope. Adjust the microscope magnification to 16X to 20X. Use your right hand to control the joystick and vertical positioning knob; use your left hand to control slit height and width (Fig. 1). Narrow the illumination beam to form an optic section. Position the corneally focused optic section at the temporal limbus of the right eye. With the optic section focused on the cornea, subjectively assess the width of the black space formed by the anterior chamber angle interval relative to the width of the corneal optic section (Fig. 2). Assess the nasal angle by using your left hand to gently swing the illumination beam to the right (nasally) of the microscope. Switch your left hand to the joystick and your right hand to the illumination housing. Ask the patient to fixate toward your left ear or over your left shoulder.

Repeat the procedure to evaluate the temporal and nasal angles of the left eye. Record your findings.

Interpretation. Anterior chamber angles assessed with the Van Herick technique are graded 1 to 4, with Grade 4 considered a wide open angle incapable of closure and Grade 1 a very narrow angle (Fig. 3).

Many clinicians will abbreviate the recording of the Van Herick grading as "V-H 4" for a Grade 4 angle, for example. To designate slight variations between gradings, an angle may be recorded as "V-H 2+" if it is slightly larger than a Grade 2, or "V-H 4−" if it is slightly less than a Grade 4. If the grades of the nasal and temporal angles are judged to be different, both readings should be recorded.

Although the Van Herick technique is not a foolproof predictor of angle size, angles that are identified as being very narrow with the Van Herick technique should be further evaluated by three-mirror or four-mirror gonioscopy (see pp. 72 and 80) prior to pupillary dilation. Frequently, angles will be found to be larger with gonioscopy than the Van Herick technique indicated. Gonioscopy is also necessary to definitively diagnose acute-angle closure glaucoma.

Complications/Contraindications. Peripheral corneal conditions such as arcus senilis may make it difficult to gauge if the optic section is positioned correctly at the limbus, or may make visualization of the anterior chamber interval difficult. Gonioscopy may then be necessary to fully evaluate the anterior chamber angle. In the unusual instance of a plateau iris, it is possible to overestimate the size of the angle with the Van Herick technique.

Potentially serious errors in angle estimation may also occur if the patient's eyes are not in primary gaze. The most common mistake that will result in angle overestimation is if the optic section is not placed far enough peripherally at the corneo-scleral junction.

V-H ANGLE ESTIMATION

Click stop:	In
Beam angle:	60
Beam width:	Optic section
Beam height:	Maximum
Filter:	None
Illumination:	Medium
Magnification:	16–20X

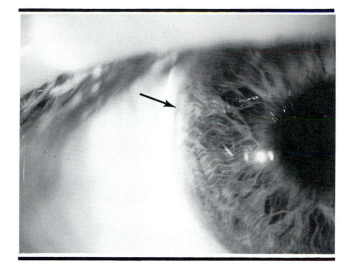

1. The slit lamp setup for Van Herick angle estimation.

2. Photograph of Van Herick estimation of the temporal angle OD. The anterior chamber appears as a black space between the cornea and iris (arrow).

3. (below) Van Herick angle Grades 1 through 4.

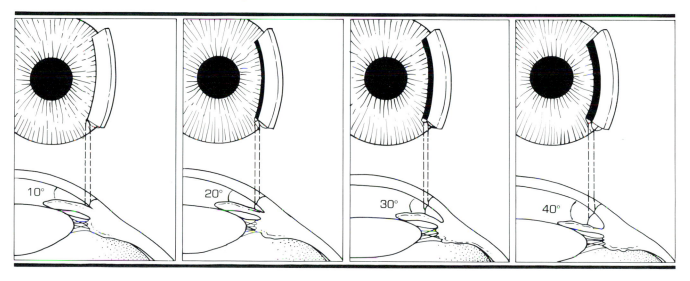

Grade 1: The width of the chamber interval is less than ¼ the width of the corneal optic section. The angle is extremely narrow and will probably close with full pupillary dilation.

Grade 2: The width of the chamber interval is approximately ¼ the width of the corneal optic section. The angle is narrow and is capable of closure.

Grade 3: The width of the chamber interval is ¼ to ½ the width of the corneal optic section. The angle is unlikely to close.

Grade 4: The width of the chamber interval is equal to or greater than the width of the corneal optic section. This is a wide-open angle.

11 Tear Meniscus Evaluation

Description/Indications. The tear layer is comprised of the outermost oily layer, the middle aqueous layer, and the innermost mucin layer. In addition to the lacrimal lake in the medial canthal area, strips of tear fluid are located at the posterior margins of both the upper and lower eyelids. The inferior marginal strip is more easily visualized and gives off a mirror-like reflection. This tear strip is actually wedge or meniscus-shaped as it simultaneously contacts the lid margin and the bulbar conjunctiva with the lid in the normal position.

In addition to diagnostic tests such as tear breakup time (p. 15), Schirmer testing (p. 108), and lactoferrin testing (p. 112), the quality of the tear layer may be assessed by inspection with the slit lamp biomicroscope. This technique may be added to the overview slit lamp examination (p. 24) and is indicated for patients with symptoms suggestive of keratitis sicca and for contact lens patients. If keratitis sicca is suspected following the patient history, tear meniscus evaluation should be the initial component of the slit lamp evaluation so that the effect of the lights on tearing is minimized.

Instrumentation. Slit lamp biomicroscope.

Technique. Position the patient comfortably at the slit lamp (see p. 22). Adjust the eyepieces to accommodate your pupillary distance and refractive error. Adjust the magnification to 10X to 16X. Make certain that the beam is in the "click" position. Use your right hand to control the joystick and vertical positioning knob; use your left hand to control the beam height and width levers. To evaluate the right eye, position the beam 60 degrees to the left (temporally) of the microscope. Turn the rheostat to its lowest setting and adjust the slit beam width to a 1 to 2-mm parallelepiped (Fig. 1). Alternatively, keep the slit beam turned off and use ambient room lighting to focus on the tear strip.

Focus the parallelepiped on the inferior tear strip near the lateral canthus. Use the joystick to scan across the tear strip, moving nasally and keeping the strip in focus (Fig. 2). At any point the beam may be narrowed to an optic section to assess the depth of the tear meniscus.

Interpretation. The tear strip will frequently exhibit superficial colored moire reflections off the outermost oily layer. Excessive tear lipids commonly occur in patients with meibomian gland oversecretion or seborrheic blepharitis. A patient who is wearing excessive eye makeup or makeup applied close to the lid margin will often exhibit colored makeup debris in the tear strip as well as in the tears covering the entire globe. A patient with bacterial conjunctivitis will exhibit exudative debris and mucus in the tear strip. A patient who has been instilling ophthalmic ointment into the conjunctival sac will exhibit oil droplets in the tear strip once the ointment has melted somewhat.

Normally the tear meniscus should be approximately 1 mm wide. In patients with keratitis sicca, the meniscus may be significantly reduced in size due to reduced quantities of the aqueous tear component. The resultant concentration of the oily and mucin tear layers may produce significant levels of mucous strands and debris in the tear strip, especially if accompanying epithelial sloughing is present, and the tear strip will appear very viscous.

Complications/Contraindications. If the patient is a suitable candidate for slit lamp examination, no risks are associated with this technique. Turning the illumination rheostat too high may induce reflex tearing and obscure the viscosity and thinning of the tear meniscus. The tear meniscus should be evaluated prior to any planned eversion of the upper lid (p. 86). Lid eversion will result in expression of the Meibomian gland secretions into the tear strip and will artifactually contribute to the appearance of debris. Lid eversion may also induce reflex tearing.

1. Slit lamp set-up for tear meniscus evaluation.

TEAR MENISCUS EVALUATION

Click stop:	In
Beam angle:	60 degrees
Beam width:	Parallelepiped
Beam height:	Maximum
Filter:	None
Illumination:	Low, or use ambient lighting only
Magnification:	10–16X

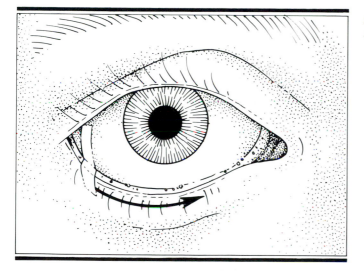

2. A parallelepiped is focused on a viscous tear strip. The arrow indicates the direction of slit lamp scanning.

12 Corneal Evaluation

Description/Indications. While using the slit lamp biomicroscope to perform an overview evaluation of the eye and adnexa (see p. 24), corneal lesions may be detected that require more thorough evaluation with additional slit lamp illumination techniques. These techniques are typically not included in routine slit lamp examination but may be easily incorporated as indicated, either singly or in combination.

Cobalt Filter Illumination: Introduction of the cobalt filter without the instillation of fluorescein will cause corneal iron lines to appear black. This technique is especially useful in detecting subtle Fleischer rings in the diagnosis of early keratoconus.

Specular Reflection: When the microscope and illumination system are set at equal angles of incidence and reflection, the anterior and posterior surfaces of the cornea will serve as reflecting surfaces. This technique is especially useful in evaluating the corneal endothelium. It may also be used for assessing the anterior and posterior surfaces of the crystalline lens.

Indirect Illumination: The microscope is focused on an area immediately adjacent to the illuminated tissue. This technique is especially useful for evaluating refractile, nonopaque corneal lesions such as microcysts and fingerprint lines.

Retroillumination: Light is reflected off the anterior surface of the iris as the cornea is focused. Lesions will be backlighted and appear black due to absorption of the reflected light.

Sclerotic Scatter: Internal reflection characteristics of the cornea are used to evaluate its transparency. This technique was invaluable for assessing central corneal clouding (CCC) that developed secondary to polymethymethacrylate (PMMA) hard contact lens wear, but may be utilized whenever corneal clarity is compromised.

Instrumentation. Slit lamp biomicroscope.

Technique. Position the patient comfortably at the slit lamp (see p. 22). Adjust the eyepieces to accommodate your pupillary distance and refractive error. Make certain that the patient's eyes are in primary gaze. To assess the right eye, ask the patient to fixate toward your right ear or over your right shoulder.

Cobalt Filter Illumination: To evaluate the right eye, position the beam 60 degrees to the left (temporally) of the microscope. Make certain that the beam is in the "click" position. Use your right hand to control the joystick and vertical positioning knob; use your left hand to control the beam height and width levers. Introduce the cobalt filter. Set the magnification to 10X and open the beam width to approximately 3 mm. Turn the illumination rheostat to its highest setting. Scan the cornea looking for subtle black linear, arcuate, or circular lines (Fig. 1).

Specular Reflection: To illuminate the central cornea of the right eye, position the microscope approximately 45 degrees to the right and the illumination system 45 degrees to the left of the visual axis. Make certain that the beam is in the "click" position. Adjust the illumination rheostat to a medium setting. Use your right hand to control the joystick and vertical positioning knob; use your left hand to control the beam height and width levers. Set the magnification to 16X to 40X and open the beam to a parallelepiped approximately 1 mm wide.

Move the joystick with your right hand to position the beam at the corneal apex. A bright reflection of the slit beam filament will be visible in one ocular of the microscope and the reflection of the endothelium will be visible through the other. With the microscope in the straight-ahead position, specular reflection will naturally occur off the curved temporal and nasal sides of the cornea when the beam is placed to the temporal and nasal sides, respectively (Fig. 2).

COBALT FILTER EVALUATION

Click stop:	In
Beam angle:	60 degrees
Beam width:	3 mm
Beam height:	Maximum
Filter:	Cobalt
Illumination:	Maximum
Magnification:	10X

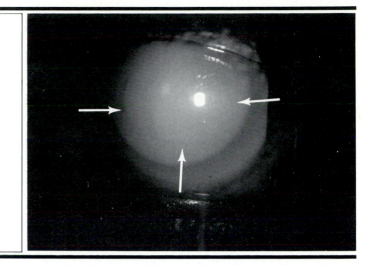

1. A. The slit lamp setup for cobalt filter illumination of the cornea.

1. B. When illuminated with the cobalt filter, the Fleischer ring of keratoconus appears black (arrows). (*See also* Color Plate 12–1.B.)

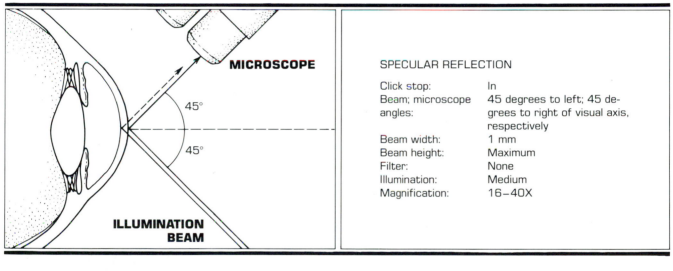

SPECULAR REFLECTION

Click stop:	In
Beam; microscope angles:	45 degrees to left; 45 degrees to right of visual axis, respectively
Beam width:	1 mm
Beam height:	Maximum
Filter:	None
Illumination:	Medium
Magnification:	16–40X

2. A. (above) The slit lamp setup for specular reflection of the cornea.

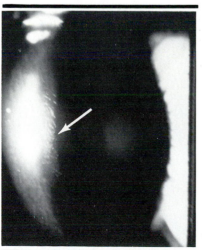

2. B. (left) Guttata are visible as an orange-peel-like disruption of the corneal endothelium (arrow).

Indirect Illumination: To evaluate the right eye, position the beam 60 degrees to the left (temporally) of the microscope. Adjust the illumination rheostat to a medium setting. Use your right hand to control the joystick and vertical positioning knob; use your left hand to control the beam height and width levers. Use your left hand to turn the beam to the left of the "click" position. Set the magnification to 10X to 16X and open the beam to a parallelepiped approximately 1 mm wide. Adjust the microscope so that the beam is focused to the left of the lesion and change your point of regard to the lesion (Fig. 3).

Retroillumination: To evaluate the right eye, po-sition the beam 60 degrees to the left (temporally) of the microscope. Adjust the illumination rheostat to a medium setting. Use your right hand to control the joystick and vertical positioning knob; use your left hand to control the beam height and width levers. Make certain that the beam is in the "click" position. Set the magnification to 10X to 16X and open the beam to a parallelepiped approximately 1 mm wide. Adjust the microscope so that the corneal lesion is in focus and positioned in front of light reflected off the anterior surface of the iris (Fig. 4). Alternatively, the beam may be moved out of "click" stop so that the cornea is viewed in light reflected off the iris.

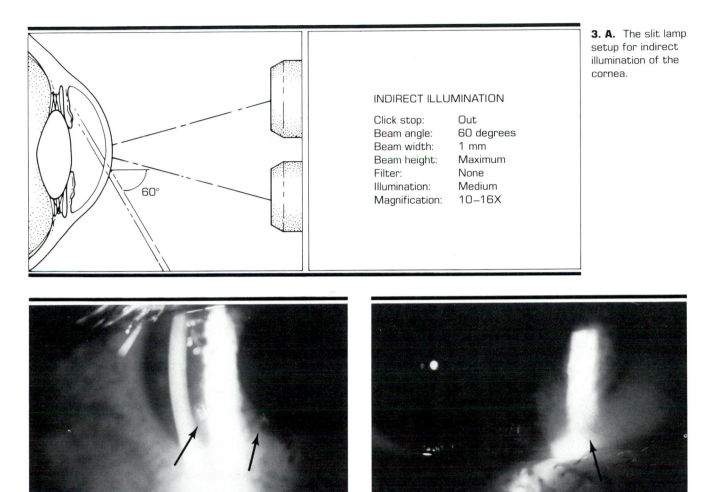

3. A. The slit lamp setup for indirect illumination of the cornea.

INDIRECT ILLUMINATION

Click stop:	Out
Beam angle:	60 degrees
Beam width:	1 mm
Beam height:	Maximum
Filter:	None
Illumination:	Medium
Magnification:	10–16X

3. B. In the photograph, two small herpes simplex dendritic ulcers are visible in indirect illumination (arrows). (*See also* Color Plate 12–3.B.)

4. A. In the photograph, a limbal neovascular tuft is seen in retroillumination. (*See also* Color Plate 12–4.A.)

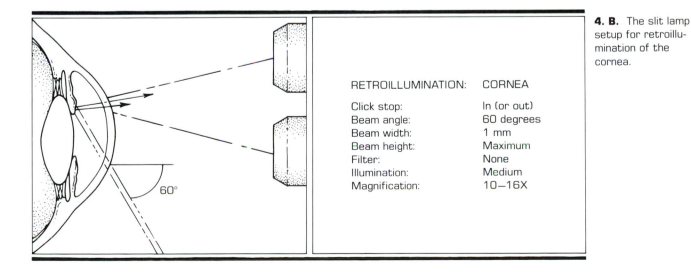

4. B. The slit lamp setup for retroillumination of the cornea.

RETROILLUMINATION:	CORNEA
Click stop:	In (or out)
Beam angle:	60 degrees
Beam width:	1 mm
Beam height:	Maximum
Filter:	None
Illumination:	Medium
Magnification:	10–16X

Sclerotic Scatter: Make certain that the beam is in the "click" position. Use your right hand to control the joystick and vertical positioning knob; use your left hand to control the beam height and width levers. To evaluate the right eye, postion the beam 60 degrees to the left (temporally) of the microscope. Adjust the rheostat illumination knob to medium.

Move the joystick to position a 1 mm parallel-epiped at the temporal limbus of the right eye. When positioned correctly the nasal limbus will exhibit a halo or glow. Looking outside the slit lamp to the nasal side, observe for areas of milky white haze in the cornea. Using the pupil as a dark background will facilitate this assessment (Fig. 5). If necessary, rotate the viewing microscope to your left so as to not obscure your view of the cornea.

Interpretation

Cobalt Filter Illumination: Iron deposits in the corneal epithelium (iron lines) will appear black with the cobalt filter. When the diagnosis of early keratoconus is suspected due to keratometer mire distortion, refractive error changes of cylinder axis and power, and slightly reduced visual acuity, a subtle partial or complete Fleischer ring may be an early corneal sign observable with the slit lamp and will aid in appropriate diagnosis. With the cobalt filter a black arc or ring will be apparent in the mid-corneal area and may be slightly decentered.

This subtle finding will be easily overlooked if the angle between the illumination system and the microscope is insufficiently large so that light reflected off the iris obscures the appearance, or if the illumination is set too low. Steroscopic appreciation that the black line is located in the cornea assists in making this assessment. The black lines are more prominent following pupillary dilation, when light reflected off the iris is less likely to interfere.

Specular Reflection: With specular reflection the normal corneal endothelium will exhibit a regular, mosaic-like appearance of polygonal cells. The higher magnification settings will be needed to fully appreciate this. When corneal guttata are present in the central cornea, areas of dimpling will appear within the corneal mosaic, similar to an orange peel (Fig. 2B). Irregularity and/or dropout of corneal endothelial cells has also been reported following intraocular lens implant surgery and prolonged soft contact lens wear.

Indirect Illumination: Corneal microcysts will appear as refractile spherical bodies in the epithelium, giving it a ground glass appearance. Fingerprint lines, a potential component of epithelial basement membrane dystrophy, will appear as sinuous, concentric refractile lines.

Retroillumination: Any corneal opacity will appear black with retroillumination. The degree of light absorption will vary with the density of the lesion.

Sclerotic Scatter: A normal clear cornea will not exhibit areas of light scatter with this technique and will appear black (Fig. 5B). If central corneal clouding (CCC) is present due to hard contact lens wear, a circular gray-white haze approximately 4 to 6 mm in diameter will be apparent in the central corneal area. Areas of significant corneal edema or white blood cell infiltration will also appear as milky areas with this technique.

Complications/Contraindications. If the patient is a suitable candidate for slit lamp examination, no risks are associated with these techniques.

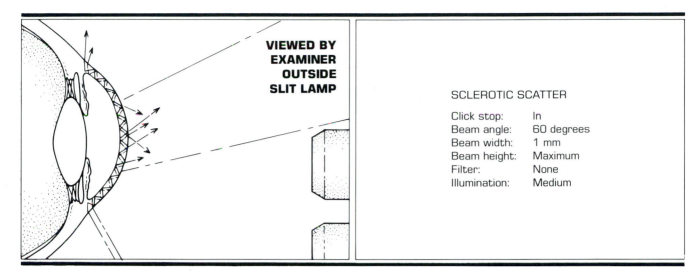

**VIEWED BY
EXAMINER
OUTSIDE
SLIT LAMP**

SCLEROTIC SCATTER

Click stop:	In
Beam angle:	60 degrees
Beam width:	1 mm
Beam height:	Maximum
Filter:	None
Illumination:	Medium

5. A. The slit lamp setup for sclerotic scatter of the cornea. Scattering of light is shown from central corneal haze.

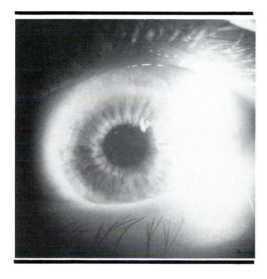

5. B. When evaluated with sclerotic scatter, the central cornea appears clear (black) against the pupillary background.

13 Anterior Chamber Evaluation

Description/Indications. The aqueous humor is normally virtually optically empty so that the anterior chamber appears black when the slit beam passes through it. In the presence of anterior uveitis, protein and white blood cells leak into the anterior chamber from inflamed blood vessels of the iris and ciliary body. The Tyndall effect will allow the visualization of these small particles as they circulate in the anterior chamber via the aqueous convection currents. Also, pigment particles from the iris pigment epithelium may be released into the anterior chamber following blunt trauma, routine pupillary dilation, and in patients with pigment dispersion syndrome. Red blood cells (erythrocytes) may be observed circulating in the anterior chamber following the development of a hyphema or microhyphema. Due to the minute size of this debris, maximum illumination and magnification obtainable with the biomicroscope are required to evaluate the anterior chamber.

Assessing the status of the anterior chamber is essential to the accurate differential diagnosis of acute ocular infections and inflammations, especially following traumatic insult. In a noninflamed eye, chronic uveitis may be suggested by keratic precipitates (KPs) on the corneal endothelium.

This technique of anterior chamber evaluation is incorporated into the biomicroscopic evaluation whenever indicated.

Instrumentation. Slit lamp biomicroscope.

Technique. Position the patient comfortably at the slit lamp and adjust the eyepieces of the microscope properly (see p. 22). Make certain that the beam is in the "click" position and that the patient's eyes are in primary gaze. To assess the right eye, ask the patient to fixate toward your right ear or over your right shoulder.

Position the light source 60 degrees to the left (temporally) of the microscope. Adjust the microscope magnification to 25X to 40X. Use your right hand to control the joystick and vertical positioning knob; place your left hand on the illumination beam housing to control slit height and width. Adjust the slit beam height and width using your left hand to form a small round spot of light (conic section) or a short parallelepiped approximately 1 mm wide and 2 mm high. Turn the slit lamp illumination rheostat to its maximum setting (Fig. 1). Turn off all ambient room lights.

Let yourself dark-adapt for approximately 30 seconds. Focus the conic section or parallelepiped on the central portion of the cornea. Move the joystick slightly forward to focus the beam on the anterior surface of the crystalline lens. As you make the forward focusing motion, carefully observe the black interval of the anterior chamber for minute particles floating vertically within the beam. Perform several of these forward and back oscillatory motions between the cornea and anterior lens surface for 30 to 60 seconds while observing for small particles reflected in the slit lamp beam (Fig. 2). Slight vertical positional changes in the beam may also be made. Debris in the anterior chamber is most easily visualized when the black pupillary area is maintained as the background. If reddish-brown particles are noted in the anterior chamber, introduce the red-free (green) filter to distinguish red blood cells from pigment particles.

1. (left) Slit lamp setup for anterior chamber evaluation.

ANTERIOR CHAMBER EVALUATION

Click stop:	In
Beam angle:	60 degrees
Beam width, height:	Conic section or parallelepiped 1 mm wide and 2 mm high
Filter:	None
Illumination:	Maximum, ambient room lights off
Magnification:	25–40X

2. A. (directly below) The short parallelepiped is first focused on the central cornea. **B.** (bottom) Focus the beam forward onto the front surface of the lens, observing the black interval of the anterior chamber. Perform several oscillatory motions for 30 to 60 seconds.

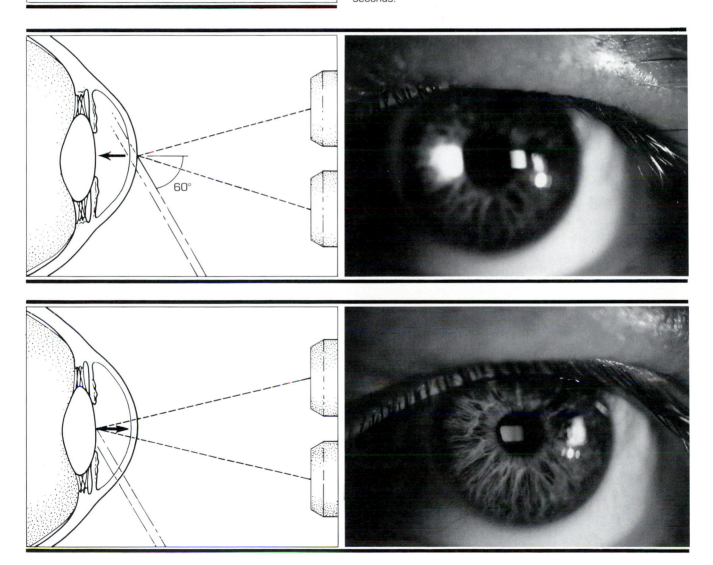

Interpretation. Evaluating the anterior chamber for "cells and flare" due to anterior uveitis refers to assessing for the presence of inflammatory white blood cells (leukocytes) and protein, respectively, that have leaked from inflamed iris and ciliary body vessels. White blood cells appear as whitish specks floating in the anterior chamber (Fig. 3A). Protein in the anterior chamber will not be visible as descrete floating particles but gives an overall milky appearance to the aqueous (Fig. 3B). Cells and flare in the anterior chamber are graded 0 to 4. The grading of cells and flare is determined by the quantity of each visible at any one time in the slit lamp beam (Fig. 4).

Using white light, red blood cells and pigment particles appear as reddish-brown specks floating in the anterior chamber. When the red-free (green) filter is introduced, the red blood cells appear black and will no longer be visible within the anterior chamber. Pigment particles will not absorb the red-free light and will still be visible.

Complications/Contraindications. The novice biomicroscopist will usually overlook mild to moderate anterior uveitis because of the subtleness of the findings. It is very important to use the maximum illumination and magnification settings of the slit lamp, to let yourself dark-adapt for a few seconds, and to take your time in scrutinizing the anterior chamber. Following the initial evaluation, pupillary dilation to increase the amount of black pupillary background area will facilitate visualization of the cells and flare.

Significant loss of corneal clarity due to conditions such as scarring, edema and white blood cell infiltration secondary to corneal healing, and large keratic precipitate (KP) formation, may make visualization of the anterior chamber difficult. In these instances, direct the conic section or short parallel-epiped beam through as clear an area of the cornea as possible. Occasionally, a difference in intraocular pressure between the two eyes, the degree of ciliary flush, and observation for fine KPs on the inferior portion of the corneal endothelium may be the only clinical signs that can be elicited to evaluate the degree of anterior chamber involvement.

When the corneal epithelium is disrupted such as following a traumatic abrasion, the anterior chamber should be evaluated prior to the instillation of fluorescein sodium (see p. 46). In this instance the fluorescein will penetrate through the cornea into the anterior chamber and will produce a green-tinged flare that may be misinterpreted as protein in the anterior chamber.

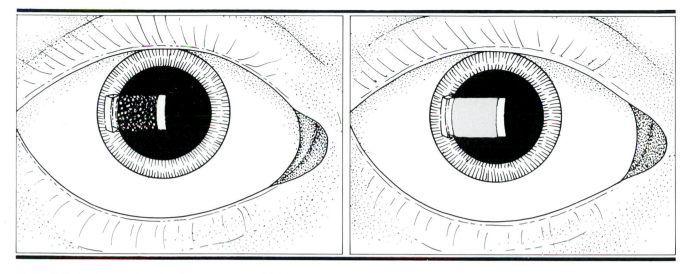

3. A. Cells in the anterior chamber appear as whitish specks.   **3. B.** Flare in the anterior chamber appears as a milky haze.

4. The grading of anterior chamber cells and flare.

GRADE	CELLS	FLARE
0	no cells	complete absence
trace (½)	any noticed	barely noticed
1	4–8	mild
2	9–15	moderate
3	too many to count	marked
4	most ever seen	severe

14   Iris Transillumination

Description/Indications. Evaluation of the iris with diffuse illumination will not reveal defects of the iris pigment epithelium (IPE). For certain clinical entities, the identification of IPE defects through iris transillumination is important for accurate diagnosis.

Iris transillumination is based on the principle of retroillumination. When the slit lamp beam is directed straight ahead through the pupil, the light will reflect off the fundus back through the pupil to form the "red reflex." When the iris is intact and the pupil undilated, the IPE will absorb all of the retroilluminated light and the iris will appear black. If localized or diffuse IPE defects are present, the red reflex will be visible through the iris in the affected areas. Areas of frank iris loss will also transilluminate.

If a Krukenberg's spindle is present on the corneal endothelium, iris transillumination will contribute to the diagnosis of pigment dispersion syndrome. Iris transillumination may help to assess the patency of surgical iridectomy or laser iridotomy performed for narrow-angle or acute-angle closure glaucoma. Diffuse iris transillumination will accompany ocular or generalized albinism and may aid in determining the etiology of nystagmus. IPE defects may follow cataract surgery or ocular trauma.

Instrumentation. Slit lamp biomicroscope.

Technique. Perform iris transillumination before pupillary dilation. Position the patient comfortably at the slit lamp and adjust the eyepieces of the microscope properly (see p. 22). Make certain that the beam is in the "click" position and that the patient's eyes are in primary gaze. To assess the right eye, ask the patient to fixate toward your right ear or over your right shoulder.

Position the light source directly in front of the microscope so that neither eyepiece is occluded. Adjust the microscope magnification to 6X to 10X. Use your right or left hand to control the joystick and vertical positioning knob. Place your opposite hand on the illumination beam housing to control slit height and width. Adjust the beam illumination to form a short, wide parallelepiped approximately 2 mm wide and 2 mm high that will fit within the pupillary area. Turn the illumination rheostat to maximum levels and turn the ambient room lighting off. Position the beam within the pupil area, focus the microscope at the plane of the iris, and observe for areas of red retroillumination (Fig. 1). Make small lateral movements with the joystick if necessary to get the brightest red reflex. If the upper and lower lids are obscuring the superior and inferior peripheral iris, respectively, instruct the patient to open the eyes more widely, or gently retract the lids to expose the entire iris.

Interpretation. Overall iris transillumination will be present in ocular or generalized albinism and will appear as a diffuse pink glow. Multiple slit or wedged-shaped areas of peripheral iris transillumination occur secondary to pigment dispersion syndrome (Fig. 2). Transillumination of the pupillary ruff develops due to exfoliation (pseudoexfoliation) syndrome or as a result of pupillary ruff atrophy in the aging process. Isolated focal peripheral iris transillumination defects result postsurgically from peripheral iridectomy or laser iridotomy.

Pronounced loss of the iris pigment epithelium will produce relatively large areas of iris transillumination postsurgically or posttraumatically. Full thickness absence of the iris secondary to conditions such as essential iris atrophy and iridodialysis will also produce transillumination defects.

Complications/Contraindications. If the patient is a suitable candidate for slit lamp examination, there are no risks associated with this technique. Subtle peripheral transillumination defects due to pigment dispersion syndrome will be overlooked if the slit lamp illumination is set too low or if the lids are blocking a substantial portion of the peripheral iris.

1. Slit lamp setup for iris transillumination.

IRIS TRANSILLUMINATION

Click stop:	In
Beam angle:	0 degrees (coaxial with microscope)
Beam width:	2 mm
Beam height:	2 mm
Filter:	None
Illumination:	Maximum, ambient room lights off
Magnification:	6—10X

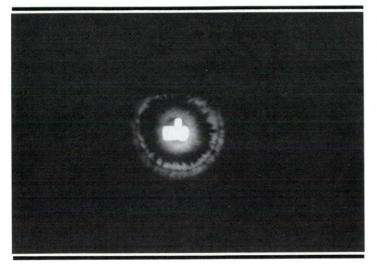

2. Extensive peripheral iris transillumination defects are present in this patient with pigment dispersion syndrome. (*See also* Color Plate 14—2.) (Courtesy of David W. Sloan, OD.)

15 Tear Breakup Time Determination

Description/Indications. Fluorescein sodium is an orange dye that fluoresces green when illuminated with a cobalt blue filter. The tear film is stained with fluorescein sodium dye and observed with a slit lamp biomicroscope as a means of assessing the integrity of the tears.

The tear layer is comprised of the outer lipid layer, middle aqueous layer, and inner mucin layer. Dissipation of the oily or mucin layer to cause tear evaporation will result in the formation of a dry area in the precorneal tear film. This dry area will appear as a black spot or streak that forms in the once uniformly fluorescent green tear film. Decreased tear secretion will also produce dry spots.

The amount of time it takes for dry areas to form in the fluorescein-sodium-stained tear layer following a blink is known as the tear breakup time (BUT). For most patients with normal tear film integrity, the BUT is sufficiently long so that blinking approximately every 15 to 30 seconds will result in the redistribution of an intact tear layer over the globe. Although BUT testing may be of questionable reliability or repeatability, a greatly reduced BUT is probably indicative of dry eye problems (keratitis sicca).

BUT testing is usually performed following a complete slit lamp examination (see p. 24) and is added when the patient has signs or symptoms suggestive of keratitis sicca, or as part of the ocular health evaluation prior to contact lens fitting.

Instrumentation. Slit lamp biomicroscope, sterile fluorescein sodium strips, sterile ophthalmic saline solution, facial tissues.

Technique. Hand the patient a fresh facial tissue. Remove a sterile fluorescein sodium strip from the package, taking care not to contaminate the fluorescein-sodium-impregnated end. Holding the strip in one hand over a wastebasket or sink, use the other hand to squeeze a drop of sterile ophthalmic saline solution onto the fluorescein end of the strip (Fig. 1A). Ask the patient to look up. Gently retract the right lower lid with the index finger or thumb of the left hand. Holding the strip in your right hand, dab the moistened fluorescein dye from the end of the strip onto the inferior bulbar conjunctiva (Fig. 1B). Alternatively, ask the patient to look down, gently retract the upper lid, and dab the fluorescein onto the superior bulbar conjunctiva. Using the same fluorescein strip, repeat this procedure for the left eye. If an anterior segment infection is present, however, instill fluorescein sodium into the uninvolved eye first or use a separate strip for each eye. Discard the fluorescein strip(s). Advise the patient that the saline solution may momentarily sting slightly. The patient may use the tissue to dab away excess fluid but should not forcefully wipe the eyes.

Position the patient comfortably at the slit lamp and adjust the eyepieces of the microscope properly (see p. 22). Make certain that the beam is in the "click" position and that the patient's eyes are in primary gaze. To assess the right eye, ask the patient to fixate toward your right ear or over your right shoulder.

Position the light source 60 degrees to the left (temporally) of the microscope. Introduce the cobalt filter into the illumination beam. Adjust the microscope magnification to 6X to 10X. Use your right hand to control the joystick and vertical positioning knob; use your left hand to widen the slit to approximately 3 mm. Increase the slit lamp illumination rheostat to its highest setting (Fig. 2).

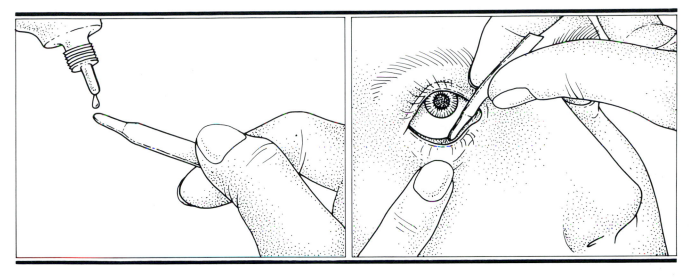

1. A. Squeeze a drop of sterile ophthalmic saline solution onto the fluorescein-sodium impregnated end of the strip.

1. B. Retract the right lower lid with the index finger or thumb of your left hand and dab the strip onto the inferior bulbar conjunctiva.

BREAKUP TIME DETERMINATION

Click stop:	In
Beam angle:	60 degrees
Beam width:	3 mm
Beam height:	Maximum
Filter:	Cobalt
Illumination:	Maximum
Magnification:	6–10X

2. Slit lamp setup for tear BUT determination.

Ask the patient to blink fully and then to refrain from blinking until instructed to do so. Begin counting mentally to yourself in 1-second intervals. While counting, manipulate the joystick with your right hand to continually scan all portions of the fluorescein-stained precorneal tear film (Fig. 3). The appearance of one or more black dry spots in the precorneal tear film marks the end of the test (Fig. 4). Record the number of seconds that elapsed as the tear breakup time (for example, BUT = 8 sec). Repeat the procedure for the left eye.

Interpretation. A normal breakup time is considered to be 10 to 15 seconds or greater. A low breakup time may be indicative of keratitis sicca. Other tests that may be performed to assess for keratitis sicca include Schirmer tear testing (p. 108), lactoferrin assay testing (p. 112), and collagen punctal plug insertion (p. 122). Focal areas initially appearing as black spots in the tear film that persist even with repeated blinks probably represent areas of "negative" fluorescein staining due to epithelial elevation rather than tear breakup (see p. 48).

Complications/Contraindications. BUT testing should be performed prior to the instillation of topical ophthalmic anesthetic solution because the BUT may be artificially lowered and corneal staining may be induced. If the patient has difficulty in refraining from blinking, gently retract the lids with your fingers with the hand not controlling the slit lamp joystick.

That portion of the bulbar conjunctiva that is touched with the fluorescein strip will stain densely and should not be interpreted as an abnormality. If the patient exhibits a Bell's reflex while the fluorescein strip is touched to the superior bulbar conjunctiva, linear staining of the cornea may be induced. Care should be taken to avoid applying too much saline solution to the fluorescein strip and inadvertently dripping fluorescein dye onto the patient's clothing. Reassure the patient that the orange discoloration of the tear film covering the cornea and conjunctiva will dissipate.

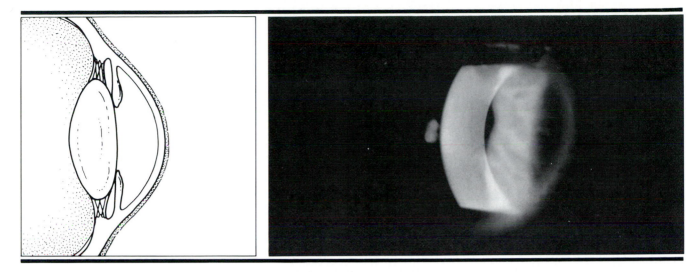

3. The intact precorneal tear film (schematic, left) appears uniformly green when stained with fluorescein sodium and illuminated with cobalt filter of the slit lamp (right). (*See also* Color Plate 15–3.)

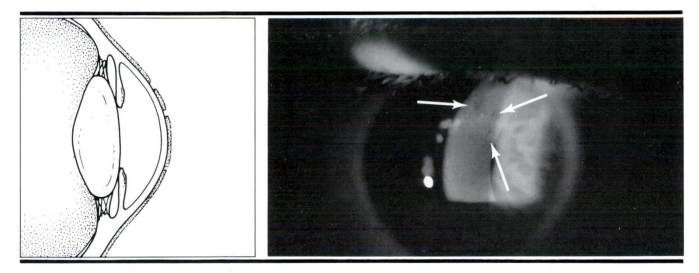

4. Dry areas appear as black spots or streaks in the fluorescein-stained precorneal tear film (arrows). (*See also* Color Plate 15–4.)

16   Vital Dye Staining

Description/Indications. Fluorescein sodium or rose bengal vital dyes are routinely used in the diagnosis of corneal and conjunctival conditions. Fluorescein sodium is an orange dye that fluoresces green when illuminated with a cobalt filter. Areas of corneal or conjunctival epithelial loss will exhibit fluorescein dye uptake and will appear bright green. This positive fluorescein staining will help to identify the extent and distribution of epithelial loss. Fluorescein staining is assessed whenever epithelial loss is suspected, such as following corneal or conjunctival trauma, contact lens removal, gonioscopy (see p. 72), or foreign body removal (see pp. 132 and 146), and to assess corneal involvement secondary to conjunctival, lid, lash, and lacrimal disorders.

The conjunctival epithelium will exhibit fluorescein staining as a result of trauma. Focal inflammatory involvements, such as nodules in nodular episcleritis or phlyctenules in phlyctenular keratoconjunctivitis, will also show positive fluorescein staining. Fluorescein dye will also tend to pool in the topographical undulations of the bulbar and palpebral conjunctiva.

Fluorescein staining will also help to assess areas of corneal epithelial elevation as occurs in a healing corneal abrasion or recurrent corneal erosion, in microcystic corneal edema, and in the geographic mapping areas of epithelial basement membrane dystrophy. The elevated epithelium causes a thinning of the precorneal tear film to produce black areas within the tear layer fluorescence.

In contrast, rose bengal staining will highlight corneal and epithelial cells that are devitalized but have not desquamated and are still intact. Rose bengal staining of the inferior cornea and bulbar conjunctiva is especially indicative of keratitis sicca.

Instrumentation. Slit lamp biomicroscope, sterile fluorescein sodium strips, sterile rose bengal strips, sterile ophthalmic saline solution, facial tissues.

Technique. Hand the patient a fresh facial tissue. Remove a sterile strip of the desired vital dye from the package, taking care not to contaminate the dye-impregnated end. Holding the strip in one hand over a wastebasket or sink, use the other hand to squeeze a drop of sterile ophthalmic saline solution onto the dye end of the strip (Fig. 1A). Ask the patient to look up. Gently retract the right lower lid with the index finger or thumb of the left hand. Holding the strip in your right hand, dab the moistened dye from the end of the strip onto the inferior bulbar conjunctiva (Fig. 1B). Alternatively, ask the patient to look down, gently retract the upper lid, and dab the dye onto the superior bulbar conjunctiva. Using the same strip repeat this procedure for the left eye. If anterior segment infection is present, however, instill vital dye into the uninvolved eye first or use a separate strip for each eye. Discard the strip(s). Advise the patient that the saline solution may momentarily sting slightly. The patient may use the tissue to dab away excess fluid but should not forcefully wipe the eyes.

Position the patient comfortably at the slit lamp and adjust the eyepieces of the microscope properly (see p. 22). Make certain that the beam is in the "click" position and that the patient's eyes are in primary gaze. To assess the right eye, ask the patient to fixate toward your right ear or over your right shoulder.

Position the light source 60 degrees to the left (temporally) of the microscope. Adjust the microscope magnification to 6X to 10X. Use your right hand to control the joystick and vertical positioning knob; place your left hand on the illumination beam housing to set the slit width at 3 to 4 mm and slit height to maximum for diffuse illumination.

Fluorescein Sodium Staining: Introduce the cobalt filter into the illumination beam and increase the slit lamp illumination rheostat to its highest setting (Fig. 2). Allow the fluorescein dye to diffuse for approximately 30 seconds. Scan the cornea and bulbar conjunctiva for areas of dye uptake that appear bright green. To assess the topography of the palpebral conjunctiva, gently retract the lower lid as the patient looks up, or evert the upper lid (see p. 86).

Rose Bengal Staining: Use diffuse white light illumination of medium intensity (Fig. 3). Scan the cornea and bulbar conjunctiva for areas of dye uptake that appear as rosy red areas.

Repeat the procedure for the left eye.

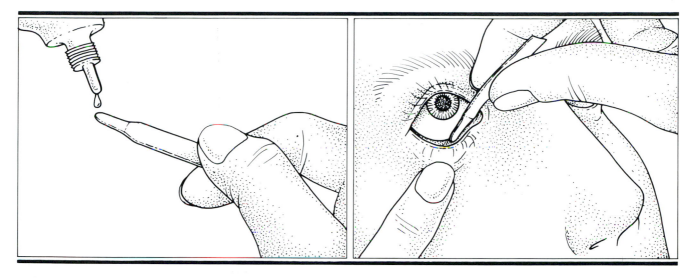

1. A. Squeeze a drop of sterile ophthalmic saline solution onto the vital dye-impregnated end of the strip.

1. B. Retract the right lower lid with the index finger or thumb of your left hand and dab the strip onto the inferior bulbar conjunctiva.

FLUORESCEIN SODIUM STAINING

Click stop:	In
Beam angle:	60 degrees
Beam width:	3–4 mm
Beam height:	Maximum
Filter:	Cobalt
Illumination:	Maximum
Magnification:	6–10X

2. Slit lamp setup for fluorescein sodium staining.

ROSE BENGAL STAINING

Click stop:	In
Beam angle:	60 degrees
Beam width:	3–4 mm
Beam height:	Maximum
Filter:	None
Illumination:	Medium
Magnification:	6–10X

3. Slit lamp setup for rose bengal staining.

Interpretation

Fluorescein Sodium Staining: Areas of missing corneal epithelium will take up fluorescein stain and appear bright green (Fig. 4). These areas are said to exhibit positive corneal staining. The extent and distribution of this staining will be dependent upon the etiology of the epithelial disruption. Mucus or epithelial debris in the tear film will also stain brightly with fluorescein.

In contrast, areas of epithelial elevation cause thinning of the fluorescein-stained tear layer. These areas will appear as black spots within the tear film and are said to exhibit negative fluorescein staining (Fig. 5). These areas present as persistent black spots in contrast to the dry spots of tear breakup, which transiently appear within the tear layer as the blink reflex is suppressed (see p. 42).

Fluorescein dye will pool in the normal topographical undulations of the bulbar and palpebral conjunctiva. On the bulbar conjunctiva this pooling of dye will appear as a subtle cross-hatching effect. On the palpebral conjunctiva, the fluorescein will pool around focal elevations of this tissue, and will accentuate the appearance of palpebral conjunctival follicles and papillae. In addition to this normally observed pooling effect, the conjunctiva will also exhibit frank fluorescein staining when the epithelium is disrupted.

Rose Bengal Staining: Rose bengal staining will appear as rosy red areas of dye uptake, indicative that epithelial cells are intact but devitalized (Fig. 6). Rose bengal will also stain mucus and keratin.

Complications/Contraindications. Vital dye staining should be performed prior to the instillation of topical ophthalmic anesthetic solution since corneal staining may be induced. That portion of the bulbar conjunctiva that is touched with the vital dye strip will stain densely and should not be misinterpreted as an abnormality. If the patient exhibits a Bell's reflex while the vital dye strip is touched to the superior bulbar conjunctiva, linear staining of the cornea may be induced.

If the fluorescein in the tear film is not allowed to diffuse slightly, the excess fluorescein may obscure areas of positive corneal staining. Conversely, excessive diffusion of the fluorescein will prevent visualization of areas of negative staining. With significant corneal epithelial disruption, the anterior chamber should be evaluated prior to the instillation of fluorescein (see p. 36). In this instance the fluorescein will penetrate through the cornea into the anterior chamber and will produce a green-tinged flare that may be misinterpreted as protein in the anterior chamber.

Care should be taken to avoid applying too much saline solution to the fluorescein or rose bengal strip and inadvertently dripping dye onto the patient's clothing. Reassure the patient that the orange or red discoloration of the tear film covering the cornea and conjunctiva will dissipate. Fluorescein sodium will discolor soft contact lenses if instilled while the lens is in the eye. Fluorexon is less likely to penetrate most soft lenses due to a higher molecular weight and may be used for vital dye staining when reinsertion of soft lenses is necessary.

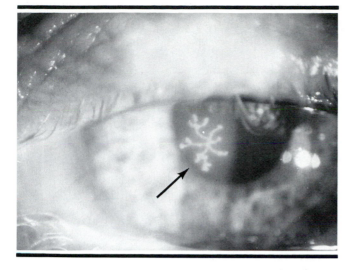

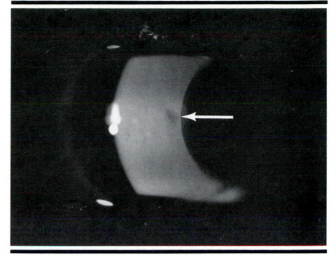

4. The cornea exhibits positive fluorescein sodium staining secondary to a herpes simplex dendritic ulcer (arrow). (*See also* Color Plate 16—4.)

5. The cornea exhibits negative fluorescein sodium staining centrally secondary to epithelial bullae resulting from Fuchs' endothelial dystrophy (arrow). (*See also* Color Plate 16—5.)

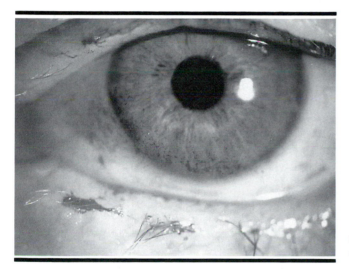

6. The bulbar conjunctiva and cornea exhibit rose bengal staining secondary to keratitis sicca. (*See also* Color Plate 16-6.)

17 Applanation Tonometry: Goldmann

Description/Indications. Measurement of the intraocular pressure (IOP) is an essential component of all routine eye examinations, is integral to assessing the efficacy of therapeutic agents for glaucoma, and is necessary to differentially diagnose acute anterior segment involvements.

Goldmann applanation tonometry is the technique for IOP measurement against which all other techniques are judged. The IOP is determined by measuring the amount of force necessary to flatten a constant corneal surface area. Compared with other techniques, the effects of intraocular volume change, surface tension, and corneal rigidity are negligible so that the applanation pressure corresponds well to the true IOP. Most Goldmann applanation tonometers are mounted on a slit lamp. The corneal area flattened by applanation will be visible through either the right or left eyepiece. A hand-held applanation tonometer (Perkins tonometer) is also available for patients who cannot be positioned in the slit lamp (see p. 56).

The three basic components of the Goldmann tonometer are the applanating probe, the probe arm mounted into a spring-loaded control box, and the measuring drum (Fig. 1). The probe is a prism that optically doubles the applanation image, displacing it into two halves. The radius of the front surface of the probe is 3.06 mm and corresponds to the flattened portion of the corneal surface. The tear layer, which appears yellow-green with fluorescein viewed with a cobalt filter, is used to demarcate the flattened corneal area. Where the probe contacts the cornea, the fluorescein-stained tears are pushed to the periphery of the applanation area to form a well-defined yellow-green ring. The inside border of the ring represents the line of transition between the area of the cornea flattened by applanation and that which is not. The knob on the measuring drum reads in grams of applanation force; one gram of force corresponds to 10 mm Hg of IOP.

Instrumentation. Slit lamp biomicroscope with Goldmann tonometer, asepticized applanation probe, fluorescein sodium–benoxinate ophthalmic solution or sterile fluorescein sodium ophthalmic strips with topical ophthalmic anesthetic solution, facial tissues.

Technique. Following slit lamp examination of the anterior segment (see p. 24), ask the patient to sit back from the slit lamp. Hand the patient a clean facial tissue. Instill a drop of fluorescein sodium–benoxinate ophthalmic solution into each eye, or instill a drop of topical ophthalmic anesthetic and fluorescein sodium vital dye (Fig. 2, see also p. 2). Advise the patient that a mild, transient burning may occur and that he or she may blot the excess fluid from the eyes with the tissue. Swing the entire Goldmann tonometer to the forward position into which the clean and dry, asepticized probe has been inserted. If the patient has less than three diopters of corneal cylinder as measured by keratometry, align the probe so that the white mark on the probe holder is continuous with the 180-degree line on the probe. Align the red mark on the probe holder with the line on the probe corresponding to the minus cylinder axis if more than three diopters of corneal cylinder are present. The probe arm should rock back freely when the measurement drum is on "zero." Make sure the probe "clicks" laterally into the straight-ahead position when the tonometer is positioned for measurement.

Position the slit lamp source approximately 60 degrees from the eyepieces. Open the slit beam to its widest setting and introduce the cobalt filter. Set the slit lamp magnification to 6X to 10X, and turn the rheostat to its maximum setting so that the probe tip is brightly illuminated (Fig. 3). Turn the knob on the measuring drum to "1," corresponding to 10 mm Hg, causing it to rock forward slightly.

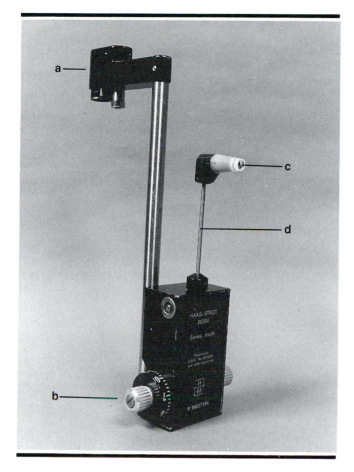

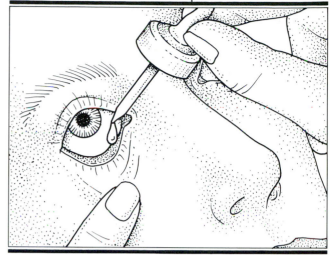

2. Instill a drop of fluorescein sodium—benoxinate solution into each eye.

1. The components of the slit-lamp-mounted Goldmann applanation tonometer. (a) Slit lamp mounting arm. (b) Measuring drum. (c) Applanation probe. (d) Probe arm.

GOLDMANN APPLANATION TONOMETRY

Click stop:	In
Beam angle:	60 degrees
Beam width:	Maximum
Beam height:	Maximum
Filter:	Cobalt
Illumination:	Maximum
Magnification:	6–10X

3. Slit lamp setup for Goldmann applanation tonometry.

Ask the patient to place the head on the chin and forehead rests of the slit lamp. Correct positioning of the patient's head against the forehead rest is important. Occasionally an assistant or family member may need to gently hold the patient's head in place. Instruct the patient to fixate straight ahead or adjust the fixation light so that the right eye is in primary gaze. Looking outside the slit lamp, grossly center the probe approximately ¾ inch from the right corneal apex (Fig. 4A). If large slit lamp movement is necessary, move the base toward the patient while keeping the joystick vertical, making subsequent finer movements with the joystick. Looking through the slit lamp, use the joystick to move the probe slightly forward. Approximately ½ inch before corneal contact is made, the reflection of the probe off the cornea will appear as two pale blue semicircles (Fig. 4B). Use the joystick and vertical positioning knob to adjust the lateral and vertical position of the slit-lamp-mounted probe so that the pale blue semicircles are centered in the field of view and equally divided, making movements in the direction of the larger semicircle.

Ask the patient to blink fully and to keep the lids wide open, looking straight ahead. Use the joystick to move the probe toward the corneal apex while maintaining centration of the pale blue semicircles as visualized through the slit lamp. After contacting the cornea you will see two steadily pulsating fluorescent green semicircles. The width of the fluorescein semicircles should be approximately one-tenth of the diameter of the flattened area. Make small adjustments with the joystick in the direction of the larger semicircle to exactly center and equally divide the fluorescein semicircles (Fig. 5). An alternative approach for achieving corneal contact is to sight outside of the slit lamp as the probe is positioned on the corneal apex. The limbus will exhibit a blue glow when contact is made. While using the joystick to carefully maintain corneal contact, resume sighting through the slit lamp and proceed with the technique.

While maintaining applanation with one hand on the joystick, quickly use the opposite hand to turn the measuring drum until the inner borders of the two fluorescein semicircles just touch each other. If significant pulsation is present, adjust the measuring drum so that the semicircles pulsate equally to either side of the correct endpoint (Fig. 6). Pull back on the joystick to remove the probe from the cornea. Note the IOP measurement in mm Hg by multiplying the figure on the drum by 10. Repeated measurements should be within a range of ± 0.5 mm Hg. Repeat the technique for the left eye, swinging the slit lamp illumination beam to the temporal side if desired. Swing the tonometer out from the forward position and check both corneas with the slit lamp for induced epithelial staining (see p. 48).

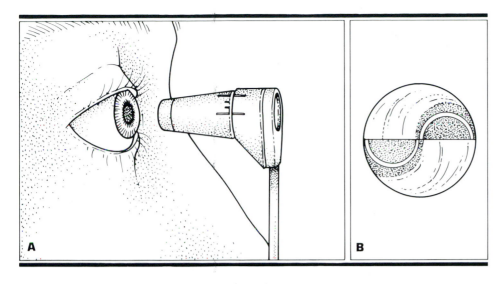

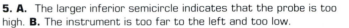

4. A. Looking outside the slit lamp, grossly center the probe approximately ¾ inch from the corneal apex. **B.** Approximately ½ inch before corneal contact is made, the reflection of the probe will appear as two pale blue semicircles, which are used to center the probe. (*See also* Color Plate 17–4.B.)

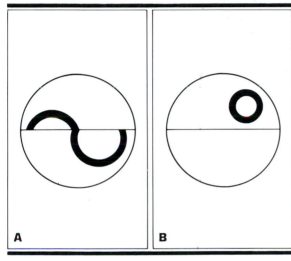

5. A. The larger inferior semicircle indicates that the probe is too high. **B.** The instrument is too far to the left and too low.

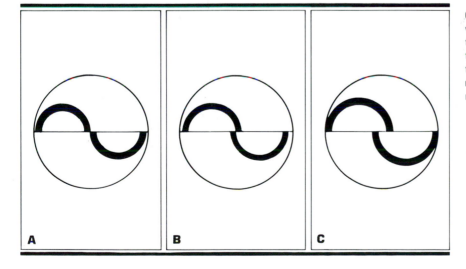

6. While maintaining corneal contact with the joystick, use the opposite hand to quickly turn the measuring drum until the inner borders of the semicircles just touch. **A.** More probe pressure is needed. **B.** Correct endpoint. **C.** Too much probe pressure.

Occasionally a patient may have difficulty keeping the lids open or may have a narrow palpebral fissure so that lid retraction is needed. Just before aligning the probe, ask the patient to look down. Use the forefinger of your left hand to gently retract the upper lid. Ask the patient to look straight ahead and use the thumb of your left hand to gently retract the lower lid. Be certain to hold the lids against the orbital rims so that pressure is not applied to the globe (Fig. 7). Proceed with the technique as described using your right hand to control the joystick. Release your right hand from the joystick to adjust the knob on the measurement drum when corneal contact is made. Since neither hand is maintaining applanation with the joystick, corneal contact is frequently lost. After adjusting the measurement drum, use your right hand on the joystick to reapplanate the cornea. Repeat this process to bracket to the applanation endpoint.

If the fluorescein semicircles are too wide, too much fluorescein is in the conjunctival sac or the lids contacted the probe during measurement. Draw back the probe, dry the probe tip with a clean tissue, ask the patient to gently blot the eyes with a tissue, and repeat the measurement. Conversely, rapid dissipation of the tears will produce semicircles that are too narrow. Draw back the probe, instill more fluorescein, and repeat the measurement (Fig. 8).

Interpretation. If the fluorescein semicircles are too wide, the IOP measurement will be artificially high. Semicircles that are too narrow yield IOP measurements that are artificially low. Most practitioners consider normal intraocular pressures as measured by applanation to be 21 mm Hg or less, with the difference in readings between the two eyes expected to be no greater that 3 to 4 mm Hg. However, because of diurnal IOP fluctuation, along with many other factors, it is extremely important that the practitioner not rely solely on the IOP reading to rule out a diagnosis of glaucoma. Careful optic nerve head assessment, anterior segment evaluation including gonioscopy, and visual field analysis are needed to determine whether the IOP is normal for that individual.

Complications/Contraindications. The examiner must be familiar with any contraindications that may preclude using any of the diagnostic agents needed for applanation tonometry. Applanation tonometry is usually avoided in the presence of conjunctival infection to prevent probe contamination, large central corneal abrasions to prevent further epithelial disruption, and significant epithelial basement membrane dystrophy to avoid inducing a corneal abrasion. Care should be taken to avoid over-manipulating eyes that have sustained severe ocular trauma. Corneas that are extremely distorted or scarred will produce irregular mires that may prevent an accurate reading.

To minimize anxiety, it is best to avoid detailing to the patient that actual corneal contact will occur. Patient anxiety tends to artificially elevate the IOP. Continual coaxing of the patient to open both eyes widely will help to minimize interference by the lids. Touching of the lids or lashes by the probe will induce a blink reflex and should be avoided. If the examiner puts pressure on the globe while retracting the lids the IOP will be artificially elevated.

It is common to induce some superficial corneal epithelial disruption following applanation tonometry. This will occur following topical anesthetic use, due to movements of the probe on the cornea, desiccation of the cornea surrounding the contact area, and unanticipated patient eye movements. Usually no treatment is required for these minor tissue disruptions. The examiner should avoid, however, large repositioning movements of the probe when it is in contact with the cornea. If the appearance of the fluorescein semicircles indicates that major repositioning is needed, use the joystick to pull the probe back from the cornea and reposition before applanating again. Rarely, poor examiner technique or sudden head or eye movements by the patient while the probe is in contact with the cornea may induce a corneal abrasion.

A patient may rarely experience vasovagal syncope during this technique. Should this occur, basic first-aid measures are taken.

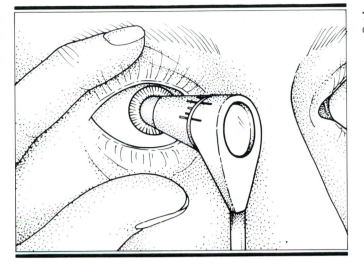

7. Gently retract the upper and lower lids against the orbital rims if necessary.

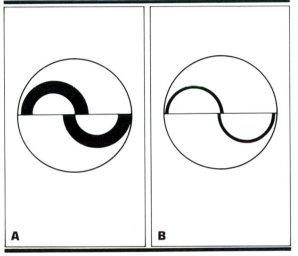

8. A. Wide semicircles indicate that too much fluorescein is present.
B. Narrow semicircles indicate insufficient fluorescein is present.

18 Applanation Tonometry: Perkins

Description/Indications. Measurement of the intraocular pressure (IOP) is an essential component of all routine eye examinations, is integral to assessing the effect of therapeutic agents for glaucoma, and is necessary to differentially diagnose acute anterior segment involvements.

Goldmann applanation tonometry is the technique for IOP measurement against which all other techniques are judged. The IOP is determined by measuring the amount of force necessary to flatten a constant corneal area. Compared with other techniques, the effects of intraocular volume change, surface tension, and corneal rigidity are negligible, so that the applanation pressure corresponds well to the true IOP. Most Goldmann applanation tonometers are mounted on a slit lamp (see p. 50). For some patients with physical disabilities who cannot be positioned in the slit lamp, when a slit lamp is not available, or for wheelchair-bound or bedridden patients, a hand-held applanation tonometer (Perkins tonometer) may be used to obtain accurate IOP measurements. The prism arm is counterbalanced so that the instrument may be used in the horizontal or vertical position.

The applanating probe is mounted into a spring-loaded holder controlled by a measurement knob. The cobalt illumination source is self-contained in the handle of the unit and turns on when the measurement knob is turned past the zero mark. An adjustable forehead rest helps to support the instrument in place (Fig. 1). The probe is a prism that optically doubles the applanation image, displacing it into two halves. The diameter of the front surface of the probe is 3.06 mm and corresponds to the flattened portion of the corneal surface. The tear layer, which appears yellow-green with fluorescein viewed with a cobalt filter, is used to demarcate the flattened corneal area. Where the probe contacts the cornea, the fluorescein-stained tears are pushed to the periphery of the applanation area to form a well-defined yellow-green ring. The inside border of the ring represents the line of transition between the area of the cornea flattened by applanation and that which is not. The knob on the measuring drum reads in grams of applanation force; 1 g of force corresponds to 10 mm Hg of IOP.

Instrumentation. Perkins tonometer with aseptized applanation probe, fluorescein sodium–benoxinate ophthalmic solution or sterile fluorescein sodium ophthalmic strips with topical ophthalmic anesthetic solution, facial tissues.

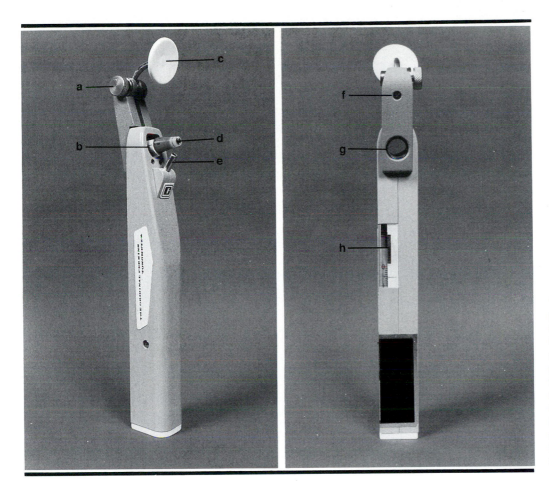

1. A. (far left) The components of the Perkins applanation tonometer. (a) Forehead rest set screw. (b) Applanating probe holder. (c) Patient forehead rest. (d) Applanating probe. (e) Illumination source. **B.** (left) (f) Examiner forehead rest mount (optional). (g) Eyepiece. (h) Measurement knob.

Technique. Insert the clean and dry, asepticized probe into the tonometer holder. If the patient has less than three diopters of corneal cylinder as measured by keratometry or as interpolated from the spectacle prescription, align the probe so that the white mark on the probe holder is continuous with the 180-degree line on the probe. Align the red mark on the probe holder with the line on the probe corresponding to the minus cylinder axis if more than three diopters of corneal cylinder are present. Adjust the length of the forehead rest by loosening the locking screw and sliding the arm in or out. Tighten the locking screw at the estimated length of the arm so that when the rest is placed on the forehead the tonometer can be angled and pivoted into a position that is parallel with the front of the face (Fig. 2).

Hand the patient a clean facial tissue. Instill a drop of fluorescein sodium–benoxinate ophthalmic solution into each eye, or instill a drop of topical ophthalmic anesthetic and fluorescein sodium vital dye (Fig. 3). Advise the patient that a mild, transient burning may occur and that he or she may blot the excess fluid from the eyes with the tissue. Position the patient's line of sight so that the eyes are in primary gaze.

To measure the patient's right eye, position yourself standing or sitting in front of and slightly temporally to the right eye. Turn the measuring knob so that the cobalt illumination turns on and the dial is set at 1 (10 mm Hg). Place the forehead rest approximately in the middle of the patient's forehead and gently hold it in position with your left hand. Looking outside the instrument, pivot the handle toward the patient so that the tip of the probe is approximately ¾ inch from the corneal apex (Fig. 4).

Sighting through the viewing lens with your right eye, the reflection of the probe off the cornea before contact is made will appear as two pale blue semicircles (Fig. 5). Move the instrument handle toward the patient while maintaining centration of the pale blue semicircles. After contacting the cornea you will see two steadily pulsating fluorescent green semicircles. The width of the fluorescein semicircles should be approximately one-tenth of the diameter of the flattened area. Make small adjustments with the handle to exactly center and equally divide the fluorescein semicircles, moving toward the larger semicircle (Fig. 6).

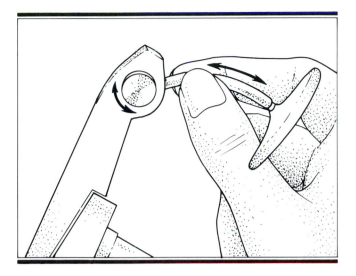

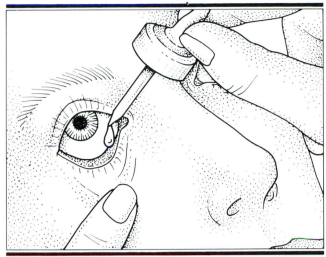

2. (above left) Loosen the locking screw, slide the forehead rest arm in or out as needed, then tighten the locking screw.

3. (above right) Instill a drop of fluorescein sodium—benoxinate solution into each eye.

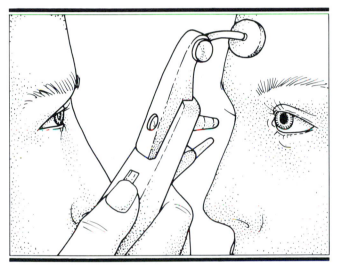

4. (left) Place the forehead rest in the middle of the patient's forehead, holding it gently with your left hand. Position the probe approximately ¾ inch from the cornea.

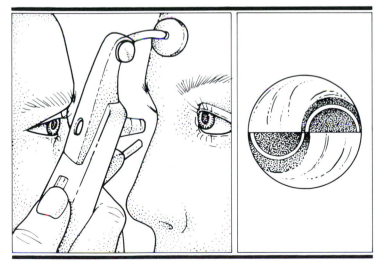

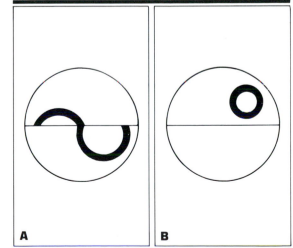

5. Looking through the instrument, the reflection of the probe off the cornea will appear as two pale blue semicircles. Move the instrument forward until two green semicircles appear. (*See also* Color Plate 17–4.B.)

6. A. The larger inferior circle indicates that the probe is too high. **B.** The instrument is too far to the left and too low.

An alternative approach for achieving corneal contact is to sight outside of the tonometer as the probe is positioned on the corneal apex. The limbus will exhibit a blue glow when contact is made. While using good hand control to carefully maintain corneal contact, resume sighting through the tonometer and proceed with the technique.

Use the thumb of your right hand to turn the knurled knob controlling the measuring drum until the inner borders of the two fluorescein rings just touch each other (Fig. 7). If significant pulsation is present, adjust the measuring drum so that the rings pulsate equally to either side of the correct endpoint. Lift the instrument off the cornea. Note the IOP measurement in mm Hg by multiplying the figure on the drum by 10. Repeated measurements should be within a range of ± 0.5 mm Hg. Repeat the technique for the left eye, using opposite hands and positioning yourself to the patient's left.

Occasionally a patient may have difficulty holding the lids open, or may have a narrow palpebral fissure requiring lid retraction. Once the forehead rest is in place, the thumb and forefinger of your left hand may be used to gently retract the lids (see p. 54). Be certain to hold the lids against the orbital rims so that pressure is not applied to the globe. Proceed with the technique as described.

If the fluorescein semicircles are too wide, too much fluorescein is in the conjunctival sac or the lids contacted the probe during measurement (Fig. 8). Draw back the probe, dry the probe tip with a clean tissue, ask the patient to gently blot the eyes with a tissue, and repeat the measurement. Conversely, rapid dissipation of the tears will produce semicircles that are too narrow. Draw back the probe, instill more fluorescein, and repeat the measurement.

Interpretation. If the fluorescein semicircles are too wide, the IOP measurement will be artificially high. Semicircles that are too narrow yield IOP measurements that are artificially low. Most practitioners consider normal intraocular pressures as measured by applanation to be 21 mm Hg or less, with the difference in readings between the two eyes expected to be no greater than 3 to 4 mm Hg. However, because of diurnal IOP fluctuation, along with many other factors, it is extremely important that the practitioner not rely solely on the IOP reading to rule out a diagnosis of glaucoma. Careful optic nerve head assessment, anterior segment evaluation including gonioscopy, and visual field analysis, are needed to determine whether the IOP is normal for that individual.

Complications/Contraindications. Good, steady technique on the part of the examiner is important to produce corneal applanation with appropriate pressure. The examiner must be familiar with any contraindications that may preclude using any of the diagnostic agents needed for applanation tonometry. Reassure the patient that the orange discoloration of the tear film will dissipate. Applanation tonometry is usually avoided in the presence of conjunctival infection to prevent probe contamination, large central corneal abrasions to prevent further epithelial disruption, and significant epithelial basement membrane dystrophy to avoid inducing a corneal abrasion. Care should be taken to avoid overmanipulating eyes that have sustained severe ocular trauma. Corneas that are extremely distorted or scarred will produce irregular mires that may prevent an accurate reading.

To minimize anxiety, it is best to avoid detailing to the patient that actual corneal contact will occur. Patient anxiety tends to artificially elevate the IOP. Continual coaxing of the patient to widely open the eyes will help to minimize interference by the lids. Touching of the lids or lashes by the probe will induce a blink reflex and should be avoided. If the examiner puts pressure on the globe while retracting the lids the IOP will be artificially elevated.

It is common to induce some superficial corneal epithelial disruption following applanation tonometry. This will occur following topical anesthetic use, due to movements of the probe on the cornea, desiccation of the cornea surrounding the contact area, and unanticipated patient eye movements. Usually no treatment is required for these minor tissue disruptions. The examiner should avoid, however, large repositioning movements of the probe when it is in contact with the cornea. Rarely, poor examiner technique or sudden head or eye movements by the patient while the probe is in contact with the cornea may induce a corneal abrasion.

A patient may rarely experience vasovagal syncope during this technique. Should this occur, basic first-aid measures are taken. These include elevating the feet above the level of the head, passing a broken ammonia inhalant ampule beneath the nostrils, and monitoring the basic vital signs.

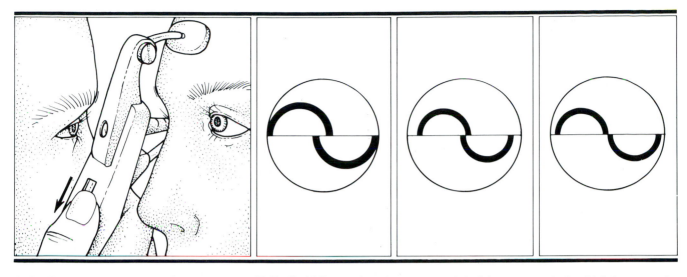

7. A. While maintaining corneal contact, use your thumb to turn the knurled knob until the inner borders of the semicircles just touch.

7. B. (Left) Too much probe pressure; (middle) correct endpoint; (right) more probe pressure is needed.

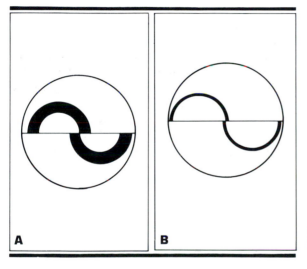

8. A. Wide semicircles indicate that too much fluorescein is present.
B. Narrow semicircles indicate insufficient fluorescein is present.

19 Crystalline Lens Evaluation

Description/Indications. The crystalline lens consists of the nucleus, cortex, and capsule. The nucleus may be further subdivided into the most clinically distinguishable components: the embryonic nucleus, seen as a dark vertical band in the center of the lens; the fetal nucleus, bounded by the anterior and posterior "Y" sutures; and the adult nucleus, most visible after the age of 30. The zones of optical discontinuity visible with the slit lamp demarcate the various layers of the crystalline lens. Any zone of the crystalline lens may exhibit a loss of transparency due to age-related changes, trauma, ocular infections or inflammation, medications, or congenital opacities. Examination with the slit lamp biomicroscope allows for detailed assessment of these congenital or acquired cataracts. Since many of these changes are acquired and progressive, periodic crystalline lens evaluation is needed.

Slit lamp examination of the crystalline lens is most accurately and easily done following pupillary dilation. During routine examination, crystalline lens evaluation with the slit lamp generally follows refractive analysis, undilated slit lamp examination, tonometry, and dilated fundus evaluation. Two types of slit lamp illumination are most frequently used to assess the crystalline lens, direct focal illumination and retroillumination.

Direct focal illumination refers to coincident focusing of the light beam and the microscope. It does not refer to coaxial placement of the light source with the microscope. The parallelepiped and optic section are two commonly used types of direct focal illumination. The parallelepiped produces a three-dimensional section of the lens and is useful for initial lens evaluation. An optic section illuminates a two-dimensional lens area that is viewed obliquely, similar to examining a histological section. The procedure is the same as parallelepiped illumination except that the beam width is narrowed until it is almost extinguished. When evaluating the lens, the optic section is sharply focused to localize lens opacities. Since the entire depth of the lens cannot be in focus at one time with direct focal illumination, systematic scanning of the lens must be performed.

When the slit lamp beam is directed straight ahead through the pupil, the light will reflect off the fundus back through the pupil to form the "red reflex" of *retroillumination*. Any frank lens opacities will absorb the reflected light and will appear as black or darkened areas in the red reflex, depending upon their density. Areas of fluid within the lens will appear as vacuolated or cleft-shaped areas of irregularity in the red reflex. This technique is especially useful to determine where the opacity lies relative to the visual axis and to assess what portion of the pupillary area is obscured by the opacity. Retroillumination used alone, however, will not definitively localize the lens opacity.

Instrumentation. Slit lamp biomicroscope, diagnostic pharmaceutical agents for pupillary dilation.

Technique

Direct Focal Illumination: Position the patient comfortably at the slit lamp (see p. 22). Adjust the eyepieces to accommodate your pupillary distance and refractive error. Adjust the slit lamp rheostat to a medium setting and the magnification to 10X to 16X. Position the microscope directly in front of the eye and the light source at approximately 60 degrees temporally from the microscope. Make certain that the beam is in the "click" position and that the patient's eyes are in primary gaze. To assess the right eye, ask the patient to fixate toward your right ear or over your right shoulder. With your left hand adjust the beam to its maximum height and narrow the beam to 1 to 2 mm in width to illuminate a parallelepiped-shaped section of the lens (Fig. 1). Use your right hand on the joystick to sharply focus the microscope and parallelepiped simultaneously.

Starting at the temporal border of the dilated right pupil, use the joystick to focus the parallelepiped on the anterior half of the lens. Keep this portion of the lens in focus while scanning across the lens to the nasal border of the pupil. Move the joystick forward to focus on the posterior half of the lens, scanning across it to the temporal pupil border (Fig. 2).

1. Slit lamp setup for parallelepiped examination of the crystalline lens.

DIRECT FOCAL: PARALLELEPIPED

Click stop:	In
Beam angle:	60 degrees
Beam width:	1–2 mm
Beam height:	Maximum
Filter:	None
Illumination:	Medium
Magnification:	10–16X

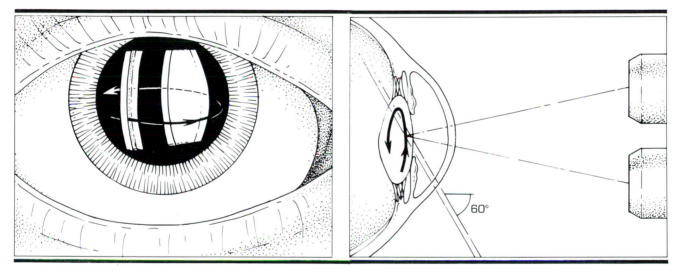

2. Focus a parallelepiped on the anterior half of the lens while scanning from the temporal pupil border to the nasal pupil border. Move the joystick forward slightly to reverse the scan while focused on the posterior half of the lens.

If a lens opacity is detected, use an optic section to localize it to a specific lens layer. Use your left hand to narrow the slit lamp beam just to the point of extinguishing it (Fig. 3). Focus the optic section sharply on the lens opacity (Fig. 4). Repeating this technique with the light source positioned nasally will ensure that the lens is thoroughly assessed.

Retroillumination: Position the light source directly in front of the microscope so that neither eyepiece is occluded. Adjust the microscope magnification to 6X to 10X. Use your right or left hand to control the joystick and vertical positioning knob; place your opposite hand on the illumination beam housing to control slit height and width. Adjust the beam illumination to form a short parallelepiped approximately 1 mm wide and 3 mm high that will fit within the central pupillary area (Fig. 5). Position the beam within the pupil area, focus the microscope at the plane of the iris, and observe for areas of black opacity or irregularity within the red reflex. If an opacity is noted, the slit lamp may be moved forward to bring it into focus (Fig. 6). Repeat the procedure for the left eye using direct focal and retroillumination.

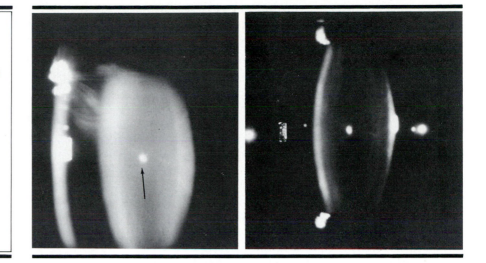

DIRECT FOCAL: OPTIC SECTION

Click stop: In
Beam angle: 60 degrees
Beam width: Nearly
                   extinguished
Beam height: Maximum
Filter: None
Illumination: Medium
Magnification: 10—16X

RETROILLUMINATION: LENS

Click stop: In
Beam angle: 0 degrees
Beam width: 1 mm
Beam height: 3 mm
Filter: None
Illumination: Medium
Magnification: 6—10X

3. (above left) Slit lamp setup for optic section examination of the crystalline lens.

4. A. (above center) An anterior axial embryonal cataract is detected using a parallelepiped (arrow). **B.** (above right) Using an optic section the opacity is localized to just anterior of the embryonic nucleus.

5. (left) Slit lamp setup for retroillumination of the crystalline lens.

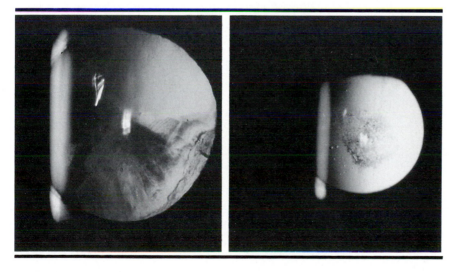

6. A. A cortical cataract as seen using retroillumination. (*See also* Color Plate 19-6.A.)

6. B. A posterior subcapsular cataract as seen using retroillumination. (*See also* Color Plate 19-6.B.)

Interpretation. The shape and location of the lens opacity will help diagnose its etiology. With direct focal illumination, most cataracts will appear white; in retroillumination they will appear black. Many vacuoles or pockets of fluid within the lens will not be visible with direct focal illumination but will be detected as round or oblong irregularities with retroillumination.

The three most common age-related cataracts are nuclear sclerosis, cortical spoking, and posterior subcapsular cataracts (Fig. 7). Depending upon its degree, nuclear sclerosis will appear as a yellow, orange, or brownish haze toward the posterior half of the lens in direct focal illumination. When pronounced, the edge of the sclerosed nucleus will create an "oil droplet" effect in the red reflex of retroillumination. Cortical spoking (cuneiform cataract) will appear as wedged-shaped opacities in the anterior or posterior cortex. Posterior subcapsular changes (cupuliform cataract) will appear as vacuolated, ground glass opacities just beneath the posterior capsule. These age-related lens changes may occur singly or in combination. The recently proposed Lens Opacities Classification System, version II (LOCS II), uses color slit lamp and retroillumination transparencies to grade nuclear opalescence and color (four standards), cortical opacities (five standards), and posterior subcapsular cataract (four standards).

It is very important that the examiner learn to estimate the effect of cataract formation on best corrected visual acuity (VA) based on the appearance of the lens. If the VA is monocularly reduced and the crystalline lens changes are judged to be symmetric, then other causes must be sought to account for the VA difference.

Complications/Contraindications. If the patient is a suitable candidate for slit lamp biomicroscopy, there are no contraindications to performing this specific examination of the crystalline lens. The routine precautions for pupillary dilation should be followed (see p. 2). The novice biomicroscopist may have a tendency to set the slit lamp illumination rheostat too high, which may produce some discomfort for the patient due to the pupillary dilation.

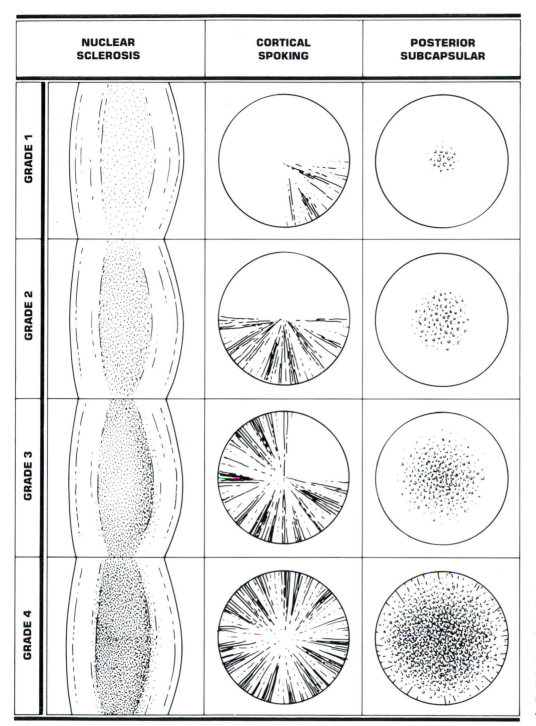

	NUCLEAR SCLEROSIS	CORTICAL SPOKING	POSTERIOR SUBCAPSULAR
GRADE 1			
GRADE 2			
GRADE 3			
GRADE 4			

7. A grading system for senile cataracts. The nuclear sclerotic changes are shown in cross-section with the anterior surface to the left. The cortical spoking and posterior subcapsular changes are seen in retroillumination. (*See also* Color Plate 19–7.)

20 Vitreous Evaluation

Description/Indications. Although the vitreous is comprised of approximately 99% water, the solid components that compose the remaining 1% reflect light sufficiently well to allow for evaluation of the vitreous using the slit lamp biomicroscope. The focal length of the slit lamp allows for observation of approximately the anterior one-third of the vitreous body. Use of auxilliary instrumentation such as the Hruby lens (see p. 208), retinal three-mirror lens (see p. 204), and the 90-D lens (see p. 210) will extend the focal range of the slit lamp further into the posterior chamber for more extensive examination of the vitreous.

Routine observation of the vitreous performed in conjunction with evaluation of the crystalline lens following pupillary dilation (see p. 62) will allow the practitioner to distinguish normal vitreous appearance from abnormal. Other indications for slit lamp examination of the vitreous include symptoms of floaters and light flashes (photopsia), to diagnose posterior vitreous detachment (PVD) with or without retinal complication, and to assess vitreous involvement in intraocular segment inflammation.

Examination of the vitreous with the slit lamp is best performed following pupillary dilation. The most useful illumination technique to evaluate the vitreous is direct focal illumination. Direct focal illumination refers to the focusing of the light beam and the microscope in the same specific area. It does not refer to coaxial placement of the light source with the microscope. The parallelepiped and optic section are two commonly used types of direct focal illumination. The parallelepiped produces a three-dimensional section of the vitreous and is most useful for its evaluation.

Instrumentation. Slit lamp biomicroscope, diagnostic pharmaceutical agents for pupillary dilation.

Technique. Position the patient comfortably at the slit lamp (see p. 22) following pupillary dilation (see p. 2). Adjust the eyepieces to accommodate your pupillary distance and refractive error. Adjust the slit lamp rheostat to a medium to medium-high setting and the magnification to 10X to 16X. Position the microscope directly in front of the eye and the light source at approximately 45 to 60 degrees temporally from the microscope. Make certain that the beam is in the "click" position and that the patient's eyes are in primary gaze. To assess the right eye, ask the patient to fixate toward your right ear or over your right shoulder. With your left hand adjust the beam to its maximum height and narrow the beam to 1 to 2 mm in width to illuminate a parallelepiped-shaped section of the vitreous. Use your right hand on the joystick to sharply focus the microscope and parallelepiped simultaneously (Fig. 1).

Starting at the temporal border of the dilated right pupil, move the joystick forward to focus the parallelepiped into the anterior vitreous. Keep this portion of the vitreous in focus while scanning across the vitreous to the nasal border of the pupil. Move the joystick further forward so as to focus into the vitreous as far as possible and scan across it to the temporal pupil border (Fig. 2). Repeating this technique with the beam positioned nasally will ensure that the vitreous is thoroughly examined.

Interpretation

Normal Vitreous: The vitreous is adherent to the lens in a 9-mm diameter arcuate or circular area known as the ligament of Wieger. Within this 9-mm diameter area is the optically empty retrolental space. Frequently a small corkscrew like fibril may be seen dangling from the central portion of the posterior lens surface. This is a remnant of the hyaloid artery and may be accompanied by a Mittendorf dot.

The anterior portion of the vitreous appears as milky folds of gossamer-like texture separated by optically empty spaces. These folds appear wavy and oscillate with eye movements. In the very young patient the collagen fibrils are difficult to distinguish. In the older patient, however, the folds are seen to be composed of individual crisscrossing fibrils. Small white dots or nodosities may be seen at the intersection of two fibrils. The spaces between the fibrils are otherwise optically empty in the normal vitreous.

1. Slit lamp setup for slit lamp examination of the vitreous.

PARALLELEPIPED: VITREOUS

Click stop: In
Beam angle: 45–60 degrees
Beam width: 1–2 mm
Beam height: Maximum
Filter: None
Illumination: Medium to medium-high
Magnification: 10–16X

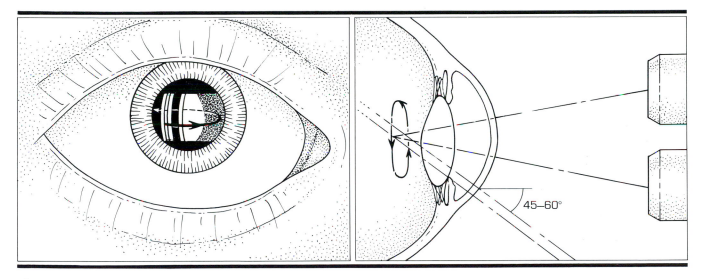

2. Focus the parallelepiped into the anterior vitreous. Beginning at the temporal pupil border, scan toward the nasal pupil border. Focus as far into the vitreous as possible and reverse the direction of scan. Repeat the scan with the beam positioned nasally.

Vitreous Cells: Multiple conditions involving the posterior segment may result in a spewing of inflammatory cells, red blood cells, or pigment cells into the vitreous. These cells will appear as small punctate opacities (Fig. 3) suspended or slowly floating within the optically empty spaces between the fibrils and in the retrolental space (space of Berger). These cells are not to be confused with nodosities that may be present at the intersection of two fibrils.

If the cells are white in color, they are probably inflammatory white blood cells (leukocytes) that are the result of posterior segment inflammation such as pars planitis, toxocara canis, or active ocular toxoplasmosis. Inflammatory white blood cells may also appear in the anterior vitreous as spillover from a significant anterior uveitis. If the vitreous cells are red-brown in color they are usually red blood cells (erythrocytes) and/or retinal pigment epithelial cells (RPE cells). Known as tobacco dusting or Shaffer's sign, these red-brown cells are usually an indication that a retinal tear or detachment is present so that RPE cells have become dislodged or associated retinal vessel damage has occurred. When the red-free (green) filter is introduced, the red blood cells appear black and will no longer be visible within the vitreous. Pigment particles will not absorb the red-free light and will still be visible.

Space-occupying lesions of the posterior chamber such as retinoblastoma and malignant melanoma may also produce vitreous cells.

Vitreous Fiber Clumping: With increasing age, the vitreous fibers lose some of their normal fluid binding (gel) capacity so that the fibers and fluid become separated (syneresis). In doing so, the fibers will tend to clump together and will produce the symptom of floaters. These clumped fibers will appear as very prominent vitreous stranding when observed with the slit lamp.

Prominent vitreous stranding may also be observed following the resolution of significant poste-rior segment inflammation or hemorrhage in which the vitreous was involved.

Posterior Vitreous Detachment (PVD): With time, pockets of fluid (lacunae) will form within the body of the vitreous. Percolation posteriorly of the liquified vitreous through the vitreous cortex will result in a pulling away of the vitreous from its peripapillary attachment to produce a PVD (Fig. 4). The posterior vitreous cortex collapses forward so that a prepapillary annulus may be visible with retroillumination with a direct ophthalmoscope (see p. 186), and the posterior vitreous cortex may be within focusing range of the slit lamp (Fig. 5). Following PVD, the posterior limiting layer of the vitreous may be apparent as an undulating, white wrinkled-looking veil that separates the collapsed and condensed fibril-laden vitreous anteriorly from the fluid-filled, optically empty space posteriorly.

Asteroid Hyalosis: Spherical calcium-containing opacities may form most commonly unilaterally, or bilaterally, in the vitreous in a middle-aged or older patient. When present in the anterior vitreous within focusing range of the slit lamp, they will appear as very bright, yellow, reflective bodies suspended in the vitreous.

Complications/Contraindications. There are no contraindications to performing this specific slit lamp examination of the vitreous. The routine precautions for pupillary dilation should be followed (see p. 2). The novice biomicroscopist may have a tendency to set the slit lamp illumination rheostat too high, which may produce some discomfort for the patient due to the pupillary dilation.

Significant cataract formation can obscure the various vitreous landmarks. A good deal of observational skill development is needed to accurately assess the presence of vitreous cells. Likewise, the collapse of the posterior limiting layer of the vitreous in PVD can be easily overlooked if the slit lamp is not focused well into the posterior chamber.

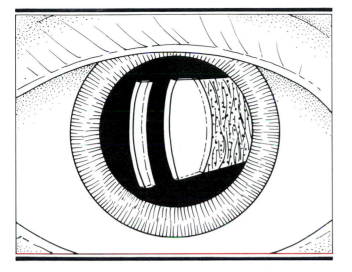

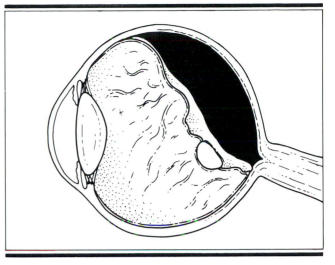

3. Cells in the anterior vitreous appear as small punctate opacities floating between the fibrils.

4. Percolation posteriorly of liquefied vitreous results in a PVD.

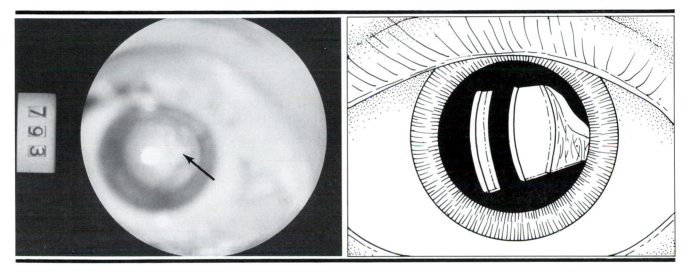

5. Clinically, a PVD may be detected by the large vitreous floater visible with distal direct ophthalmoscopy formed by the prepapillary annulus (left; *see also* Color Plate 20–5), and by the collapsed posterior vitreous limiting layer visible with the slit lamp (right).

21 Gonioscopy: Three-Mirror Lens

Description/Indications. Gonioscopy is the technique used to visualize and assess the anterior chamber angle. The gonioscopic lens is a plastic cone-shaped contact lens containing reflecting mirrors that is used in conjunction with the slit lamp biomicroscope to indirectly evaluate the anterior chamber angle. Gonioscopic lenses come in various sizes and designs, containing one, two, or three mirrors. The most commonly used lens is the three-mirror lens, which allows for evaluation of the angle, as well as the posterior pole and the mid and far peripheral retina (see p. 204).

Indications for gonioscopy include the evaluation of glaucoma suspects to accurately diagnose open, narrow, or closed-angle glaucoma; to assess angle pigmentation; to accurately assess the angle as suitable for pupillary dilation; to diagnose suspected angle recession; to evaluate for angle neovascularization, tumors, congenital anomalies, or foreign bodies; and to assess peripheral anterior synechiae.

Instrumentation. Three-mirror gonioscopic contact lens (goniolens), slit lamp biomicroscope, gonioscopic solution, topical ophthalmic anesthetic solution, sterile ophthalmic irrigating solution, facial tissues.

Technique. Storing the bottle of gonioscopic fluid in its container upside down along with proper lens filling technique will reduce the amount of bubbles that may form in it. Instill gonioscopic fluid into the concave end of the goniolens by initially squeezing gonioscopic fluid onto a clean facial tissue. While continuing to squeeze, move the tip of the gonioscopic fluid bottle over the concave surface of the goniolens and fill it approximately halfway (Fig. 1).

Hand the patient a clean facial tissue. Instill two drops of topical ophthalmic anesthetic solution in each eye (see p. 22). Advise the patient that a mild, transient burning sensation may occur and that he or she may blot excess fluid from the eyes with a tissue.

Position the patient comfortably at the slit lamp (see p. 22). Adjust the eyepieces to accommodate your pupillary distance and refractive error. Adjust the slit lamp rheostat to a medium setting and the magnification to 10X. Position the microscope straight ahead and the light source directly in front of the microscope so that neither eye is occluded. Adjust the beam width to approximately 2 mm. Make certain that the beam is in the "click" position (Fig. 2). Advise the patient that once in place the goniolens will feel awkward but not uncomfortable. The patient should make every effort to keep the chin and forehead completely in the slit lamp and to try not to squeeze the lids shut.

To insert the goniolens in the right eye, position yourself slightly to the patient's right and move the slit lamp all the way to the patient's left. Ask the patient to look up and use the forefinger or thumb of your left hand to gently retract the patient's lower lid. With your right hand place one edge of the slightly tilted goniolens into the inferior fornix and release the lower lid (Fig. 3A). Use the thumb of your left hand to gently but firmly grasp the right upper lid as the patient continues to look up (Fig. 3B). Ask the patient to look straight ahead (Fig. 3C). Quickly pivot the goniolens onto the cornea and release the upper lid. Exchange hands so that the thumb and forefinger of your left hand are holding the edge of the goniolens (Fig. 3D).

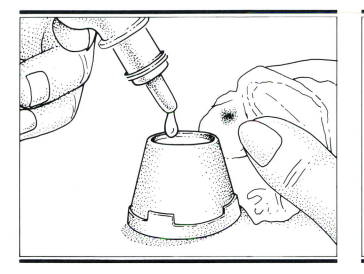

GONIOSCOPY: THREE-MIRROR

Click stop:	In
Beam angle:	0 degrees
Beam width:	2 mm
Beam height:	Maximum, may be shortened
Filter:	None
Illumination:	Medium
Magnification:	10–16X

1. Instilling the gonioscopic fluid.

2. Slitlamp setup for three-mirror gonioscopy.

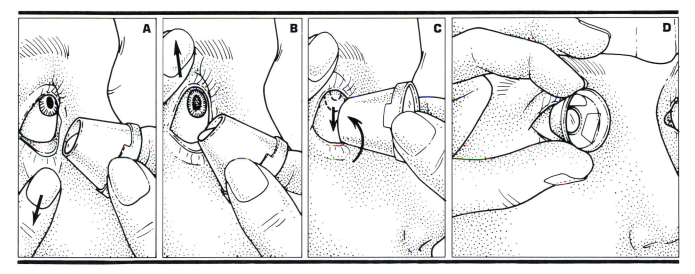

3. A. As the patient looks up, retract the lower lid and place on edge of the slightly tilted goniolens in the inferior fornix. **B.** Use your thumb to grasp the upper lid, and (**C**) ask the patient to look straight ahead. The arrow indicates pivoting of the lens into position. **D.** Hold the lens with the thumb and forefinger of your left hand, suspending your remaining fingers from the forehead strap.

Support your left hand firmly by suspending your remaining fingers from the forehead strap, by resting the heel of your hand on a support rod attached to the upright bar of the slit lamp when available, or by resting your elbow on the slit lamp table. If the length of your forearm is too short to reach the slit lamp table, an inverted facial tissue box or similar item may be placed under your elbow. With your right hand, use the joystick to move the slit lamp in front of the patient. Instruct the patient to look straight ahead or at the fixation light, which has been positioned in front of the left eye.

Use the joystick to position the slit lamp beam onto the center of the semicircular angle mirror. With the joystick move the slit lamp forward to focus on the reflected mirror image of the angle (Fig. 4). Increase the magnification to 16X to assess the angle structures. If desired, the slit beam illumination may be positioned approximately 45 degrees from the microscope and the beam narrowed to an optic section. The angle between the reflection of the beam off the anterior iris surface and the corneal endothelium may be estimated (Fig. 5).

To assess all areas of the angle, the three-mirror goniolens must be rotated into different locations. To do so, gently rotate the goniolens between your thumb and forefinger while maintaining good corneal contact (Fig. 6). With each repositioning of the goniolens, relocate the slit lamp beam onto the angle mirror. It is usually helpful to use the right hand to hold the goniolens in place so that the thumb and forefinger of the left hand may be repositioned to allow for further lens rotation.

To remove the goniolens, ask the patient to squeeze the lids shut and the lens should pop off the eye. If not, while the patient is squeezing the lids shut, hold the lens in your right hand and use the forefinger of your left hand to gently push on the globe through the lower lid just temporal to the lens to break the suction between the goniolens and the cornea (Fig. 7). Use sterile ophthalmic saline solution to irrigate the gonioscopic solution from the conjunctival sac as the patient holds multiple paper towels around the eye (see p. 130).

Repeat the procedure for the opposite eye, reversing the hands used.

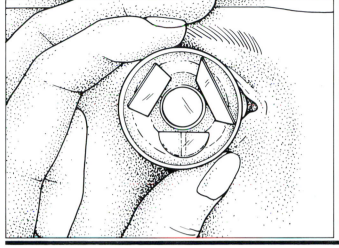

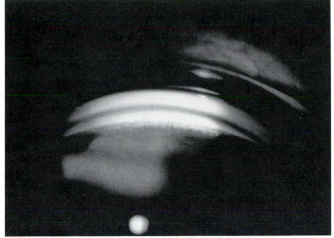

4. (above left) Position the slit beam onto the center of the semicircular mirror and focus forward onto the reflected image (above right; *see also* Color Plate 21—4).

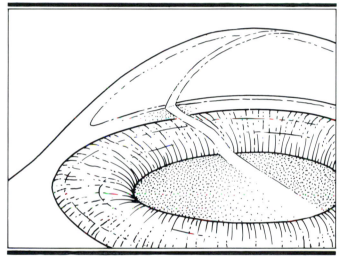

5. (left) An optic section placed at 45 degrees from the microscope may be used to estimate the size of the angle utilizing reflections off the corneal endothelium and anterior iris.

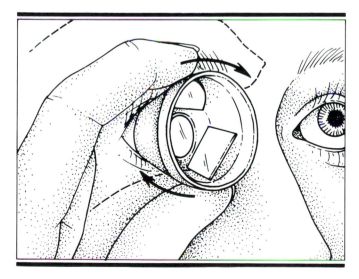

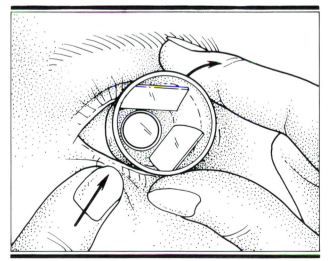

6. Rotate the goniolens between your thumb and forefinger to visualize all areas of the angle.

7. To remove the goniolens, use the forefinger of your left hand to gently push on the globe through the lower lid as the patient squeezes the eyes closed.

Interpretation. Since the three-mirror goniolens uses a mirror to indirectly visualize the angle, the gonioscopic image will be of the angle 180 degrees away from the mirror position.

Multiple methods of interpreting and recording the gonioscopic findings have been proposed. All techniques involve determining to what extent the various anterior chamber angle structures are visible. Some techniques also include an assessment of the angle made between the anterior surface of the iris and the posterior surface of the cornea, the configuration of the iris, and the insertion point of the iris root.

The most commonly used angle grading system is that of Becker-Shaffer (Fig. 8). The Van Herick technique of angle assessment using a slit lamp optic section corresponds well with this technique (see p. 26).

Iris pigment epithelial (IPE) cells may dislodge and collect in the anterior chamber angle. The pigmentation will be densest overlying Schlemm's canal and may be secondarily prominent at Schwalbe's line. The pigmentation is also described with a system of Grades 0 to 4, although much subjective interpretation is involved (Fig. 9).

Although all pigment in the angle will be dark brown, the interpretation of the pigment grading usually takes into account the iris color. A dark brown iris would be expected to release some pigment particles, whereas a blue iris would not. As a result, a given amount of pigment may be assessed as Grade 1 with a brown iris and Grade 2 with a blue iris. The novice gonioscopist should avoid confusing the granular, dark brown pigment overlying Schlemm's canal with the smooth, gray-brown ciliary body.

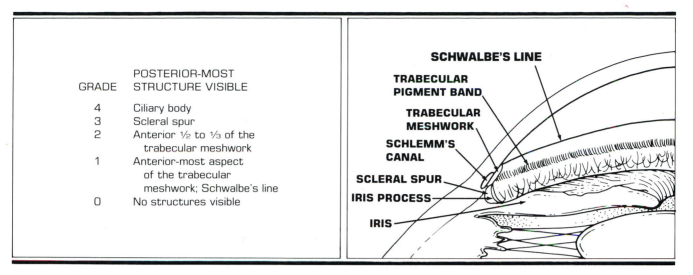

8. The Becker-Shaffer system of angle grading.

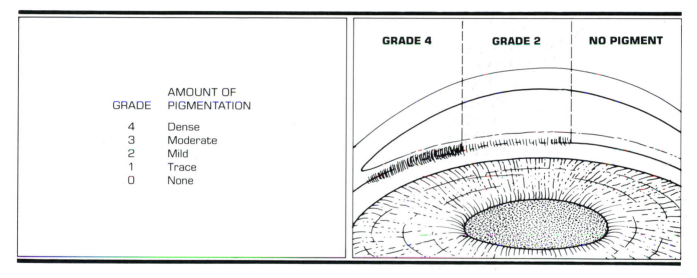

9. Grading system for angle pigmentation.

Several techniques for recording the information obtained via gonioscopy have been described. The two most straightforward methods involve using two crossed lines representing the four quadrants into which the appropriate grade is entered (Fig. 10). The angle is largest inferiorly and narrowest superiorly. This same technique can be used to record angle pigmentation in each quadrant, which is usually densest inferiorly. Another technique uses a circle to diagrammatically represent the 360 degrees of the anterior chamber angle (Fig. 11). Labeled arrows are used to illustrate the extent of each angle finding as they correspond to the hour markings on a clock. With this technique it is relatively easy to indicate areas of angle recession, iridodialysis, peripheral anterior synechiae, and so on.

A myriad of normal variations or frank abnormalities may be observed by gonioscopy. For example, blood in Schlemm's canal will appear as a pale pink, indistinct band, often due to excessive lens pressure. Dense iris processes may obscure the ciliary body. Angle recession may appear as a focal shearing off of iris processes or a frank clefting in the anterior ciliary body. Comparison of the different angle areas of the same eye as well as the opposite eye will help in the diagnosis of subtle angle recession. Iridodialysis will allow for the visualization of the ciliary processes at the point where the iris has been torn away. Peripheral anterior synechiae (PAS) will produce a "tenting" of the iris, usually up to Schwalbe's line.

Contraindications/Complications. For the novice gonioscopist, several errors of technique are commonly made. If too much gonioscopic solution is instilled, the excess will drip down the patient's cheek. Good support of the hand holding the gonioscopic lens is imperative to maintain steady control of the lens and to minimize patient discomfort. Putting too much pressure of the supporting hand against the patient's cheek will result in a tendency for the patient to back away from the slit lamp.

Conversely, bubbles in the gonioscopic fluid layer may indicate that inadequate pressure is being used to hold the lens in place. Gently increasing the corneal contact pressure may rectify this. If not, gentle pressure and tilting of the goniolens may eliminate trapped air bubbles. If the bubbles cannot be eliminated and the angle image is obscured, remove the goniolens and reapply it. Wiping any gonioscopic fluid from the patient's lids will facilitate lens reinsertion. Inadvertent entrapment of the patient's lower lid or lashes can usually be remedied by gently lifting the goniolens slightly and retracting the lower lid.

Tilting the lens or applying too much pressure to the globe may distort the angle appearance and result in inaccurate assessments. Failure to keep the thumb and forefinger of the hand holding the goniolens on the side of the lens rim may block the slit lamp illumination onto the mirror. If the slit lamp illumination system is not "clicked" into the straight-ahead position, one eyepiece of the microscope may be blocked and stereopsis lost.

It is very common to induce transient superficial punctate keratitis (SPK) following gonioscopy and subsequent irrigation. When significant, this corneal disruption may interfere with visualization and photography of the fundus. Usually reassurance to the patient that a transient foreign body sensation may develop is all that is necessary, although artificial tears may be dispensed and used for 12 to 24 hours. Due to the suction that is created between the lens and the cornea, it is possible that significant corneal disruption could result when underlying abnormalities are present such as epithelial basement membrane dystrophy.

Uncommonly, patient anxiety may produce significant blepharospasm, so that three-mirror gonioscopy cannot be performed. In these instances, the four-mirror technique may be a successful alternative (see p. 80). A patient may rarely experience vasovagal syncope during this technique. Should this occur, basic first-aid measures are taken. These include elevating the feet above the level of the head, passing a broken ammonia inhalant ampule beneath the nostrils, and monitoring the basic vital signs.

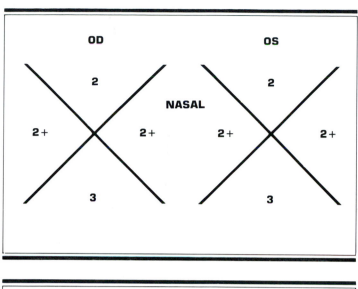

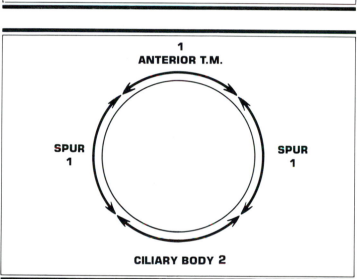

10. For recording angle size or pigmentation, two crossed lines create spaces for entering numerical gradings for the superior, inferior, nasal, and temporal angles.

11. The circle represents the 360 degrees of the angle, with the arrows indicating the visible extent of each structure. The numbers indicate pigment grading.

22 Gonioscopy: Four-Mirror Lens

Description/Indications. Gonioscopy, the evaluation of the anterior chamber angle, may be performed with a four-mirror lens such as the Zeiss goniolens. The Zeiss lens is a symmetrical, truncated polished pyramid with four mirrored sides, all inclined to view the anterior chamber angle. The Zeiss lens is mounted in a removable Unger holder. Other four-mirror lenses may have a permanently mounted handle (such as the Posner) or are hand-held (Fig. 1).

Indications for gonioscopy include the evaluation of glaucoma suspects to accurately diagnose open, narrow, or closed-angle glaucoma; to assess angle pigmentation; to accurately assess the angle as suitable for pupillary dilation; to diagnose suspected angle recession; to evaluate for angle neovascularization, tumors, congenital anomalies, or foreign bodies; and to assess peripheral anterior synechiae.

There are several advantages to four-mirror compared to three-mirror gonioscopy (see p. 72). It is performed quickly, allows for rapid comparison between the two eyes, requires no gonioscopic fluid, is smaller in size and may be better suited for patients with small palpebral apertures, and may be easier for the patient to tolerate. This technique tends to be less traumatic to the globe and may be well-suited to perform for those cases of ocular trauma when gonioscopy is indicated or to assess suspected acute-angle closure glaucoma. Indentation gonioscopy may be performed with the four-mirror lens to assess for peripheral anterior synechiae. Four-mirror gonioscopy can be readily performed on a routine basis following applanation tonometry to allow the practitioner to become familiarized with angle evaluation.

The major disadvantages to this technique are that maintaining proper positioning of the lens can be difficult to master since no suction is created between the lens and the cornea, and that errors in technique are more likely to result in inaccurate distortions of the angle.

Instrumentation. Four-mirror gonioscopic contact lens (goniolens), slit lamp biomicroscope, topical ophthalmic anesthetic solution, contact lens wetting solution or artificial tears, facial tissues.

Technique. Hand the patient a clean facial tissue. Instill two drops of topical ophthalmic anesthetic solution in each eye (see p. 2). Advise the patient that a mild, transient burning sensation may occur and that he or she may blot excess fluid from the eyes with a tissue. If desired, instill a single drop of contact lens wetting solution or artificial tears into the concave surface of the goniolens.

Position the patient comfortably at the slit lamp (see p. 22). Adjust the eyepieces to accommodate your pupillary distance and refractive error. Adjust the slit lamp rheostat to a medium setting and the magnification to 6X to 10X. Position the microscope straight ahead and the light source directly in front of the microscope so that neither eye is occluded. Adjust the beam width to approximately 2 mm. Make certain that the beam is in the "click" position (Fig. 2). Advise the patient that he or she will feel the goniolens in place but that it should not be uncomfortable. The patient should make every effort to keep the chin and forehead completely in the slit lamp and to try not to squeeze the lids shut.

To evaluate the patient's right eye, hold the handle of the goniolens with the thumb and forefinger of your left hand. Position your fingers as far up the handle as necessary to feel comfortable and to allow for excellent hand support. Using the remaining fingers of your left hand to gently support your left hand on the patient's cheek, hold the lens approximately 1 inch from the corneal apex (Fig. 3). With your right hand, use the joystick to focus the slit lamp on the front of the goniolens. Looking through the center portion of the goniolens you will see a minified image of the iris and pupil. Using this image as a guide, approach the cornea with the goniolens while moving the joystick forward to maintain focus on the lens (Fig. 4). Once the cornea is contacted with the goniolens, support the heel of your left hand on the patient's cheek or use the remaining fingers of your left hand to brace against the upright bar of the slit lamp. Alternatively, apply the lens to the cornea while looking outside the slit lamp. Hold the lens as steady as possible and return to sighting through the slit lamp. The hand-held four-mirror goniolens is used in a similar fashion except that the rim of the lens is held between your thumb and forefinger.

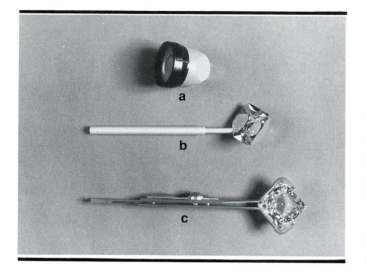

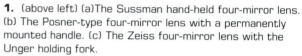

GONIOSCOPY:	FOUR-MIRROR
Click stop:	In
Beam angle:	0 degrees
Beam width:	2 mm
Beam height:	Maximum, may be shortened
Filter:	None
Illumination:	Medium
Magnification:	6–16X

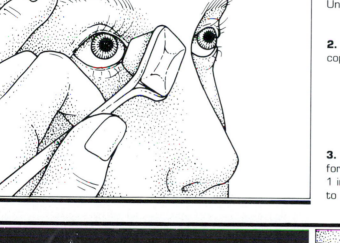

1. (above left) (a)The Sussman hand-held four-mirror lens. (b) The Posner-type four-mirror lens with a permanently mounted handle. (c) The Zeiss four-mirror lens with the Unger holding fork.

2. (above right) The slit lamp setup for four-mirror gonioscopy.

3. (left) Hold the goniolens handle between the thumb and forefinger of your left hand. Hold the lens approximately 1 inch from the corneal apex and use the remaining fingers to support your hand firmly.

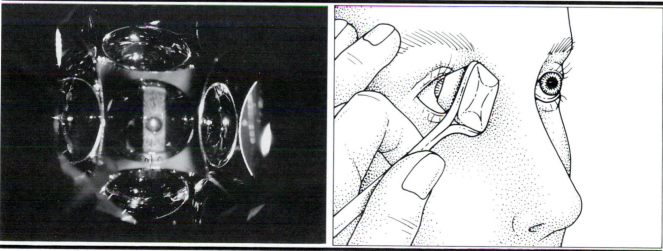

4. A. Use the minified view of the iris and pupil seen through the center of the goniolens to maintain proper lens position as the cornea is approached. (*See also* Color Plate 22–4.A.)

4. B. Support your left hand firmly once the goniolens is in position.

As the patient's eye is approached with the goniolens avoid touching the lashes and inducing a blink reflex. With narrow palpebral apertures or if the patient has difficulty keeping his or her lids wide open, tilt the top of the lens slightly forward to lift up and under the upper lid as the cornea is approached (Fig. 5).

Once the goniolens is properly positioned, instruct the patient to look straight ahead or at the fixation light, which has been positioned in front of the left eye. Use your right hand to control the joystick and vertical positioning knob to move the slit lamp beam onto the center of one of the four mirrors. Increase the magnification to 16X to assess the angle structures. Move the slit lamp forward with the joystick to focus on the reflected mirror image of the angle. Move the slit lamp beam to each of the four mirrors to assess the major quadrants of the angle.

It is common to induce corneal wrinkling during this technique, an indication that too much pressure is being applied. This is likely to occur if the goniolens is inadvertently tilted. Maintain just enough pressure so that no gaps in the tear film result as visualized in the center of the goniolens but without inducing corneal wrinkling. Keep the goniolens as straight as possible.

To remove the goniolens simply lift it off the corneal apex. No irrigation of the patient's eye is necessary. Repeat the procedure for the opposite eye, reversing the hands used.

Interpretation. Since the four-mirror goniolens uses a mirror to indirectly visualize the angle, the gonioscopic image will be of the angle 180 degrees away from the mirror position.

One unique feature of the four-mirror goniolens is the ability to perform indentation gonioscopy. Since the four-mirror lens has such a small diameter contact surface, increasing pressure on the lens will indent the central cornea. The resultant increase in aqueous pressure will cause the iris root to fall away from the angle. If the angle is assessed to be very narrow or closed without indentation, this technique will allow the practitioner to distinguish between appositional and synechial closure in acute angle closure glaucoma (Fig. 6). If corneal edema develops secondary to an acute intraocular pressure elevation, the instillation of topical ophthalmic anesthetic solution followed by 1 to 2 drops of topical ophthalmic glycerin solution will temporarily clear the cornea to allow for angle evaluation.

Other aspects of angle interpretation and recording of results are identical to those of three-mirror gonioscopy (see p. 76).

Complications/Contraindications. Maintaining adequate corneal contact without excess pressure is the most difficult aspect of four-mirror gonioscopy for the novice. Tilting the lens or applying too much pressure to the globe will distort the angle appearance and result in an overestimation of its size. If the slit lamp illumination is not "clicked" into the straight-ahead position, one eyepiece of the microscope may be blocked and stereopsis lost.

It is very common to induce transient superficial punctate keratitis (SPK) following gonioscopy, especially if the lens is tilted or moved excessively on the cornea. When significant, this corneal disruption may interfere with visualization and photography of the fundus. Usually reassurance to the patient that a transient foreign body sensation may develop is all that is necessary, although artificial tears may be dispensed and used for 12 to 24 hours. It is possible that significant corneal disruption could result when underlying abnormalities are present such as epithelial basement membrane dystrophy, although this is less likely to occur than with three-mirror gonioscopy since no suction is created between the goniolens and the cornea.

Uncommonly, patient anxiety may produce significant blepharospasm, so that four-mirror gonioscopy cannot be performed. A patient may rarely experience vasovagal syncope during this technique. Should this occur, basic first-aid measures are taken. These include elevating the feet above the level of the head, passing a broken ammonia inhalant ampule beneath the nostrils, and monitoring the basic vital signs.

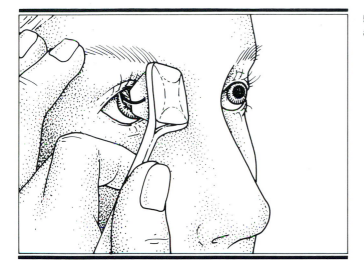

5. If necessary, tilt the top of the goniolens slightly forward and lift up and under the upper lid.

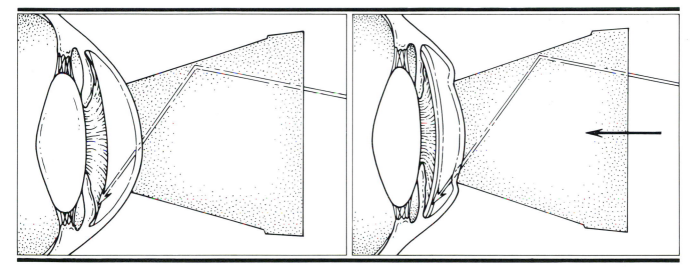

6. A. With the goniolens in its normal position, only the trabecular meshwork is visible in this narrow angle.

6. B. Indentation of the corneal apex with the goniolens allows for visualization of all structures, indicating that peripheral anterior synechiae are not the cause of the narrow angle.

II Suggested Readings

Alexander LJ: *Primary Care of the Posterior Segment.* Norwalk, CT, Appleton & Lange, 1989.

Amos JF: Age-related cataract, in Amos JF (ed): *Diagnosis and Management in Vision Care.* Boston, Butterworths, 1987, pp 601–637.

Brandreth R: *Clinical Slit Lamp Biomicroscopy.* Berkeley, University of California Multimedia Communications Center, School of Optometry, 1978.

Catania LJ: Diagnoses of the anterior chamber, iris, and ciliary body, in *Primary Care of the Anterior Segment.* Norwalk, CT, Appleton & Lange, 1988, pp 183–213.

Chylack LT, Leske C, McCarthy D, et al: Lens opacities classification system II (LOCS II). *Arch Ophthalmol* 1989;**107**:991–997.

Farris RL: Abnormalities of the tears and treatment of dry eyes, in Kaufman HE, Barron BA, McDonald MB, Waltman SR (eds): *The Cornea.* New York, Churchill Livingstone, 1988.

Fingeret M, Potter JW: Uveitis, in Bartlett JD, Jaanus SD (eds): *Clinical Ocular Pharmacology,* ed 2. Boston, Butterworths, 1989, pp 623–638.

Garston MJ: Light flashes and floaters . . . Making a differential diagnosis. *Contemporary Optometry* 1988; **7**:19–30.

Gray LG: Fundamentals of gonioscopy. *Rev Optometry* 1977;**114**:51–60.

Jaanus SD: Dyes, in Bartlett JD, Jaanus SD (eds): *Clinical Ocular Pharmacology,* ed 2. Boston, Butterworths, 1989, pp 323–335.

Locke LC: Conjunctival abrasions and lacerations. *J Am Optom Assoc* 1987;**58**:488–493.

Terry JE: Slit lamp biomicroscopy (Chapter 7), Tonometry and tonography (Chapter 5), and Gonioscopy and fundus contact lens (Chapter 9), in Terry JE (ed): *Ocular Disease Detection, Diagnosis and Treatment.* Springfield, IL, CC Thomas, 1984.

Van Herick W, Shaffer RN, Schwartz A: Estimation of width of angle of anterior chamber. *Am J Ophthalmol* 1969;**68**:626–629.

Warwick R: The eyeball (Chapter 2), The ocular appendages (Chapter 3), and Normal appearances as seen with the slit-lamp and corneal microscope (Chapter 4), in Last RJ (ed). *Wolff's Anatomy of the Eye and Orbit,* ed 7. Philadelphia, Saunders, 1976.

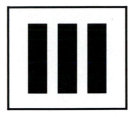

Eyelid Procedures

23 Eyelid Eversion: Single

Description/Indications. Single eversion of the upper eyelid should be performed whenever evaluation of the superior palpebral conjunctiva is needed. Indications for this procedure include, but are not limited to, a history of ocular foreign body or symptoms of foreign body sensation, the evaluation of contact lens patients during the prefitting assessment as well as during follow-up care, and the diagnosis of palpebral vernal conjunctivitis or superior limbic keratoconjunctivitis. Eyelid eversion is typically included as part of the basic "red eye" workup.

The goal is to evert or "fold" the upper lid upon itself at the uppermost aspect of the superior tarsal plate (Fig. 1). Since the tarsal plate is fibrous and relatively rigid, attempts to evert the lid within the body of the plate itself will generally be unsuccessful. This technique may be performed with or without a slit lamp biomicroscope depending upon the degree of magnification needed. Lids can be everted using your fingers alone (digital technique) or in conjunction with a cotton-tipped applicator. For patients with tight lids, the applicator technique will be easier to perform than the digital technique.

Instrumentation. Slit lamp biomicroscope (optional), cotton-tipped applicators (optional).

Technique. Position the patient behind the slit lamp biomicroscope if desired (see p. 22). Use your left hand to evert the patient's right lid; your right hand to evert the patient's left lid.

Digital Method: Instruct the patient to look downward. Actual closure of the eyes should be avoided as the technique then becomes more difficult. Grasp a central section of lashes of the upper lid or the lid margin itself between your thumb and forefinger. Gently pull the lid down and out, away from the globe (Fig. 2A). Simultaneously, place your middle finger at the superior margin of the tarsal plate. Using slight downward pressure at this point along with upward rotation of the margin, "flip" or evert the lid (Fig. 2B).

Applicator Method: Follow the same technique outlined above except position a cotton-tipped applicator at the superior edge of the tarsal plate with your unused hand. After the lid has been gently pulled away from the globe, use slight downward pressure to evert the lid (Fig. 3). Once the lid is everted gently slide the swab out from the lid so as to free your opposite hand. When everting smaller, tighter lids this same technique may be facilitated by using the "stick" end of the applicator placed tangentially against the lid.

While evaluating the everted lid use your thumb to hold the lashes against the superior orbital rim with moderately firm pressure. Instruct the patient to continue to look downward (Fig. 4). Once the examination is complete, release the lashes, instruct the patient to look upward, and the lid should snap back into position. Reversal of the eversion may be facilitated if you provide a gentle "unfolding" movement with your thumb or forefinger as the patient looks upward.

Interpretation. The normal superior palpebral conjunctiva will appear as a glossy, smooth, well-vascularized mucous membrane. Moderately sized papillae are usually present at the superior border of the tarsal plate, medially and laterally. Lid eversion may reveal deviations from normal such as foreign bodies, follicles, small papillae, or giant cobblestone papillae.

Contraindications/Complications. Some patients may exhibit minor anxiety about this procedure. Usually reassurance that the procedure feels awkward but is not painful is all that is required. Should the patient back away while the technique is performed, the resultant pulling on the lashes and lid may cause some mild discomfort.

Loss of a few lashes following this technique is not uncommon. Should the patient have very short lashes or scanty lashes, gentle grasping of the lid margin itself may be necessary. Eversion of the upper lid will naturally cause expression of the Meibomian glands so that a transiently oily tear layer may result.

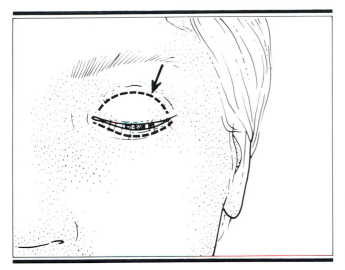

1. The superior aspect of the tarsal plate (arrow) is the pivot point for lid eversion.

2. A. (below left) As the patient looks downward, grasp the lashes between your thumb and forefinger, and gently pull the lid down and out. **B.** (below right) Place your middle finger at the superior edge of the tarsal plate (dashed line). Use pressure as shown and evert the lid.

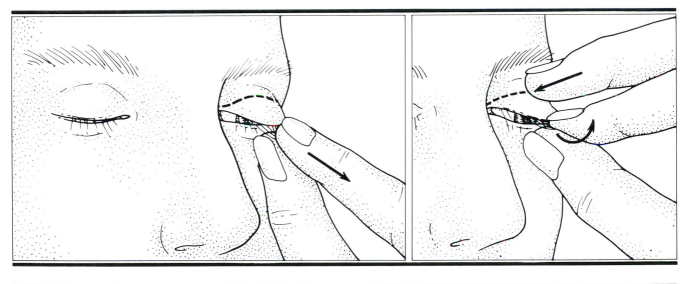

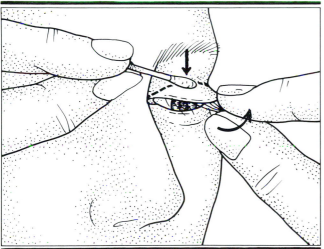

3. Place the cotton tipped applicator at the superior edge of the tarsal plate (dashed line) with your unused hand. Use pressure as shown and evert the lid.

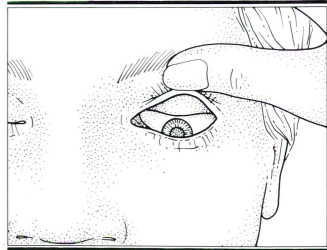

4. Using relatively firm pressure, hold the lashes against the superior orbital rim during examination of the everted lid. Instruct the patient to continue looking down.

24 Eyelid Eversion: Double

Description/Indications. Double eversion of the upper lid is performed when access to the superior fornix area is required. Two common indications for this procedure include examining for one or more hard-to-find foreign bodies, such as a displaced contact lens, and performing conjunctival irrigation (see p. 130). The term *double eversion* is somewhat of a misnomer, as the technique does not actually result in two folds of the upper lid. This technique is usually performed using a lid retractor (Fig. 1) with the patient positioned outside of the slit lamp biomicroscope.

Instrumentation. Lid retractor, cotton-tipped applicators (optional).

Technique. Instill topical ophthalmic anesthetic solution (see pp. 2–3) and perform single lid eversion (Fig. 2A; see also pp. 86–87). Grasping the handle of the retractor between the thumb and forefinger of the unused hand and supporting the heel of this hand and/or wrist on the patient's forehead, position the retractor to "hook" the superior edge of the tarsal plate of the everted lid (Fig. 2B). As the patient continues to look downward, use the retractor to lift the upper lid gently but firmly in an upward and outward direction away from the globe to expose the superior fornix, which now may be visualized and evaluated (Fig. 3).

Once the retractor is in position, the hand that originally grasped the lashes may be removed to perform other techniques, or the hand holding the retractor may be exchanged.

Interpretation. The most common abnormality of the superior fornix region is locating a foreign body. Frequently, however, the foreign body or suspected debris cannot be visualized and irrigation will help to dislodge it.

Contraindications/Complications. Instructing the patient to continue looking downward will avoid the possibility of inducing a corneal abrasion from use of the retractor. The patient may experience symptoms of mild foreign body sensation for several hours following this procedure, which may be relieved by artificial tears.

1. The lid retractor used in double eversion.

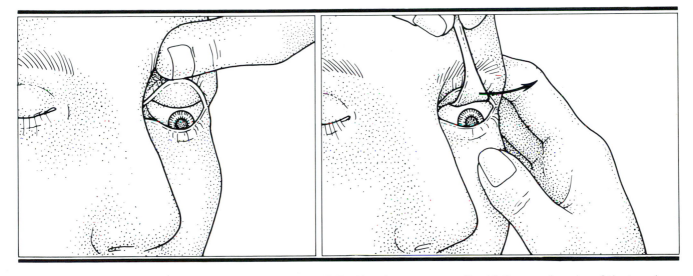

2. A. First singly evert the upper lid.

2. B. Use the retractor to "hook" the superior edge of the tarsal plate. Lift the lid gently but firmly upward and slightly outward to expose the superior fornix.

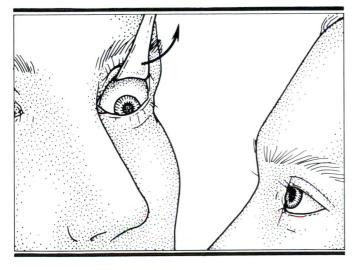

3. Through double eversion the superior fornix may be directly visualized and evaluated.

25 Speculum Insertion

Description/Indications. In the operating room an ophthalmic speculum is used to immobilize the eyelids during surgical procedures such as cataract extraction. A speculum may be used in-office for certain ophthalmic techniques when definitive lid immobilization is required, such as during suture cutting (see p. 282), or when the patient is unable to voluntarily control lid movements or exhibits a tendency toward blepharospasm, such as during corneal foreign body removal (see p. 146). The spring-type (Barraquer) speculum is one of the easiest types available for in-office use (Fig. 1).

Instrumentation. Barraquer speculum, topical ophthalmic anesthetic solution.

Technique. Instill 2 drops of topical ophthalmic anesthetic solution in each eye (see p. 2–3). To insert the speculum into the right eye, hold the speculum between your right thumb and forefinger so that the handle is oriented temporally. Ask the patient to look up. Use the forefinger of your left hand to gently retract the lower lid, then "hook" the medial portion of the lower lid with the inferior arm of the speculum (Fig. 2). Ask the patient to look down and use your left forefinger to gently retract the upper lid. Squeeze the speculum slightly, and "hook" the upper lid (Fig. 3). Ask the patient to look straight ahead keeping both eyes open and proceed with the necessary procedure (Fig. 4).

To remove the speculum, gently grasp the handle of the speculum between your right thumb and forefinger. Position your left thumb gently on the right upper lid. Simultaneously spread the lids apart slightly by retracting the upper lid with your left thumb and the lower lid with the remaining fingers of your right hand. Ask the patient to look down, squeeze the speculum and "unhook" the upper lid; ask the patient to look up and "unhook" the lower lid. In-office instillation of a prophylactic antibiotic drop following speculum removal is recommended.

To insert the speculum into the left eye, repeat the procedure, using opposite hands if desired.

Complications/Contraindications. Some patients may be quite bothered by the awkward feeling of a speculum in place. A speculum should not be inserted when manipulation of the globe is contraindicated, such as in the immediate postoperative period or when penetrating ocular injury is suspected. Poor insertion technique or a strong Bell's reflex on the part of the patient may induce a corneal abrasion, which should be treated appropriately. It is conceivable, but rarely encountered, that one or more small subconjunctival hemorrhages may be induced.

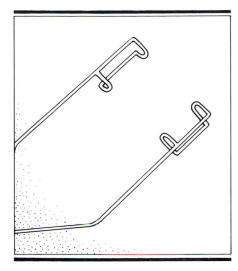

1. The spring-type (Barraquer) speculum.

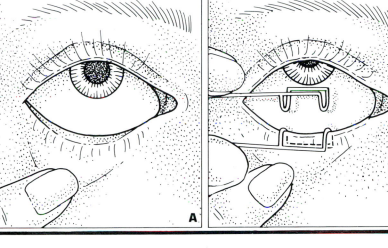

2. A. (above left) Use the forefinger of your left hand to gently retract the lower lid as the patient looks up, then **B.** (above right) "hook" the medial portion of the lower lid with the inferior arm of the speculum.

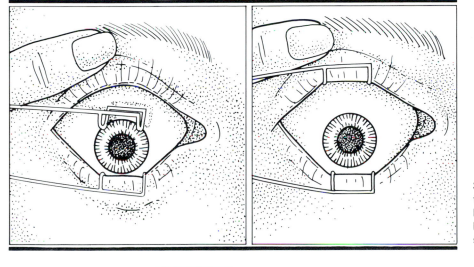

3. A. (far left) Use your left forefinger to gently retract the upper lid as the patient looks down, then **B.** (left) squeeze the speculum slightly and "hook" the upper lid.

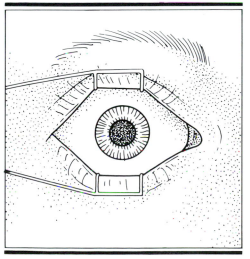

4. The patient is looking straight ahead with the speculum in place.

26 Epilation

Description/Indications. Epilation is performed when a lash (cilium) or lashes (cilia) requires mechanical removal, usually because of induced ocular irritation from contact with the globe. Indications for this procedure include, but are not limited to, trichiasis and entropion. In the latter condition epilation of multiple lashes may serve as a temporary presurgical treatment measure. Less commonly, the epilation technique may be used to remove a lash that has become lodged in the inferior punctum or in a meibomian gland orifice.

Epilation may be performed with the patient positioned outside of or in the slit lamp biomicroscope. If the lash to be removed is relatively long and dark in color, epilation is easily performed without use of the slit lamp. Conversely, if the lash is short and/or light in color, epilation is difficult unless the slit lamp is utilized.

Several types of surgical-quality forceps are available for epilation (Fig. 1). The jewelers-type forceps has tapered, rather pointed tips or jaws. The cilia forceps has wider jaws, similar to a familiar tweezers, and may be squared-off, angled, tapered, or rounded. The jewelers-type forceps is useful for grasping the lash to be epilated when it is located in an area of numerous or closely spaced lashes. In this instance the wider cilia forceps may result in the inadvertent epilation of adjacent normal cilia. Use of the jewelers-type forceps is also helpful when the targeted lash is short or broken off.

Instrumentation. Desired forceps type, slit lamp biomicroscope (optional).

Technique.

Slit Lamp Technique: Position the patient comfortably in the slit lamp (see p. 22). No topical anesthetic is required. If the lash to be removed is on the lower lid, instruct the patient to look upward so that the cornea may not be inadvertently abraded during the procedure. Firmly support the heel of your hand holding the forceps on the patient's cheek, the bridge of the nose, or the upright bar of the slit lamp. Looking first outside of the slit lamp, position the tips of the forceps approximately 1 inch away from the lower lid (Fig. 2A). Using low slit lamp magnification (6X to 10X) and a wide illumination beam, observe the illuminated tips of the forceps through the slit lamp as the lid is approached. Grasp the base of the lash with the forceps and use a gentle "plucking" motion to epilate (Fig. 2B).

For epilation of the upper lid, instruct the patient to look downward. It may be helpful to slightly retract the lid to more accessibly position the upper lid lash for epilation (Fig. 3). So that you can use your free hand to control the slit lamp joystick, retraction of the upper lid may be facilitated with the help of an assistant.

External Method: Position the patient's head comfortably on the headrest of the examining chair and illuminate his or her face with the stand lamp. The techniques of patient fixation are the same as those for the slit lamp technique. You may find it helpful to rest the heel of your hand holding the forceps on the patient's cheek (Fig. 4). If difficulties are encountered localizing the cilium or cilia to be epilated, the slit lamp technique may then be used.

Interpretation. During epilation slight resistance will be felt as the lash is plucked from the follicle. If the lash is actually lodged in the orifice of the meibomian gland or punctum, the lash will glide out smoothly.

Contraindications/Complications. Successful epilation for the cooperative patient will generally have no contraindications or complications. The examiner should take reasonable care when performing epilation with the pointed jewelers forceps. If repeat epilation is necessary it should be performed in approximately 2 to 4 months to coincide with the cilia growth rate. Permanent follicle destruction may be considered when repeat epilation is performed on multiple occasions.

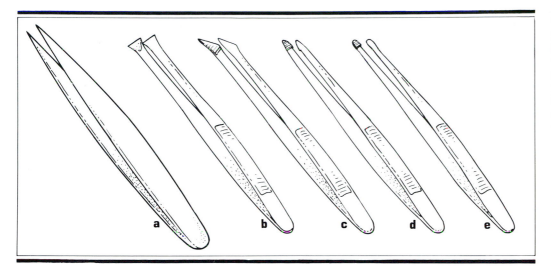

1. The surgical-quality jewelers forceps (a) has pointed tips; cilia forceps may be squared off (b, Littauer), angled (c, Bergh), tapered (d, Zeigler), or rounded (e, Beer).

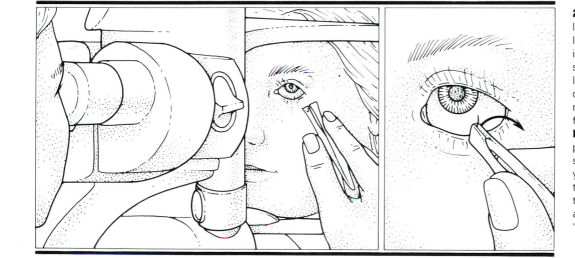

2. A. (far left) To epilate a lash on the lower lid, position the patient in the slit lamp and instruct him or her to look up. Place the tips of the forceps approximately 1 inch away from the lower lid.
B. (left) Having approached the lower lid, support the heel of your hand on the patient's cheek. Grasp the lash near its base and use a gentle "plucking" motion.

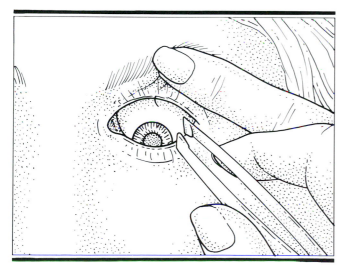

3. To epilate the upper lid, an assistant is retracting the upper lid slightly and the patient is looking downward.

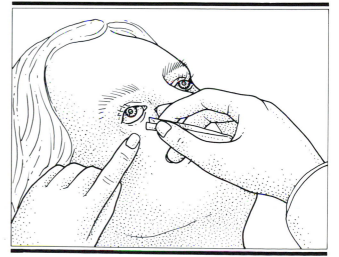

4. Epilation without the use of a slit lamp. The patient's head is positioned on the headrest, the stand lamp illuminates his or her face, and your hand is supported on the patient's cheek.

27 Meibomian Gland Expression

Description/Indications. The meibomian glands, the sinuous sebaceous glands located within the tarsus of the upper and lower lids, may become clogged by an overproduction of sebum and other noninflammatory debris (Fig. 1). This nonacute mechanical blockage may involve a single gland or multiple glands; the latter condition is known as chronic meibomianitis. Occlusion of the gland(s) by the cheesy sebaceous material may cause gland distention that is visible as a yellow "streaking" of the palpebral conjunctiva in the area of the affected gland(s) (Fig. 2). Occlusive plugs may also be visible in the gland orifices. Mild hyperemia and edema of the corresponding lid margin may be present, apparent especially when only a single gland is involved. Mild irritation of the lid margin may be reported and an irritative conjunctivitis or keratoconjunctivitis may result.

Meibomian gland expression is indicated to relieve chronic meibomianitis or to open a single clogged meibomian gland that is causing irritation. The small, waxy, nonirritative meibomian gland orifice plugs that are often noted during routine examination generally do not require expression. Another potential etiology of an isolated clogged meibomian gland that may be alleviated by expression is the residual inflammatory debris that may persist in the gland orifice following resolution of an internal hordeolum. However, gland expression is not indicated for acute internal hordeolum, nor is it included in the therapeutic regimen for chalazion.

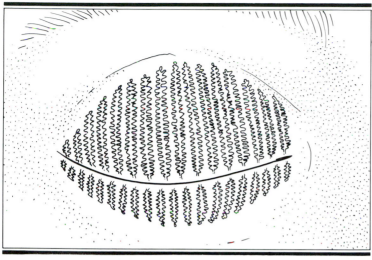

1. The meibomian glands are the sinuous sebaceous glands located within the tarsus of the upper and lower lids.

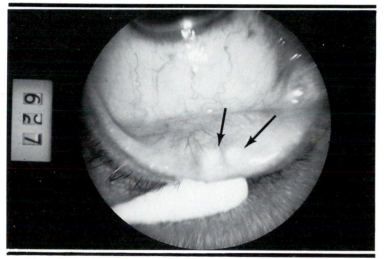

2. Occlusive sebaceous distention of the gland is visible as yellow "streaking" through the overlying palpebral conjunctiva (arrows). (*See also* Color Plate 27–2.)

Instrumentation. Topical ophthalmic anesthetic solution, sterile cotton-tipped applicators.

Technique. Instill topical anesthetic drops (see pp. 2–3). Advise the patient that a mild, transient burning may occur. Position the patient's head comfortably on the headrest of the examining chair, and illuminate his or her face with the stand lamp. For meibomian gland expression of the lower lid, instruct the patient to look up. Horizontally place one sterile cotton-tipped applicator that has been moistened with sterile saline in the inferior cul-de-sac in the region of the gland to be expressed (Fig. 3). Moistening the applicator will allow for smoother contact with the mucous surface of the palpebral conjunctiva. Using the other hand, place a second dry cotton-tipped applicator on the outside of the lid, just opposed to the applicator in the cul-de-sac, and with the handle oriented in the opposite direction. Lightly support the heels of the your hands on the patient's face. Gently but firmly squeeze the applicators against each other as you roll the applicators upward along the length of the gland toward the lid margin (Fig. 4). Wipe away any expressed sebaceous material with a third sterile applicator. Continue the procedure until the material can no longer be expressed.

Meibomian gland expression of the upper lid is probably easiest to perform if the lid is first singly everted using a dry cotton-tipped applicator (see pp. 86-87). Hold the applicator in place behind the everted lid and instruct the patient to continue looking down. Place a second moistened cotton-tipped applicator on the palpebral conjunctiva of the everted lid just opposite to the applicator on the skin side of the lid and with the handle of the applicator oriented in the opposite direction. Gently but firmly squeeze the applicators against each other, as you express upward along the length of the gland and approach the lid margin (Fig. 5). Wipe away any expressed sebaceous material with a third sterile applicator.

Interpretation. Expression of normal meibomian glands will produce a clear, fluid material. In meibomianitis expression will produce a semisolid, yellow-white material that exudes like toothpaste squeezed from a tube, which may be voluminous (Fig. 4B). For a clogged gland orifice, expression will produce a single waxy solid plug.

Once expression is completed, a treatment regimen of hot compresses, lid hygiene measures (see pp. 104–105), lid massage, and/or prophylactic ophthalmic antibiotic drops may be recommended. Repeated in-office meibomian gland expression may be needed for chronic meibomianitis.

Contraindications/Complications. Since the lids and lid margins are richly innervated, meibomian gland expression may produce a mild to moderate amount of discomfort for the patient. The examiner should judge the degree of pressure he or she is able to use during the procedure by the comfort level of the patient. Rarely, meibomian gland expression may precipitate an acute internal hordeolum.

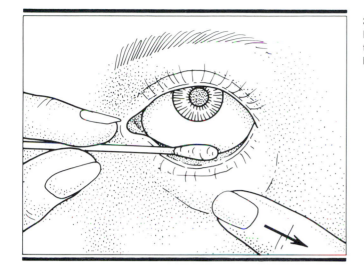

3. To express the lower lid, ask the patient to look upward. Place a moistened sterile cotton-tipped applicator horizontally in the inferior cul-de-sac in the region of the gland(s) to be expressed.

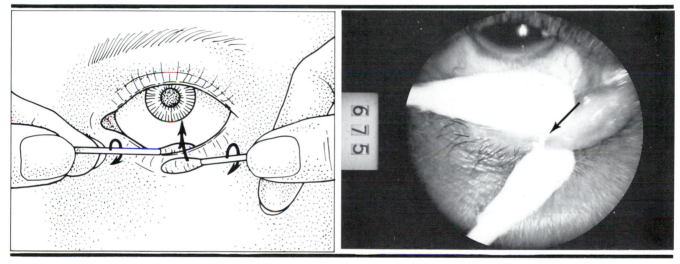

4. A. Using the other hand, place a second dry cotton-tipped applicator on the outside of the lid just opposite to the applicator in the cul-de-sac. Gently but firmly squeeze the applicators against each other, rolling them upward toward the lid margin (arrow).

4. B. Cheesy sebaceous material (arrow) is being expressed from a meibomian gland in the right lower lid. The position of the swab on the outside of the lid is slightly different than described due to examiner positioning at the camera. (*See also* Color Plate 27–4.B.)

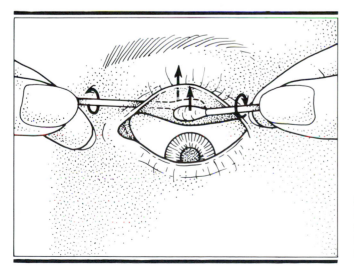

5. To express the superior glands, singly evert the upper lid, keeping the dry applicator in place. Place a second moistened applicator on the opposing palpebral conjunctiva. Gently but firmly squeeze the applicators against each other, rolling them upward.

28 Sebaceous Cyst Evacuation

Description/Indications. Sebaceous retention cysts due to duct blockages may occur on the skin of the lids just as they occur on other skin areas. They appear as well-demarcated smooth, round, noninflamed, nontender nodules, and one or more capillaries may surround or overlie the lesions. They occur singly or in multiples. When the lesions are superficial they are creamy white in color; cysts located deeper within the skin appear pinker or more flesh-toned in color (Figs. 1, and 2).

A superficial sebaceous cyst may be evacuated when it is sufficiently large so that a patient expresses concern about the cosmetic appearance of the lesion. Cyst evacuation is generally not indicated for lesions noted during routine examination of the asymptomatic patient.

Instrumentation. Sterile disposable 25G needle, sterile cotton-tipped applicators, topical ophthalmic anesthetic solution (optional).

Technique. Position the patient's head comfortably on the headrest of the examining chair, and illuminate his or her face with the stand lamp. If the cyst to be removed is on the lower lid, instruct the patient to look up; when the cyst is on the upper lid, instruct the patient to look down. Use an alcohol pad to clean the skin overlying and surrounding the cyst and allow the skin to air dry. Topical anesthesia is generally not necessary, but if desired, you may hold a cotton-tipped applicator saturated with topical ophthalmic anesthetic drops in contact with the cyst for approximately 30 seconds. Pull the skin adjacent to the cyst taut. With the heel of your hand supported on the patient's face, use a sterile 25G needle to score or puncture the top of the cyst, in a nonvascularized area if possible (Fig. 3). The wall of the cyst may be fairly tough so that repeated scoring may be necessary, or the original scoring may need to be enlarged to facilitate expression.

Using two sterile cotton-tipped applicators positioned at opposite sides of the base of the lesion, gently but firmly evacuate the cyst by rolling the applicators toward each other until the sebaceous material is completely expressed (Fig. 4). Use additional sterile applicators to wipe away the sebaceous material (Fig. 5). It is usual for a minute amount of bleeding to occur during and following expression.

Instruct the patient to apply antibiotic ointment as prophylaxis against infection three or four times daily for several days until a small scab forms and the area heals. If the sebaceous cyst is located away from the lid margin, a nonophthalmic antibiotic ointment may be used for prophylaxis.

Interpretation. During sebaceous cyst evacuation, cheesy, yellow-white sebaceous material will be expressed.

Contraindications/Complications. This technique is *not* appropriate for the removal of deep sebaceous cysts that required incision through skin tissue. The examiner should warn the patient to monitor for the unlikely onset of secondary bacterial infection following removal of the cyst.

When the cyst is located on the lid margin, care should be taken when swabbing the skin with alcohol so as not to contaminate the eye. This might best be accomplished by using a cotton tipped applicator moistened with isopropyl alcohol. Care should be taken when scoring the lid margin cyst with the needle, and manipulation with the applicators in this area can be awkward. The patient should be informed that the sebaceous cyst may occasionally recur.

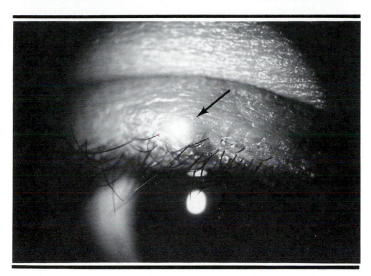

1. The superficial sebaceous cyst appears as a well-demarcated, creamy white, smooth, round nodule (arrow). (*See also* Color Plate 28–1.)

2. The deeper sebaceous cyst is more flesh-toned in color and less well demarcated (arrow). (*See also* Color Plate 28–2.)

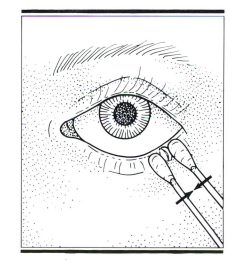

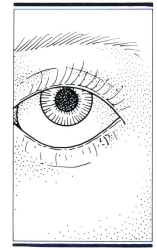

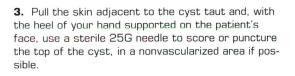

3. Pull the skin adjacent to the cyst taut and, with the heel of your hand supported on the patient's face, use a sterile 25G needle to score or puncture the top of the cyst, in a nonvascularized area if possible.

4. Place the two sterile applicators at opposite sides of the base of the lesion, and gently but firmly express the cyst until the cheesy sebaceous material is completely evacuated.

5. The evacuated sebaceous cyst.

29 Sudoriferous Cyst Evacuation

Description/Indications. Retention cysts of the sweat glands of Moll, known as sudoriferous cysts, appear as one or more small, noninflamed, avascular, clear, fluid-filled cysts on the anterior portion of the lid margin (Fig. 1). When sufficiently large, a sudoriferous cyst may be evacuated for cosmetic reasons if the patient so desires. Cyst evacuation is generally not indicated for lesions noted during routine examination of the asymptomatic patient.

Instrumentation. Slit lamp biomicroscope, sterile 25G needle.

Technique. Position the patient comfortably in the slit lamp (see p. 22), and instruct him or her to keep the head firmly against the chin and forehead rests. No topical anesthetic is needed. If the cyst is located on the lower lid margin, instruct the patient to look upward so that the cornea may not be inadvertently abraded during the procedure. Support the heel of your hand holding the needle firmly on the patient's cheek or on the upright bar of the slit lamp. Looking first outside of the slit lamp, position the needle approximately 1 inch away from the lower lid (Fig. 2A). Using low slit lamp magnification (6X to 10X) and a wide illumination beam, observe the illuminated tip of the needle through the slit lamp as the lid is approached. Use the tip of the needle to "puncture" the sudoriferous cyst (Fig. 2B). Use a tissue or cotton-tipped applicator to wipe away the clear exudate.

When the cyst is located on the upper lid margin, instruct the patient to look down. To more accessibly expose the cyst it may be helpful to slightly retract the upper lid. In order for you to continue using your free hand to control the slit lamp joystick, retraction of the upper lid may be facilitated with the help of an assistant (Fig. 3).

Generally no topical antibiotic prophylactic treatment is required following evacuation of a sudoriferous cyst, but a one-time application of ophthalmic antibiotic ointment may be used. Advising the patient that the cyst may reform or that other cysts may appear is helpful.

Interpretation. As the sudoriferous cyst is evacuated, a minute amount of clear, watery fluid will appear.

Contraindications/Complications. Successful evacuation of a sudoriferous cyst for the cooperative patient will generally have no contraindications or complications.

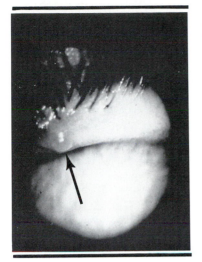

1. Sudoriferous cysts appear as one or more small, noninflamed, avascular, clear fluid-filled cysts on the anterior lid margin (arrow). (*See also* Color Plate 29-1.) (Courtesy of Primary Eyecare Educational Services, Inc.)

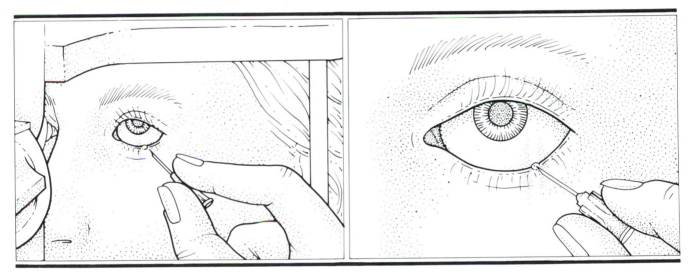

2. A. Position the patient in the slit lamp and ask him or her to look up. Place the tip of the needle approximately 1 inch away from the lower lid.

2. B. Use the tip of the needle to "puncture" the sudoriferous cyst.

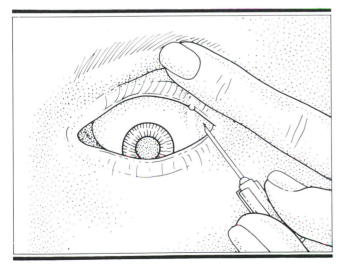

3. To evacuate a sudoriferous cyst of the upper lid, an assistant is retracting the upper lid slightly and the patient is looking downward.

30 Verruca, Papilloma Removal: Chemical

Description/Indications. Verrucae and papillomas (Fig. 1) may involve the skin of the lids and adnexa. The lesions may be chemically removed for cosmetic reasons if the patient so desires.

Bichloracetic acid (dichloroacetic acid), an effective chemical keratolytic and cauterizing agent, may be used to remove verrucae and papillomas. It is available in a treatment kit that includes a bottle of acid, a micro-dropper, acid receptacles, petrolatum, and pointed wooden applicator sticks. This technique is usually performed with the patient positioned outside of the slit lamp biomicroscope.

Instrumentation. Bichloracetic acid treatment kit.

Technique. Position the patient's head comfortably on the headrest of the examining chair, and illuminate his or her face with the stand lamp. Using a cotton-tipped applicator, apply a thin layer of petrolatum to the normal tissue surrounding the lesion to protect it from treatment (Fig. 2A). Transfer a small amount of bichloracetic acid to one of the acid receptacles with the micro-dropper to prevent contamination of the solution. Dip the applicator stick into the acid in the receptacle to moisten it, and remove excess acid by drawing the applicator over the lip of the receptacle. Apply a small amount of bichloroacetic acid to each lid lesion by touching it with the acid-moistened applicator stick (Fig. 2B). Usually only one application is necessary; however, retreatment may be performed as needed.

Interpretation. With application of bichloracetic acid to a verruca or papilloma, the area will immediately turn white (Fig. 2C), followed several days later by a gray-white appearance (Fig. 2D). The lesion will typically desquamate in 7 to 10 days (Fig. 3).

Complications/Contraindications. Bichloracetic acid should not be applied to lesions on the lid margin as chemical keratoconjunctivitis may result. Care should be taken that excess bichloracetic acid does not drip from the applicator stick onto areas of the skin not intended for treatment. Acid that is accidently spilled onto normal tissue should immediately be removed by wiping with a cotton-tipped applicator or cotton pledget and rinsing with water.

Bichloracetic acid should not be used to treat malignant or premalignant lesions. Other clinical techniques used to remove verrucae and papillomas of the eyelids include cryopexy, and curettage and cautery. If the lid lesions are not adequately treated by bichloracetic acid, removal by an alternative technique may be necessary.

1. A papilloma is present on the upper lid.

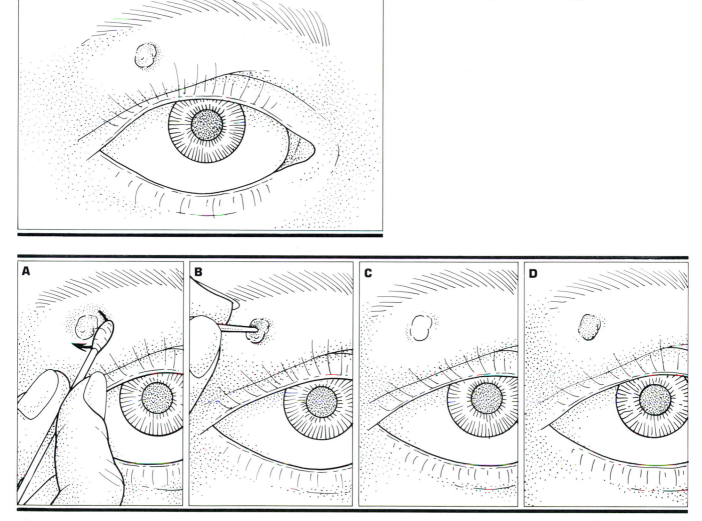

2. A. Using a cotton-tipped applicator, apply a thin layer of petrolatum to the normal tissue surrounding the papilloma. **B.** Apply a small amount of bichloracetic acid to the papilloma with a wooden applicator stick. **C.** The papilloma immediately turns white due to chemical cauterization by the acid. **D.** In several days the treated papilloma is gray-white in appearance.

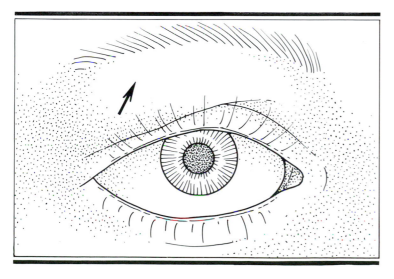

3. The papilloma has desquamated in 7 to 10 days (arrow). When necessary, retreatment may be performed.

31 Eyelid Scrubs

Description/Indications. Lid hygiene measures ("lid scrubs") may be used to treat and/or control a number of disease processes that involve the lid margin. The conditions for which lid scrubs may be indicated include, but are not limited to, marginal blepharitis, *Demodex* blepharitis, contact dermatitis, and control of recurrent hordeola or chalazia. The examiner usually recommends to the patient that this procedure be done at home once or twice daily.

This technique may be performed in a variety of ways. The two common components to this procedure, however, include a solution for cleaning the lids and a mechanical technique for doing so. In past years, water-diluted baby shampoo was recommended since it was considered least likely to burn or irritate the eyes. More recently, commercially prepared antiseptic lid scrub solutions have become available complete with patient instructions and gauze pads. Lid scrubs have also been performed using ophthalmic antibiotic ointments.

Instrumentation. Lid hygiene solution, clean facecloth, gauze pads or cotton-tipped applicators.

Technique

Washcloth/Gauze Pad Technique: Instruct the patient to apply a small amount of the recommended lid scrub solution to either a clean facecloth that has been moistened with warm water or to a clean gauze pad. Rubbing together two portions of the facecloth or gauze pad that are moistened with the solution will create a mild lather. Instruct the patient to close the eyes and, using firm but gentle pressure in a horizontal motion, rub the cloth or pad along the lid margins (Fig. 1). A gentle rinsing of the lid area with warm water followed by drying with a clean face towel completes the procedure.

Cotton-Tipped Applicator Method: Instruct the patient to dip a clean cotton-tipped applicator into the recommended lid scrub solution. The procedure should be done while looking into a mirror so as to carefully monitor the placement of the applicator. To clean the lower lid margin, instruct the patient to tilt the chin down slightly, causing the globe to roll upward, and retract the lower lid slightly with the index finger of one hand to expose the lid margin.

Holding the cotton-tipped applicator in the opposite hand, the patient should gently but firmly rub the applicator in a horizontal motion along the base of the lashes for the length of the lower lid (Fig. 2). To clean the upper lid margin, instruct the patient to elevate the chin slightly so that the globe rolls downward. While the upper lid is retracted slightly with the index finger of one hand, and holding the cotton-tipped applicator in the opposite hand, the patient gently but firmly rubs the applicator in a horizontal motion along the base of the lashes for the length of the upper lid (Fig. 3). A clean applicator may be used for each eye.

To help ensure compliance it is useful to give definitive guidelines as to the duration of the procedure, such as 10 seconds per eye or 10 scrubs per eye. Dispensing prepared written instructions outlining the recommended lid scrub technique is also helpful.

Interpretation. If the patient is compliant and performing the technique correctly, a diminution or complete resolution of lid margin debris should be noted following lid hygiene measures.

Contraindications/Complications. When compliance is problematic, it is helpful to simplify the procedure as much as possible so that it may be easily incorporated into the daily hygiene regimen.

Should lid irritation develop in the course of this therapy, the patient may be performing the technique too vigorously or too frequently. Patients who may be susceptible to this complication include those with very delicate lid tissues, such as accompanies acne rosacea. If the patient is inappropriately performing lid scrubs with a nonrecommended product, ocular and/or lid irritation may result.

Patients who are performing lid scrubs using cotton-tipped applicators should be advised to carefully position the applicator on the lid margin while looking in a mirror. Mechanical irritation of the globe may result if inadvertent slipping of the applicator occurs. Patients susceptible to this complication may include presbyopes and patients with manual dexterity difficulties.

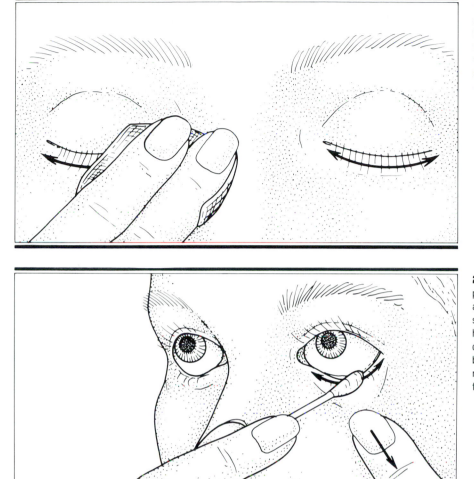

1. The patient is performing lid scrubs using a clean gauze pad that has been moistened with the recommended lid hygiene solution. Using firm but gentle pressure in a horizontal motion, the pad is rubbed along the lid margins.

2. While looking into a mirrow, the patient has tilted the chin down, and the lower lid is retracted slightly with the index finger of one hand. Holding the applicator in the opposite hand, the patient is gently but firmly rubbing in a horizontal motion along the base of the lashes for the length of the lower lid.

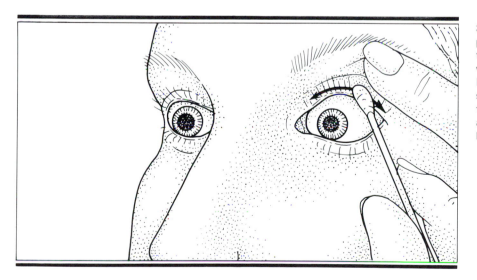

3. While looking into a mirror, the patient has tilted the chin up, and the upper lid is retracted slightly with the index finger of one hand. Holding the applicator in the opposite hand, the patient is gently but firmly rubbing in a horizontal motion along the base of the lashes for the length of the upper lid.

III Suggested Readings

Bartlett JD: Diseases of the eyelids, in Bartlett JD, Jaanus SD (eds): *Clinical Ocular Pharmacology,* ed 2. Boston, Butterworths, 1989, pp 455–489.

Catania LJ: Diagnoses (by SOAP) of the eyelids and adnexa, in *Primary Care of the Anterior Segment.* Norwalk, CT, Appleton & Lange, 1988, pp 15–47.

Kut LJ, Moran DD: Examination of the emergency eye patient, in Wilensky JT, Read JE (eds). *Primary Ophthalmology.* Orlando, Grune & Stratton, 1984, pp 3–18.

McCulley JP: Meibomitis, in Kaufman HE, Barron BA, McDonald MB, Waltman SR (eds): *The Cornea.* New York, Churchill Livingstone, 1988, pp 125–138.

Polack FM, Goodman DF: Experience with a new detergent lid scrub in the management of chronic blepharitis. *Arch Ophthalmol* 1988;**106**:719–720.

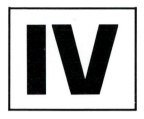

Lacrimal System Procedures

32 Schirmer Tear Test

Description/Indications. The Schirmer tear test is a gross measure of the aqueous volume (quantity) of the tears. It is an indirect indicator of tear production. While not extremely sensitive, it is easy to perform, and when used in conjunction with other tear tests (see p. 42), a slit lamp evaluation (see p. 20), corneal stain evaluations (see p. 46), lactoferrin immunoassay test (see p. 112), and a history, valuable information concerning a tear deficiency state (keratoconjunctivitis sicca, or KCS) is obtained. The test is useful in any patient complaining of dry-eye type symptoms. Examples of such symptoms are stinging, burning, foreign body sensation, tearing, and itching. The test is also helpful in documenting pseudo-epiphora, excess tearing due to a dry eye with secondary lacrimal stimulation.

There are three variations of the Schirmer's test. Schirmer's test 1 measures the total reflex and basic secretory levels since topical anesthetic is not used. The basic secretion test is done after the instillation of a topical anesthetic and measures the basic secretory tear level by eliminating reflex tearing produced by corneal stimulation; this test is especially useful in individuals who find test 1 irritating or uncomfortable. It is also useful in individuals who wet the strip fully in test 1 yet complain of dry-eye-type symptoms. Schirmer's test 2 measures the reflex tear secretion and is done by instilling a topical anesthetic agent and irritating the unanesthetized nasal mucosa with a cotton-tipped applicator. An indication for test 2 is when initial Schirmer tests yield subnormal values. This test is rarely done because a lack of reflex tearing is not a typical cause of clinical problems.

Instrumentation. Schirmer filter strip papers (Whatman #41) (Coopervision) (Fig. 1), topical ophthalmic anesthetic solution, cotton-tipped applicators, millimeter ruler.

Technique

Schirmer's Test 1: While the strips are in the plastic package, prepare them by folding the terminal end at the indentation, approximately 5 mm from the end. Open the plastic package and remove one strip at a time, holding the strip from the bottom. Have the patient look up, pull the lower lid down, and insert the strip into the lower cul-de-sac, placing the fold at the lid margin (Figure 2A). Position the strip so it is in the lateral third of the eyelid. Allow the longer end to hang inferiorly over the lower eyelid. As the strip is inserted, avoid touching any part of the eye. Once inserted, the patient may gently close the eyes (Fig. 2B). Insert a strip into the other eye. The lights in the room should be dimmed to prevent reflex stimulation. Patients may blink as they wish but they should avoid forceful lid closure. The test is done for 5 minutes or until the strip is completely wet, whichever occurs first. Remove the strip from the inferior cul-de-sac and, using a millimeter rule, measure the amount of wetting, beginning the measurement at the folded notch. The measuring guide found on the Schirmer box is useful for this purpose. A template of a strip is next to a ruler. This allows for an accurate measurement of the amount of strip wetting (Fig. 3).

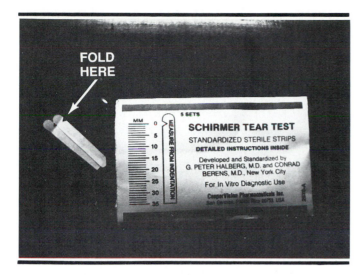

1. A package of Schirmer tear strips.

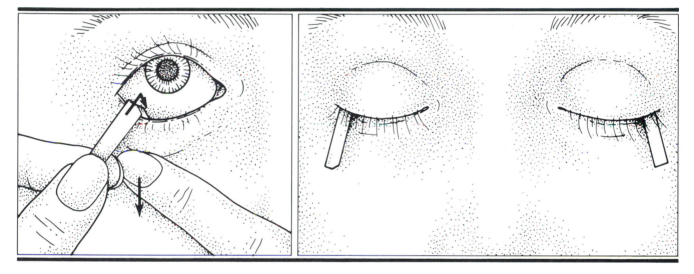

2. A. The Schirmer strip is placed at the outer third of the lid with its folded edge overlying the edge of the eyelid.

2. B. The Schirmer strips in position during the test with the patient gently closing both eyes.

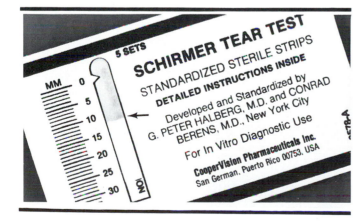

3. The wet strip is measured by using the ruler and template on the Schirmer box.

Basic Tear Secretion Test: This test is done in a similar fashion to test 1, but before commencing, a topical anesthetic agent is instilled. The test is also done for 5 minutes.

Schirmer's Test 2: This modification is done by placing a topical anesthetic in the eye. Place the strips in the eye as described for test 1, and begin timing the test. Insert a cotton-tipped applicator up the nostril, and gently irritate the ipsilateral nasal mucosa for 10 to 15 seconds (Fig. 4). This should theoretically stimulate the lacrimal gland to produce tears. This test is done for 2 minutes.

Interpretation. A normal eye will wet between 10 and 30 mm of the strip when Schirmer's test 1 or the basic secretion test is done. The basic secretion test will usually give slightly lower readings because the reflex component is eliminated, but a normal eye will still produce more than 10 mm of wetting. Values between 5 and 10 mm are considered borderline and need to be rechecked. A result of less than 5 mm is considered to be a positive finding for KCS.

If Schirmer's test 1 is abnormal with results less than 5 mm, there is no need to do the basic secretion test. If Schirmer's test 1 is negative, with the strip being wet greater than 10 mm, a basic secretion test is then indicated to determine if the strip wetting is due to reflex corneal stimulation or to the basic tear level. A normal finding on Schirmer's test 1 with reduction on the basic secretion test may also be indicative of a KCS patient with pseudo-epiphora.

Test 2 is evaluated differently. A value of less than 15 mm in 2 minutes is considered to be diagnostic of a problem in reflex secretion. There should be an increase in wetting of the strip in test 2 compared to the basic secretion test if the reflex secretors are intact.

In order to obtain consistent results, do the test the same way for every patient, every time.

Contraindications/Complications. The Schirmer's tests must be done before applanation tonometry or any other test that may irritate the cornea. Schirmer test results tend to be variable and at times difficult to reproduce. They are not sensitive tests and must be used in conjunction with other tests to obtain a diagnostic picture of KCS. When repeated over a period of time, a pattern often occurs that is diagnostic of KCS.

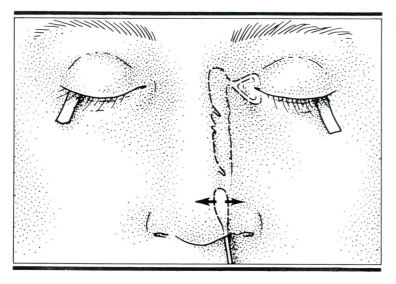

4. A cotton-tipped applicator is inserted into the nostril to irritate the nasal mucosa for Schirmer test 2. The remainder of test is similar to the basic secretion test.

33 Lactoferrin Immunoassay Test

Description/Indications. The lactoferrin tear immunological assay test (Lactoplate) measures the concentration of the tear protein lactoferrin. The concentration of lactoferrin decreases as the lacrimal gland declines in function, with the test providing an objective measure of the quality of the tears produced by the lacrimal gland. The test alone, while sensitive, may not diagnose all patients with keratoconjunctivitis sicca (KCS), but when used in conjunction with the slit lamp findings and other tear evaluation tests will detect most dry-eyed individuals. The lactoferrin test is extremely useful when signs and/or symptoms of the dry eye are present but the Schirmer test is equivocal. It may also be used in the evaluation of contact lens patients with dry-eye complaints, or to predict which contact lens patients may be at risk for dry-eye complications.

The lactoferrin immunoassay test is done by placing a tear sample into a diffusion chamber (Lactoplate) containing a gel with antibodies to human lactoferrin (Fig. 1). The lactoferrin in the tear sample diffuses into the gel. A precipitation ring is formed when the lactoferrin antigen reacts with the antibody. The ring is measured and correlated with known values of lactoferrin tear concentrations. A topical anesthetic agent may effect the results and should be avoided unless absolutely necessary.

Instrumentation. Lactoplate, paper disc, ruler, blunt forceps, conversion table.

Technique. Pull the lower lid margin down, exposing the inferior palpebral conjunctiva. Using a forceps remove a paper disc from the container, and place it in the temporal region of the inferior palpebral conjunctiva (Fig. 2). Place a disc in the other eye and have the patient relax with the eyes either open or shut, whichever is most comfortable.

Remove the disc from the inferior cul-de-sac when it is soaked with tears or at 5 minutes, whichever occurs first. It is not important how long a disc remains in the eye as long as the disc is saturated with tears. In cases of extreme dry eye, the filter disc may not be completely wet.

Blot the disc on the filter paper surrounding the gel to remove excess fluid (Fig. 3A). Once blotted, place the disc in the appropriate place on the reagent gel chamber corresponding to the eye tested (Fig. 3B). The same procedure is repeated for the second eye. Close the cover of the gel chamber, mark the patient's name and date on the cover, and place it aside. Allow it to remain at room temperature for 3 days, when it will be read. With a ruler measure the diameter of the formed antigen–antibody white ring in mm (Fig. 4). The ring, once formed, will be stable for 1 month. Using the conversion table, convert the diameter of the ring (in mm) into a lactoferrin concentration (mg/mL) (Fig. 5).

Interpretation. The average normal tear lactoferrin concentration is 1.42 mg/mL. This is equivalent to a ring diameter of approximately 11.25 mm. A reading of 1.0 mg/mL is considered a borderline figure, with readings below being abnormal. The results of the lactoferrin immunoassay test do not correlate exactly with actual lacrimal gland production but are an indicator to the gland's function or dysfunction. A severe case of KCS may lead to incomplete wetting of the filter disc and abnormally low values of lactoferrin may result. When no ring is visible after 3 days, make sure that a very large ring has not been formed that borders the edges of the gel chamber. Large rings are possible if the disc is not blotted properly or if two discs are accidently used.

Contraindications/Complications. Care must be exercised when placing or removing the paper discs from the eye.

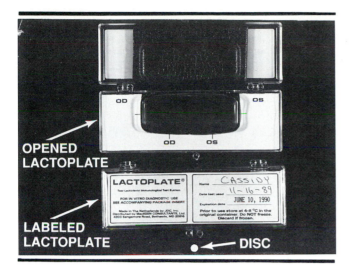

1. The paper disc and Lactoplate gel chamber.

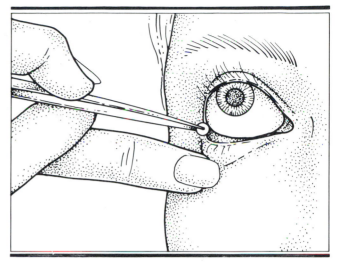

2. Using forceps, the disc is inserted onto the temporal aspect of the inferior palpebral conjunctiva.

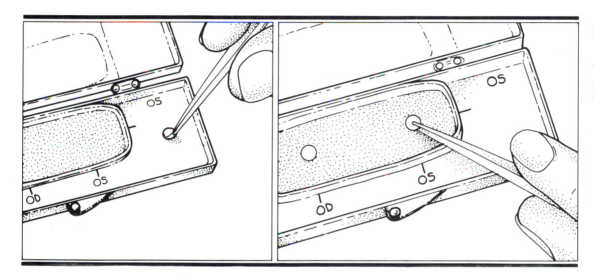

3. A. (far left) The disc is lightly blotted to remove excess tears. **B** (left) The disc is placed in position on the gel chamber and left for 3 days for the white precipitation ring to form.

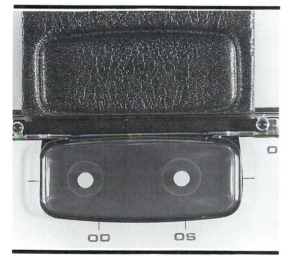

4. (far left) A precipitation ring, revealing normal tear production.

5. (left) Conversion table. The concentration of lactoferrin in each tear sample is derived from the table, using the measured ring diameter (Courtesy of Eagle Vision, Inc.).

Dia	Conc	Dia	Conc
5.0	0.28	11.0	1.36
5.5	0.34	11.5	1.48
6.0	0.40	12.0	1.6
6.5	0.47	12.5	1.8
7.0	0.55	13.0	1.9
7.5	0.63	13.5	2.0
8.0	0.72	14.0	2.2
8.5	0.81	14.5	2.4
9.0	0.91	15.0	2.5
9.5	1.01	15.5	2.7
10.0	1.12	16.0	2.9
10.5	1.23	16.5	3.0

34   Punctal Regurgitation/Lacrimal Sac Palpation

Description/Indications. An obstruction along the course of the nasolacrimal drainage system will affect the excretion of tears from the eye. Epiphora, an abnormal overflow of tears down the cheek, is the symptom indicative of malfunction in the tear drainage system. Causes of the obstruction include anatomic malformations, debris clogging the naso-lacrimal channels (dacryoliths, concretions), or infection either of adjacent tissues (cellulitis) or directly in the lacrimal sac (dacryocystitis). The resultant stasis of fluid can lead to an infection and inflammation of the lacrimal sac (acute or chronic dacryocystitis) if not already present. Since acute dacryocystitis may precede or follow an obstruction, a careful history regarding the onset of both epiphora and discharge is crucial to determining which came first. Symptoms of acute dacryocystitis include pain, tenderness, inflammation, and epiphora. Orbital cellulitis may be an accompanying condition. Chronic dacryocystitis is usually secondary to an obstruction in the tear drainage system. The signs of inflammation evident in acute cases are often absent in the chronic situations with epiphora being the lone complaint.

Palpation of the lacrimal sac is a useful test in evaluating patients with suspected dacryocystitis. It allows the examiner to feel the tear sac lying within the lacrimal fossa, exploring for masses, lumps, or nodules. Gentle pressure is applied to the sac area, looking for discharge regurgitating back through the punctum.

Instrumentation. Slit lamp, cotton-tipped applicators.

Technique. With the patient seated behind the biomicroscope, place the index finger on the medial canthal ligament so it lies over the body of the lacrimal sac (Fig. 1). If there is a question of where the lacrimal sac is, place the index finger over the inferior orbital rim and move medially until the finger is adjacent to the nose. Gently exert pressure over this region while observing the punctum for discharge (Fig. 2). A cotton-tipped applicator may be used instead of the finger to apply gentle pressure on the sac (Fig. 3). In certain instances the cotton-tipped applicator may be preferable because pressure can be more easily localized. With slight pressure a copious mucous or puslike discharge may ooze from the punctum (Fig. 4). In this situation does the sac feel or look inflamed or distended? Is the area tender to the touch?

Interpretation. Infection and/or inflammation of the lacrimal sac is diagnosed by noting a regurgitation of mucous or pus coming from the canaliculus and punctum when pressure is applied over the body of the lacrimal sac. The accompanying symptoms and history differentiate an acute from a chronic problem. In one case, epiphora has occurred acutely with a moderately red eye and mild to moderate pain in and around the eye. The pain is more intense and localized with palpation of the lacrimal sac and the sac is usually distended, warm, and inflamed, leading to a diagnosis of acute dacryocystitis. In adults acute dacryocystitis is usually accompanied by erythema overlying the sac. If after the resolution of an acute dacryocystitis, epiphora continues, a determination must be made if an obstruction has secondarily developed, which can lead to a chronic dacryocystitis. Irrigation of the nasolacrimal system (see p. 116) is indicated to relieve any persistant blockages. When epiphora has been a problem for weeks to months, chronic dacryocystitis is suspected. The sac is not distended or tender when palpated but mucoid regurgitation is common. Nodules may be felt within the body of the tear sac and are usually consistent with chronic dacryocystitis. If blood regurgitates through the punctum, especially with a palpable mass, a lacrimal sac tumor must be ruled out.

Contraindications/Complications. Patient discomfort may occur when palpation is done on a case of acute dacryocystitis. Extension of the inflammation into surrounding tissues may indicate a severe problem is developing, such as a cellulitis, which would require a more comprehensive management plan.

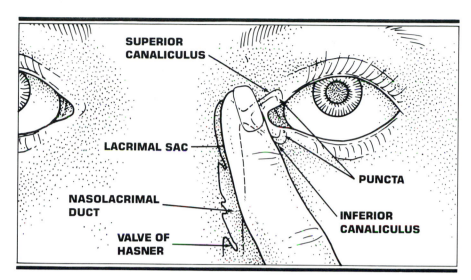

1. The index finger is placed over the lacrimal sac, pressing gently to palpate the lacrimal sac.

SUPERIOR CANALICULUS

LACRIMAL SAC

NASOLACRIMAL DUCT

VALVE OF HASNER

PUNCTA

INFERIOR CANALICULUS

2. The lacrimal sac is palpated while viewing through the biomicroscope for the regurgitation of pus or mucus.

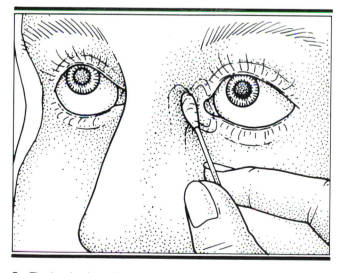

3. The lacrimal sac is palpated with a cotton-tipped applicator while the punctum is viewed with a biomicroscope.

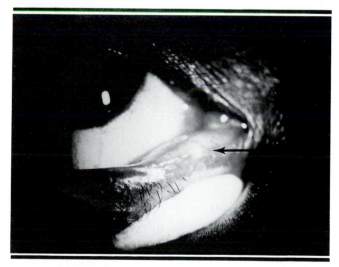

4. A mucoid discharge regurgitating from punctum (arrow) in a case of chronic dacryocystitis.

35 Lacrimal Dilation and Irrigation

Description/Indications. Epiphora, an abnormal overflow of tears down the cheek, is a common complaint that requires careful investigation. Epiphora is rarely caused by hypersecretion of tears; rather, a functional blockage occurs within the lacrimal excretory system leading to improper tear drainage. Epiphora may be constant or intermittent, and the extent of the blockage determines the frequency of tearing. A lacrimal dilation and irrigation (D&I) procedure will determine the patency of the lacrimal excretory system but will not localize the obstruction. On occasion a D&I may open a functionally blocked system by causing the release of a concretion or mucous plug that was blocking the channel. Thus the test has both diagnostic and therapeutic implications.

Instrumentation. Lacrimal dilator, lacrimal cannula, sterile disposable syringe, topical ophthalmic anesthetic (0.5% proparacaine), cotton pledget, sterile saline solution (Fig. 1).

Technique. Before starting, arrange all the instruments within easy reach. The punctum is usually small and needs to be enlarged to accommodate the lacrimal cannula. A lacrimal dilator is used to widen the orifice. Dilators are thin, cylindrical rods that taper to a narrow tip. Dilators come in different sizes, with a thin and medium tapered dilator usually required to meet the size needs of most individuals. The lacrimal cannula is a short, blunted needle that allows saline to be irrigated into the canaliculus. It is attached to a disposable sterile syringe that is filled with saline.

It is best to prepare the syringe before starting the procedure. Remove the plunger and fill the syringe with sterile saline to the top of the tube (Fig. 2A). Place the plunger back into position and slowly push the plunger down the barrel of the syringe so some of the fluid is released. The plunger is left midway down the barrel in a position so the finger(s) may reach the top of the plunger to depress it while the remaining fingers hold the syringe in place (Fig. 2B). There should not be any air bubbles evident in the barrel. If there are, remove the plunger and add more saline solution.

Anesthetize the punctum using a topical anesthetic agent. A deep anesthesia may be obtained by placing a soaked cotton pledget over the punctum and allowing it to sit for several minutes (Fig. 3). Alternately, anesthesia may be obtained by instilling the drops directly onto the punctum and waiting several minutes for maximal effect.

Gently pull the lower lid temporally to expose the inferior punctum and make the lid taut. The hand holding the lacrimal dilator is firmly supported by allowing the free fingers to be placed either on the cheek or the bridge of the nose. Place the tip of the thin dilator in the punctum (Fig. 4A), keeping it perpendicular to the lid margin. Roll the dilator between the fingers (Fig. 4B), slowly advancing the tip into the punctum until the dilator width is greater than the size of the punctal opening. The dilator will no longer easily advance into the punctum. The elastic punctum will temporarily expand as the lacrimal dilator is further rotated. Once the punctum widens, switch to a wider dilator (medium taper) if necessary (Fig. 4C), rolling it back and forth to get enough punctal enlargement to allow the easy entrance of the cannula. Do not force the dilator deep into the canaliculus.

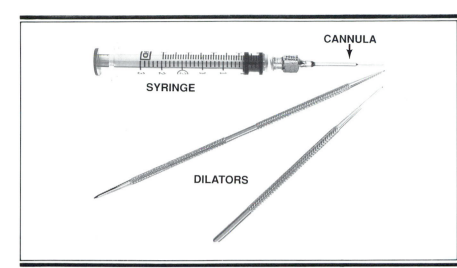

1. Instruments used for dilation and irrigation: syringe, dilators, lacrimal cannula.

2. A. (below left) To avoid air bubbles, the syringe is filled to the top with saline before the plunger is inserted.
B. (below center) During preparation, depress the plunger midway down the tube to allow the fingers to reach the plunger and depress easily.

3. (below right) A pledget of proparacaine is placed over punctum for several minutes to obtain deep anesthesia.

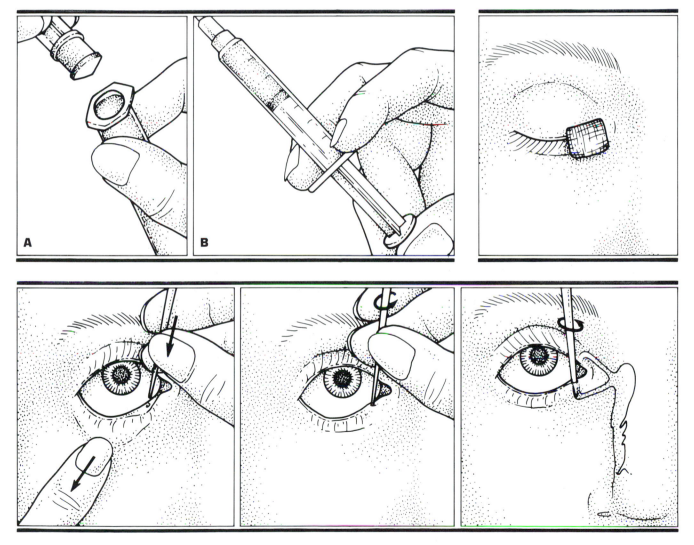

4. A. A small dilator is placed in the punctum. Dilation enlarges the punctum to allow the entrance of the lacrimal cannula. Note how the lid is pulled temporal to expose the punctum.

4. B. The dilator is held between the fingers so a rolling or twirling motion is created.

4. C. Once the punctum is enlarged with a small dilator, it is replaced with a medium tapered dilator to further increase the punctal opening. The dilator is held vertically as it is twirled, only entering the vertical canaliculus. Note how the punctal opening has enlarged.

Remove the dilator and insert the lacrimal cannula perpendicular to the lid margin (Fig. 5A). In some individuals the punctum snaps closed very quickly after the dilator is removed. If this occurs and the punctum is too small to allow entrance of the cannula, again dilate the punctum and attempt to insert the cannula more quickly after removing the dilator. An assistant may help facilitate this part of the procedure.

The hand holding the syringe needs good support. This can be provided by allowing the free fingers to rest on the cheek or the bridge of the nose. The free hand can also be used to brace the hand with the syringe. Insert the cannula into the punctum, let it slide downward for 2 mm, and gently turn the syringe sideways so the cannula is pointing nasally. Insert it another 3 to 4 mm (Fig. 5B). Keep the lid pulled taut to allow easy access. The cannula is inserted far enough into the canaliculus so it will stay in place as irrigation is performed.

Express the saline from the syringe by exerting a slow gentle pressure onto the plunger (Fig. 6). Ask the patient to swallow as the fluid is being expressed to avoid coughing when the saline hits the back of the throat. Have the patient signal when fluid is tasted or felt in the back of the throat or in the nose. Once this occurs, withdraw the cannula.

As pressure is exerted on the plunger, it may not move because of a blockage within the excretory system. A blockage may also cause fluid to regurgitate from the superior punctum as the inferior punctum is irrigated (Fig. 7A). In this instance have an assistant occlude the upper punctum with a medium-taper dilator and irrigate again (Fig. 7B). An alternate method to occlude the superior punctum is by placing, with pressure, a cotton-tipped applicator against the superior punctum. If there is still no movement of the plunger after a few seconds of gentle pressure, a significant blockage exists and the system may need to be probed to relieve the blockade. Sometimes resistance is felt as irrigation is begun that with gentle pressure applied to the plunger

for 10 to 15 seconds will cause the release of a mucous plug or a dacryolith. The release of the pressure will be felt in the ease with which the plunger can now be depressed. Most blockages are in the lower canaliculus or inferior to this, so irrigation through the superior punctum is rarely necessary.

After a D&I some irritation of the tissues lining the nasolacrimal system is possible. In difficult cases or where irritation is suspected, a topical antibiotic-steroid solution is indicated, two to four times per day for up to 3 days.

Interpretation. When irrigating the lower canaliculus, if fluid returns through the upper punctum a blockage exists in the common canaliculus or lacrimal sac (Fig. 7A). The returning fluid may be clear or mucopurulent, the latter indicating that an infection or inflammation is a cause of the blockage. If fluid enters the nose or back of the throat, the excretory system is not completely blocked. A functional blockage is possible that may create symptoms of epiphora under the low-pressure situation of normal tear drainage. The high-pressure of irrigation forces fluid down a narrow channel that may be too constricted to allow enough drainage during some situations. The Jones dye test (see p. 120) is used to differentiate functional blockages from patent systems. If fluid regurgitates from the inferior punctum as irrigation is being performed there, or if fluid is not recovered either through the upper punctum or nose with pressure being encountered, a blockage exists in the canaliculus (Fig. 8).

Contraindications/Complications. Too great a force exerted onto the syringe could create a large force within the excretory system, causing tissue damage. Patients may complain of "fullness" or discomfort if a blockage is present that will not release as the lacrimal system is irrigated. If the excretory system is completely blocked or continually becomes blocked after being opened for short periods, then surgical repair may be indicated.

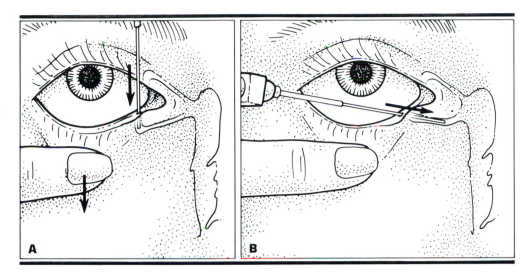

5. A. The lacrimal cannula is inserted vertically about 2 mm. **B.** Once inserted vertically, the syringe and cannula are gently guided horizontally. The cannula is now inserted about 3 mm further into the horizontal canaliculus.

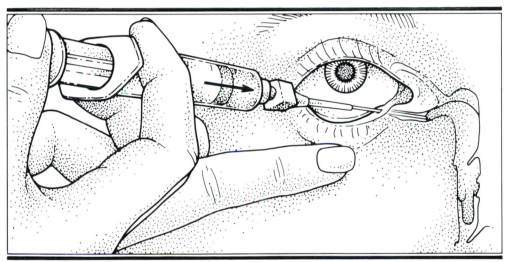

6. Gentle pressure is applied to plunger to express saline solution into the lacrimal excretory system.

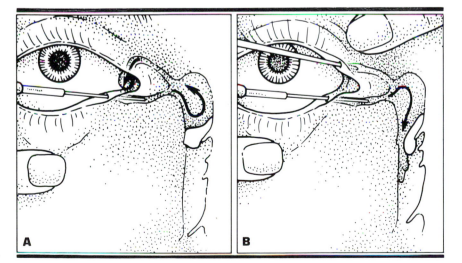

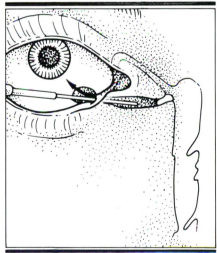

7. A. A blockage in the lacrimal sac does not allow saline solution to drain and instead solution returns through the upper punctum. **B.** An assistant plugs the upper punctum with a dilator while the lower punctum is irrigated, attempting to keep the solution within the system and create a gentle pressure to move a blockage.

8. A blockage in the canaliculus does not allow for saline to be expressed. Pressure is felt on the plunger as irrigation is attempted, and some saline may regurgitate back through the punctum being irrigated.

36 Jones Dye Tests 1 and 2

Description/Indications. The Jones dye tests 1 (primary) and 2 (secondary) are used to determine the patency of the lacrimal drainage system. The test is performed when symptoms of epiphora are present and the lacrimal dilation and irrigation test is negative (see p. 116). In this situation the Jones dye test will ascertain if there is a functional blockage of the nasolacrimal sac or duct. With a functional blockage one of the channels of the nasolacrimal drainage system is too narrow to allow for the proper flow of tears under normal conditions, producing epiphora. The Jones dye test is done by placing fluorescein into the eye and determining if it travels the length of the lacrimal drainage system.

Instrumentation. Two percent sodium fluorescein strips, cotton-tipped applicators, Burton (ultraviolet) lamp, lacrimal dilation-irrigation set, sterile saline solution, white tissue paper.

Technique

Jones Dye Test 1 (Primary Dye Test): Wet four fluorescein strips with sterile saline solution, instilling the fluorescein into the inferior cul-de-sac near the punctum (Figure 1A). Blot any excess fluorescein dripping down the lower eyelid but do not reduce the volume of the lacrimal lake. Do not use a topical anesthetic. Instruct the patient to sit quietly, blink normally with eyes open, and not rub the eyes. After 5 minutes ask the patient to occlude one nostril and using the other nostril to blow into a white tissue. Inspect the tissue for evidence of fluorescein. A Burton (ultraviolet) lamp may aid in the inspection for fluorescein. If fluorescein is evident, the test is positive and the lacrimal system is patent and functioning.

If fluorescein is not present, wait 5 more minutes and repeat the procedure. If fluorescein is still not evident, a cotton-tipped applicator is inserted approximately 1 cm. into the nose (Fig. 1B). The applicator is placed against the inferior turbinate and left in place for 10 seconds. The cotton-tipped applicator is then removed and viewed under a Burton lamp (Fig. 1C).

If dye is still not seen, gently massage the lacrimal sac and again ask the patient, with one nostril occluded, to blow into a white tissue. This may allow dye to appear, indicating a narrowing or partial obstruction of the nasolacrimal duct. If still negative, a functional blockage is possible and the Jones dye test 2 (secondary dye test) is done.

Jones Dye Test 2 (Secondary Dye Test): Jones dye test 2 is done immediately after the primary dye test by irrigating the inferior canaliculus (see p. 116) with saline solution (Fig. 2). Recover some of the saline solution by having the patient lean forward and expectorate into a basin or blow the nose into a tissue. Examine the solution or tissue using the Burton lamp.

Interpretation. The test does not quantify a defect but will have a positive or negative outcome. In a positive Jones dye test 1, fluorescein will drain through a patent lacrimal system and be retrieved (Fig. 3A). In a negative Jones dye test 1 or 2, fluorescein is never retrieved (Fig. 3B, 3C). In a positive Jones dye test 2, fluorescein is retrieved after the lacrimal system is irrigated, indicating that the system has a functional blockage (Fig. 3D). Fluorescein was able to enter the lacrimal sac and a functional blockage exists somewhere below this point. If during the Jones dye test 2 saline is recovered but is clear, a functional blockage exists that is nearer to the punctum and canaliculus, since dye never entered the excretory system.

False positive results are rare, but because of the technical problems in retrieving fluorescein, false negatives are possible. Therefore, while a positive test indicates a patent and functioning lacrimal excretory system, a negative test is inconclusive and does not always indicate the system is obstructed.

Contraindications/Complications. Care must be taken not to apply too much pressure to the drainage system when irrigation is done. The test should not be done during an episode of acute dacryocystitis.

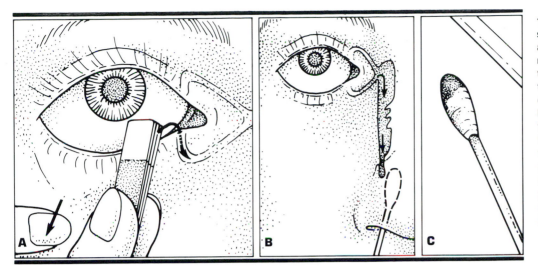

1. A. Four fluorescein strips, stacked together, are touched to the inferior palpebral conjunctiva, near the punctum, to create a lacrimal lake containing fluorescein. **B.** A secondary method to retrieve fluorescein is by placing a cotton-tipped applicator several mm up into the nose. **C.** The cotton-tipped applicator is inspected under an ultraviolet light, looking for fluorescein.

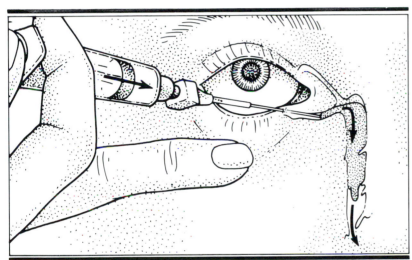

2. The Jones dye test 2 is done by irrigating the lacrimal system after fluorescein instillation. The draining fluid is inspected for fluorescein.

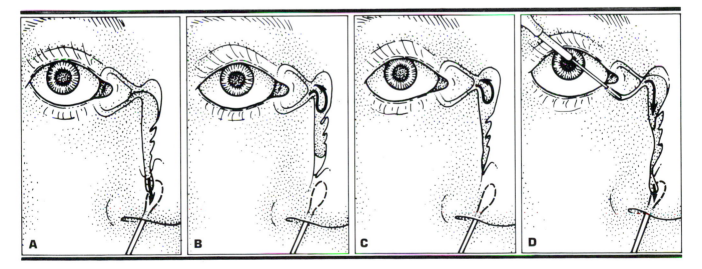

3. A. Fluorescein draining through a patent lacrimal excretory system during a Jones dye test 1. This test is positive. Fluorescein is retrieved on the cotton-tipped applicator. **B.** An example of a negative Jones dye test 1. A blockage in the nasolacrimal duct impairs the flow of dye. **C.** Another example of a negative Jones dye test 1. A stenotic nasolacrimal duct impairs the flow of dye. **D.** An example of a positive Jones dye test 2. Irrigation forces fluorescein to leave through a narrow but patent nasolacrimal duct.

37 Temporary Intracanalicular Collagen Implant

Description/Indications. The dry eye (keratoconjunctivitis sicca, or KCS) is a common problem seen in many elderly individuals. Artificial tear supplementation is often the first line of treatment. When the signs or symptoms are not relieved with artificial tears, additional treatment strategies need to be considered.

One alternative is the intracanalicular collagen implant; being small, this slides easily into the canaliculus. There it swells, expands, and decreases tear drainage before being resorbed. The implant will decrease the excretion of tears by 60 to 80%, so that more tears bathe the eye, keeping it lubricated and decreasing the signs and symptoms of KCS. The collagen implants are temporary, as they dissolve in 7 to 10 days. They are placed in all four puncta and used as a diagnostic tool to determine if a permanent or semipermanent punctal oblative procedure would be beneficial. During the trial period the benefits of punctal occlusion are weighed against adverse reactions. If signs and/or symptoms do improve, a semipermanent procedure such as the reversible punctal plug may be attempted (see p. 124).

The collagen implants are 2 mm in length; they are available in three diameters, 0.2, 0.3, and 0.4 mm.

Instrumentation. Collagen implants, jeweler's forceps, biomicroscope, topical ophthalmic anesthetic solution.

Technique. Prepare the patient by anesthetizing each punctum using a topical anesthetic agent, placing the drops onto the punctal orifice. The next step is to prepare the collagen implants for insertion. The implants come in a foam package (Fig. 1). Place the foam package under the slit lamp and with low magnification, using a jeweler's forceps, remove an implant from the packaging by grabbing an implant at one end and pulling straight out. The 0.4-mm diameter implant fits most patients and is the first choice in most cases. Use a thinner implant if the implant seems too wide for the punctal opening.

Position the patient in the slit lamp, giving him or her a suitable object to hold fixation in an upward direction. With the free hand place the index finger below the lid margin, pulling the lid taut to evert the lid margin so the punctum is exposed. Holding the implant with the jeweler's forceps, slowly approach the punctum, lining up the implant with the punctal opening (Fig. 2). Insert the narrow end into the punctum so it goes as far in as possible. The implant will be partially inside the canaliculus (Fig. 3). To position the implant all the way into the canaliculus, release the forceps so the implant is held in place by the pressure of the punctal opening. Close the forceps, and holding the tips closed, gently push the implant into the punctum until it is flush with the lid margin (Fig. 4A). Open the forceps and using one pointed end, push the implant further down into the canaliculus until it disappears from sight (Fig. 4B, C).

Place an implant into each remaining punctum, and when finished, inspect each implant while still positioned at the slit lamp to ensure that each is still in position. Patients should be reexamined about 10 to 14 days after insertion to ascertain if the implants have been beneficial.

Interpretation. Patients may report improvement in their symptoms within a few days of insertion, which indicates a semipermanent procedure should be considered. Improvement of objective signs such as a keratitis or conjunctivitis may take longer than 10 days before a change is noted. If constant epiphora occurs after insertion, remind the patient that it will be temporary since the implants will be reabsorbed in 7 to 10 days. Further punctal occlusion procedures should be avoided for these patients.

Contraindications/Complications. Implants should not be used in cases of acute or chronic dacryocystitis.

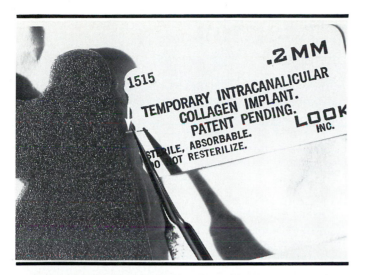

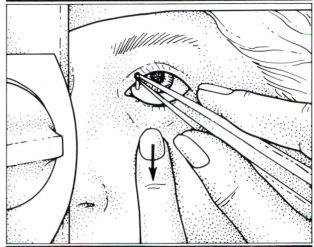

1. (above left) The collagen implants come in a foam insert. A jeweler's forceps is used to both remove an implant from the packaging and to insert the implant into the canaliculus.

2. (above right) With the patient seated at the slit lamp, the implant is held by the forceps and brought toward the punctum for insertion.

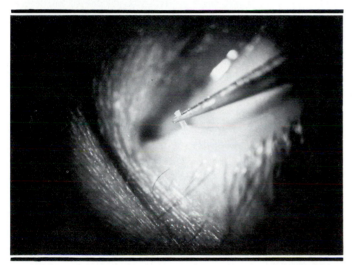

3. (left) The collagen implant as seen just after insertion, partially inserted into the canaliculus.

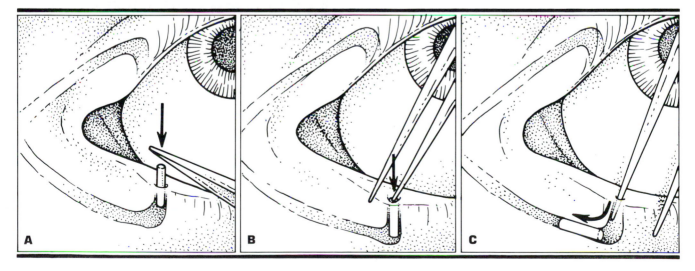

4. A. The closed ends of the forceps are used to gently push the implant down into the canaliculus so that it lies flush with the lid margin. **B.** The pointed end of the forceps is used to push the implant further down into the canaliculus into the final position. **C.** Collagen implant in resting position. The implant swells, occludes the canaliculus, and retards tear drainage.

38   Punctal Plug Insertion

Description/Indications. In the moderate to severe dry eye individual, punctal occlusion retards tear drainage and allows the scant amount of tears available to bathe the eye. In the past only permanent procedures were available to occlude the punctum. These were usually done with some form of electrocautery, leading to scar tissue formation and punctal obliteration. A temporary, resorbable collagen implant (see p. 122) is available and useful in predicting which individuals may do best with punctal occlusion. If a trial with the collagen implants is a success, a silicone plug may be inserted into the punctum for occlusion, left in place for several months, and withdrawn at any time. This reversibility is an attractive feature, especially in cases where the plug is not tolerated or if epiphora results. The plug is hollow and has flanges on the top and bottom to allow for easy insertion and stability once in place. The plugs come in three sizes: the standard 2.8-mm length, a medium plug 2.0 mm in length with a reduced dome diameter, and a small plug 1.6 mm in length (Fig. 1).

The insertion procedure is similar to a dilation and irrigation technique (see p. 116), with the punctum being dilated to allow for insertion of the punctal plug. One punctum is occluded at a time, using the other eye as a control. If satisfactory results occur with the first eye, then the second eye may be done. Since the majority of drainage occurs through the lower punctum, it is usually only necessary to occlude the inferior punctum. If the symptoms diminish when the lower punctum is blocked, a trial of occlusion for the upper punctum may be attempted.

Instrumentation. Punctal plug, dilator-inserter tool, topical ophthalmic anesthetic agent, jeweler's forceps.

Technique. Anesthetize the punctum with a topical ophthalmic anesthetic agent. This can be done by placing a saturated cotton pledget over the punctum or by instilling the drops directly into the punctum.

Allow 1 to 2 minutes for the anesthetic agent to take maximal effect. A loupe may aid in visualization of the punctum.

Start with a 2.8-mm plug, and use the smaller models if the eye and punctum appear small or if there is difficulty in inserting the larger plug. Place the sleeve over the guidewire and place the plug onto the guidewire with the pointed side facing toward the eye (Fig. 2). The plug will rest on the plastic sleeve, which will also be used to keep the plug in place after insertion as the guidewire is being withdrawn. The combination instrument does not have to be used. A blunt-end needle or cannula thin enough to allow the hollow middle of the plug to be inserted onto it is appropriate and some clinicians may be more comfortable with these instruments.

Recline the patient and gently pull the lower lid down and temporal to expose the inferior punctum. Slowly and gently dilate the punctum to a maximum 1.2-mm width (Fig. 3A). This can be done in several ways. The dilater-inserter tool that comes with the plugs has a dilating end that will lead to a 1.2-mm dilation. This may be the only tool used for dilation, but in patients with small puncta, a thin tapered dilator may be needed to first enlarge the orifice before switching to the 1.2-mm dilator. The dilator need not be inserted more than 2 mm into the canaliculus.

Once the punctum is dilated, quickly reverse the combination tool so the plug is facing the punctum. Introduce the thin wire of the inserter tool into the punctum. Push the plug into the punctum until the domed base sits on the lid margin. The body of the plug will lie within the vertical canaliculus (Fig. 3B). If the plug seems too large for the punctum, try the smaller plugs. Do not force the plug into the punctum. If the punctum constricts before the plug can be inserted, redilate the punctum and introduce the plug quicker the next time. An assistant may help facilitate this part of the procedure.

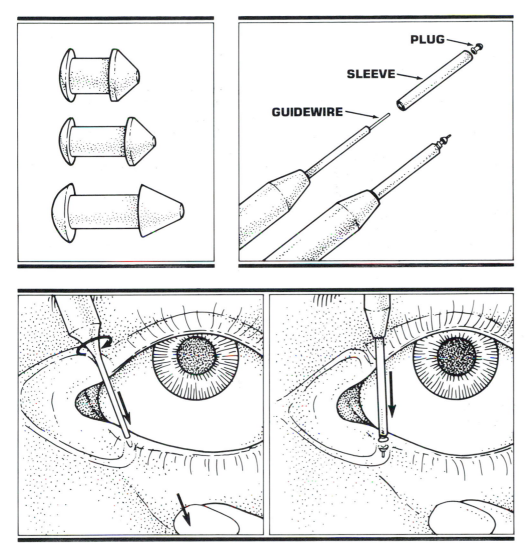

1. (far left) Three different sizes of punctal plugs.

2. (left) The inserting instrument is seen apart and with plug in place. The opposite end of the tool is used for dilating the punctum.

3. A. Dilation of the punctum. The punctum is anesthetized before dilation is begun.

3. B. The insertion of the punctal plug, trying to come in vertical to the lid margin.

Frequently a flaccid lower lid needs to be stabilized with forceps to allow the plug to be inserted (Fig. 4). Forceps are held parallel to the lid margin with the lid gently grasped just below its margin to enhance the stability of the lid margin.

To remove the tool once the plug is inserted, grasp the outer sleeve with a small forceps and let the sleeve press gently on the domed head of the plug. This pressure will keep the plug in place as the inserting tool is withdrawn (Fig. 5). Pull the tool out from the punctum, keeping it perpendicular to the lid. The guidewire of the tool should slide out of the sleeve, leaving the plug in place touched by the forceps-held outer sleeve. Remove the sleeve and verify the plug is fully inserted (Fig. 6). If using a cannula or needle for insertion, use a forceps to press on the domed plug head as you withdraw the inserting instrument.

If for any reason it is necessary to remove the plug, grip the plug with a small forceps from below the domed head and gently pull it straight out (Fig. 7).

Interpretation. One measure to assess if the plug insertion is successful is if the patient's symptoms have decreased or resolved. Wait up to 1 month before deciding if the procedure is a success. If the results are equivocal, wait awhile longer before proceeding on the second eye. Concomitant artificial tear use may be needed with the plugs to maintain corneal integrity. If a plug inserted into the inferior punctum leads to partial improvement in the signs and/or symptoms, a trial placing an additional plug in the upper punctum is warranted to assess if further improvement is feasible.

Contraindications/Complications. Care must be exercised when a punctal plug is inserted. The plug should slip into place with a minimal amount of pressure. If the plug does not enter the punctum easily, do not use it. Avoid excessive force in any circumstance. There has been a report of the migration of the smallest size plug such that it entered the canaliculi at the time of insertion in one occasion and on another occasion, migrated at a later date. Migration has only been reported with the smallest size plug, and may be an indication to only use that size when a punctal plug is clearly indicated and no other plug will work.

Irritation from the plug may be a cause for removal. If the irritation occurs after insertion, wait several days before removing the plug. The irritation may be due to the mechanical manipulation of the insertion and not the plug itself. The plug may point backward toward the eye, especially in cases of concomitant entropion, leading to conjunctival irritation. These plugs need to be withdrawn, with entropion being a relative contraindication for the use of punctal plugs. Epiphora is another indication for removal. Other contraindications to the use of punctal plugs are acute or chronic ocular infections or inflammations and individuals sensitive to silicone.

The punctal plug may be accidently removed if the eye is vigorously rubbed.

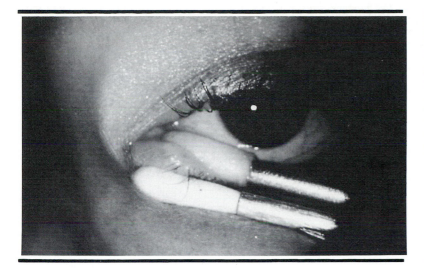

4. Forceps are used to stabilize the lower lid and punctum to facilitate insertion. (Courtesy of Eagle Vision, Inc., Memphis.)

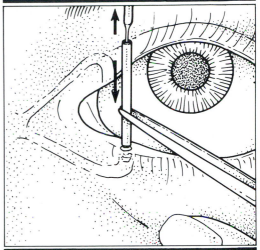

5. The punctal plug in proper position with inserting tool being removed. The plug is kept in position by the plastic sleeve until the guidewire is removed.

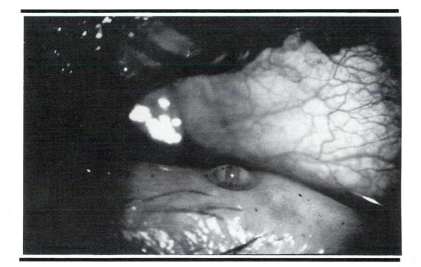

6. Punctal plug in place. (Courtesy of Eagle Vision, Inc., Memphis.)

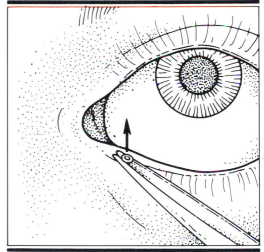

7. If needed a punctal plug can be removed with forceps. The forceps are placed below the domed head and the plug is pulled straight out.

IV   Suggested Readings

Boesma HGM, van Bijsterveld OP: The lactoferrin test for the diagnosis of keratoconjunctivitis sicca in clinical practice. *Ann Ophthalmol* 1987;**19**:152–154.

Hecht SD: Evaluation of the lacrimal drainage system. *Am Acad Ophthalmol Otolaryngol* 1978;**85**:1250–1258.

Holly FJ, Lemp MA: Tear physiology and dry eyes. *Surv Ophthalmol* 1977;**22**:69–87.

Hornblass A, Ingis TM: Lacrimal function tests. *Arch Ophthalmol* 1979;**97**:1654–1655.

Lamberts DW: Punctal occlusion. *Int Ophthalmol Clin* 1987; **27**:44–46.

Lamberts DW: Punctal occlusion in dry eye patients, in Holly FJ (ed): *The Preocular Tear Film in Health, Disease and Contact Lens Wear*. Lubbock, TX, Dry Eye Institute, 1986.

Lemp ML: Recent developments in dry eye management. *Ophthalmology* 1987;**94**:1299–1304.

Tuberville AW, Frederick WR, Wood TO: Punctal occlusion in tear deficiency syndromes. *Ophthalmology* 1982; **89**:1170.

Willis RM, Folberg R, Krachmer J, Holland EJ: The treatment of aqueous-deficient dry eye with removable punctal plugs. *Ophthalmology* 1987;**94**:514–518.

Wright MM, Bersani TA, Freuth BR, Musch DC: Efficacy of the primary dye test. *Ophthalmology* 1989;**96**:481–483.

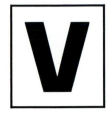

Conjunctival Procedures

39 Conjunctival/Ocular Irrigation

Description/Indications. When an acid, alkali, or other foreign substance gets into the eye, further damage can be prevented with prompt flushing. Because the damage and sequelae are different depending upon which chemical has affected the eye, a thorough history is required. On occasions when the patient does not know what substance contaminated the eye(s), have him or her bring the container into the office. While the eye is being irrigated, have an assistant review the contents in an ocular toxicology textbook (such as Grant) or with a poison control hotline.

In most emergencies, a history and examination is done before treatment is instituted. A chemical burn is the exception to this rule, where prompt treatment is of the essence and instituted immediately. Certain chemical burns are severe and will require a prompt referral to a corneal specialist for further evaluation and treatment. Signs indicating a severe burn are corneal opacification, decreased visibility of iris detail, greater than 50% epithelium loss, perilimbal ischemia, or increased intraocular pressure.

Conjunctival irrigation is also used to wash small foreign bodies from the eye (see p. 132), to wash away any discharge in patients with conjunctival infections, to periodically rinse the orbital socket in patients with prosthetic eyes, and to flush the viscous solution from the eye following gonioscopy.

Instrumentation. Sterile saline, lid speculum, emesis basin, litmus paper, topical ophthalmic anesthetic solution.

Technique

Chemical Burns: Lay the patient back in the examining chair. If the patient is in pain because of an abraded cornea or has a blepharospasm, instill a topical ophthalmic anesthetic agent.

Give the patient a point to fixate above his or her head while spreading open the eyelids (Fig. 1). Slowly but steadily instill sterile saline solution into the eye, irrigating into the upper and lower fornices in addition to the bulbar conjunctival surface. Sev-

eral bottles of sterile saline solution will usually be required for the *thirty minute minimum* procedure. A lid speculum is used if the patient cannot keep the eyes open (see p. 90).

Use an emesis basin to catch the solution draining from the eye. Have the patient or an assistant hold the basin just below the eye being irrigated so the draining solution is captured. Paper towels or tissues may be used to capture the draining fluid if a basin is not available. Hold the towels below and to the side of the eye, maintaining a tight bond with the skin so fluid will not run underneath.

Litmus paper is used as a rough guide to determine when to stop irrigation (Fig. 2A). Touch the green litmus paper to the palpebral conjunctiva, near or at the site of injury. If the paper turns a dark blue, the conjunctiva is alkaline. If it turns yellower, the conjunctiva is acidic. Any change in color from the original green means further irrigation is needed. On the label of most litmus paper bottles is a color scale used for interpreting the results to known standard colors (Fig. 2B).

A thorough slit lamp examination is required after irrigation, noting any hyperemia, chemosis, epithelial damage, or corneal edema.

Conjunctival Foreign Bodies: For superficial conjunctival foreign bodies, aim the spray at the particles' edge to dislodge and float it from the eye. A spud, loupe or needle may be required to remove embedded foreign bodies (see p. 132). Double lid eversion may be required to localize foreign bodies trapped under the eyelids (see p. 88). Once the lid is everted, inspect and irrigate, aiming the spray under the lid to get deep into the superior and inferior fornices (Fig. 3). Use a moistened cottontipped applicator (see p. 132) or a forceps to remove any remaining particles from the palpebral conjunctival surface.

Contraindications/Complications. Superficial punctate keratitis or hyperemia are common findings after irrigation. Irrigation is contraindicated in any case where a penetrating injury is suspected.

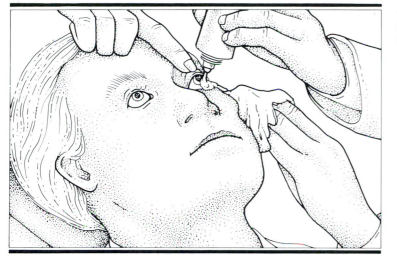

1. The eyelids are gently spread apart as the eye is irrigated, and paper towels or tissues are used to catch the draining fluid.

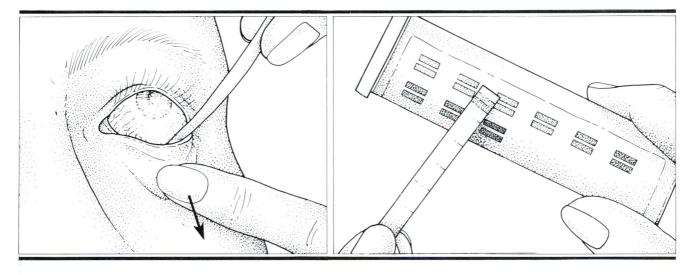

2. A. Litmus paper is used as a guide to determine when irrigation may be terminated. A small piece is touched to the conjunctiva, near or at the point of injury, watching for a change in color of the paper.

2. B. The scale on the bottle may be used for an approximation of the extent of chemical injury to the eye.

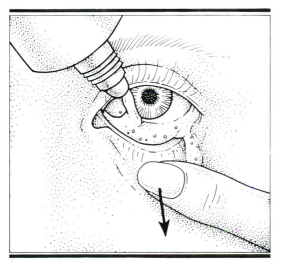

3. Irrigation into the inferior cul-de-sac to remove small particles from the eye.

40 Conjunctival Foreign Body Removal

Description/Indications. A foreign body (FB) embedded under the upper or lower lid is a common source of patient complaints. When visible the FB commonly appears as a dark speck on the pink (palpebral) or white (bulbar) conjunctival surface. The eye is usually moderately injected, with the superior palpebral conjunctiva the most common place to find conjunctival foreign bodies. At times symptoms may suggest a FB but the object may be difficult to find. Lid eversion (see p. 86) is then needed to locate the FB. Double lid eversion (see p. 88) with slit lamp magnification may be required to localize small particulate matter such as fiberglass strands, glass, or steel, especially if it is lodged in the sulcus behind the lid margins. Fine linear streaks or FB tracks on the cornea (Fig. 1) that stain with fluorescein are indicative of an embedded FB on the lid margin or superior palpebral conjunctival surface. Easier to locate are FBs embedded on the bulbar conjunctival surface within the palpebral fissure.

Assessment of conjunctival FB(s) include determining its number (single or multiple); location (superior palpebral conjunctiva, bulbar conjunctiva, or inferior palpebral conjunctiva); and whether it is superficial or embedded. Utilizing this information, the FB is removed with the appropriate procedure. A hard-to-find embedded FB may be localized by an anchored mucus tag on the superior palpebral conjunctiva or by an area of localized hyperemia or edema.

Topical anesthesia is avoided unless the patient is extremely sensitive and exhibiting significant blepharospasm. Topical anesthesia is avoided so that when the particle is located and removed, the patient will feel immediate relief, indicative that no other FBs remain in the eye. On occasion the FB has irritated the cornea sufficiently so that even with removal, the eye is still sensitive and uncomfortable with a FB-type sensation. A thorough slit lamp examination with lid eversion will confirm that no other FBs are in the eye.

Instrumentation. Spud, sterile disposable needle, spatula, jeweler's forceps, topical ophthalmic anesthetic solution, sterile saline solution, sterile cotton-tipped applicators.

Technique. The simplest method for removing a superficial conjunctival FB is with irrigation (Fig. 2). Locate the FB, using lid eversion if necessary, and forcefully irrigate, aiming the fluid spray at the edge of the particle so that it dislodges and washes away.

If irrigation has not dislodged the superficial conjunctival FB, use a sterile cotton-tipped applicator that has been moistened with sterile saline. Work under the slit lamp and if necessary evert the lid to make the FB accessible. Gently dislodge the particle, using small strokes tangential to the plane of the eyelid (Fig. 3). As with the lavage maneuver, this method works best on superficial FBs, especially those in the cul-de-sac and on the superior tarsus.

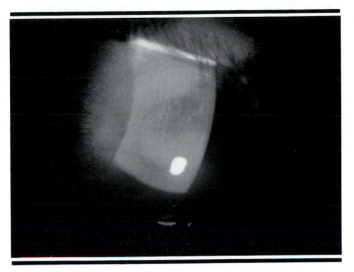

1. Linear streaks on the cornea staining with fluorescein, indicative of a FB under the superior eyelid.

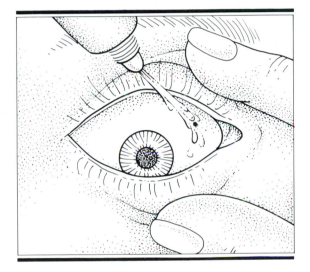

2. An irrigating spray is directed at the edge of the FB to wash it off the surface.

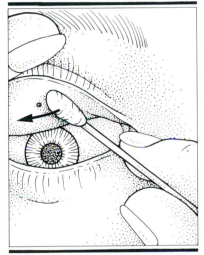

3. A cotton-tipped applicator wiping the superior conjunctival surface to eliminate a FB.

Foreign matter embedded in the conjunctiva not dislodged by lavage or swabbing will require a sterile spud or disposable sterile needle for removal. The technique is similar to the removal of a corneal FB (see p. 146). Using the slit lamp and following the instillation of topical anesthesia, give the patient a suitable object for fixation to expose the FB. Medium magnification (10X) is used with diffuse white light. Align the spud close to the eye by viewing outside the slit lamp, and once aligned, use the slit lamp for greater magnification. Utilize a handrest or rest the elbow on the slit lamp table to achieve greater stability. Hold the spud or needle so it is tangential to the conjunctival plane and slowly loosen the edges of the FB (Fig. 4A). Once the peripheral excavation is complete, bury the spud underneath the FB (Fig. 4B) and in a flicking-like motion, elevate the buried spud. If the edges have been sufficiently loosened, the FB should lift off (Fig. 4C). Copiously irrigate the eye following removal to flush any remaining pieces of matter. Residual particulate matter is removed using the slit lamp with a blunt spatula or jeweler's forceps (Fig. 5). The spatula is used to scoop up loose pieces of material while the forceps is used to individually grasp pieces of matter before removing them from the eye.

Jeweler's forceps may be needed to locate suspected conjunctival foreign bodies covered by a mucus tag. The tag is pulled away with the forceps, often leaving a visible burr embedded underneath. The burr is removed utilizing the procedure of choice to remove embedded particles.

When, after thorough examination, a FB cannot be identified, saline irrigation of the superior tarsal region and inferior cul-de-sac, followed by blind wiping of the anesthetized palpebral conjunctival surfaces with a moistened cotton-tipped applicator (as if removing an FB), may be successful in removing the hard-to-find microscopic FB.

For prophylaxis, an antibiotic ointment or drop is instilled after the procedure. If there is considerable tissue disruption, antibiotics may be required for longer use. Cycloplegia and pressure patching are rarely needed, since the conjunctiva heals quickly, usually within 12 to 24 hours for most epithelial disruptions. Whenever antibiotic prophylaxis is used, have the patient return for a follow-up examination in 24 to 48 hours. Remind the patient to return sooner if symptoms of a FB persist.

Contraindications/Complications. Monitor for secondary infection in the days after removal, especially if the FB is embedded and a spud is required for removal. Any FB, particularly those on the bulbar conjunctiva, may be a sign of perforating injury. This is especially true if a history of hammering metal-on-metal or working around high-speed machinery (such as a grinder's wheel) is elicited. A perforating injury is easily masked by a subconjunctival hemorrhage, and the Seidel test (see p. 290) aids in this differential diagnosis. Radiologic studies of the eye and orbit may also be indicated in these circumstances. If signs of a penetrating injury are present, referral is indicated for further exploration and closure of the globe.

Reassure the patient that a small subconjunctival hemorrhage may occur following the removal technique and that it is not a sign of the eye getting worse. A small amount of superficial punctate keratitis is inevitable after the eye is irrigated due to the mechanical irritation from the fluid on the cornea.

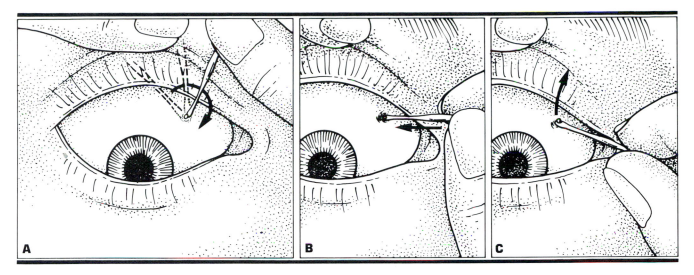

4. A. A spud being used to begin the excavation around the edges of an FB leading to its removal. **B.** The spud is buried underneath the FB. **C.** The head of the spud is flicked upward to remove the FB.

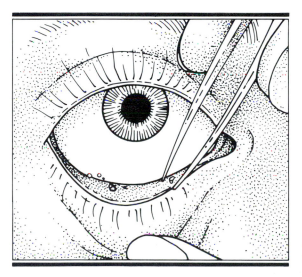

5. Forceps can be used to grasp particles in the inferior cul-de-sac and eliminate them from the eye.

41 Lymphatic Cyst Drainage

Description/Indications. Lymphatic conjunctival cysts are relatively common, often presenting acutely as a ''blister'' (Fig. 1) or as a foreign body sensation that alarms the patient. The cysts, which may be several millimeters in length, are associated with a preexisting conjunctival lymph vessel whose ends collapse, leading to the formation of a lymphatic cyst, which may appear alone or in multiples. The caliber may be irregular, with lobulations appearing along their route. They move freely with the conjunctiva over the sclera. Aside from the occasional cosmetic concern, patients with lymphatic cysts are usually asymptomatic. In situations where the cyst is large and the patient desires removal, remind him or her that as the cyst may recur, unless it is noticeable it may best be left alone. If a cyst does become cosmetically obvious or irritated, it can be lanced and drained.

Inflamed lymphatic cysts or recurrent cysts may require surgical excision and biopsy to rule out a lymphangioma or other conjunctival tumors.

Conjunctival epithelial retention cysts may resemble lymphatic cysts but are on the palpebral conjunctival surface. They are small, from 2 to 5 mm in size, and vary in color from clear to yellow in appearance. They are associated with the accessory lacrimal glands and occur after trauma, surgery, or inflammation. Lymphangectasias are dilated lymph channels with segmental dilations on the bulbar conjunctival surface. They are patent and may also look like a lymphatic cyst. Lymphangectasias are usually longer than 3 to 4 mm and rarely become inflamed or require drainage.

Instrumentation. Sterile disposable needle, topical ophthalmic anesthetic solution, biomicroscope, sterile cotton-tipped applicators, sterile saline solution.

Technique. Instill several drops of a topical anesthetic agent directly onto the cyst, waiting 1 minute for the drops to take effect. Seat the patient behind the slit lamp and give the patient a suitable target to ensure optimal fixation and to expose the lymphatic cyst. At one end, puncture the cyst with a sterile disposable needle, making a short stabbing-like motion into the cyst to create a hole (Fig. 2A). Work tangentially to the eye, trying to angle the needle so it points away from the ocular surface as the cyst is lanced. The cyst will often collapse after penetration is made (Fig. 2B). If the cyst does not collapse, make a second puncture. Gentle massage through the closed lids (Fig. 3) may help flatten the cyst. Using two fingers, a gentle back-and-forth movement is made on the lids near the site of the cyst. If the cyst has not deflated after massage and a patent puncture is visible, use a sterile cotton-tipped applicator moistened with sterile saline solution to level the cyst (Fig. 4). Apply pressure to the end opposite the puncture site. Gently roll the cotton-tipped applicator over the cyst, forcing fluid through the puncture site.

Instill a topical broad-spectrum antibiotic solution into the eye, advising the patient to use antibiotic eyedrops four times per day for 2 days. Instruct the patient to gently massage the collapsed cyst through closed eyelids twice a day to prevent a recurrence. Have the patient continue massage until returning in 2 weeks for a followup reexamination.

Interpretation. Reexamine the eye at 2 weeks, checking the area where the cyst was located. Any hyperemia, edema, or new tissue growth requires further investigation. If the cyst has not recurred at the 2-week examination, chances are good the cyst will not recur. Remind the patient that cysts tend to recur, so have the patient check the eye with a mirror every few weeks. If the cyst recurs, a second procedure can be done. Recurrence after a second procedure warrants a referral for the entire cyst to be excised and a pathologic diagnosis made.

Contraindications/Complications. A secondary infection is a possibility after any procedure and must be monitored. Do not lance a cyst when a bacterial conjunctivitis is present. Conjunctival tumors need to be ruled out for any growth on the conjunctiva, especially if the growth is recurrent, inflamed, large, or possesses a feeder vessel.

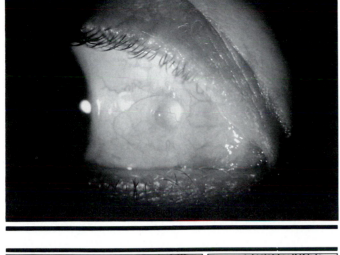

1. A bulbar conjunctival lymphatic cyst.

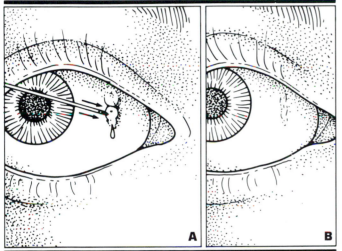

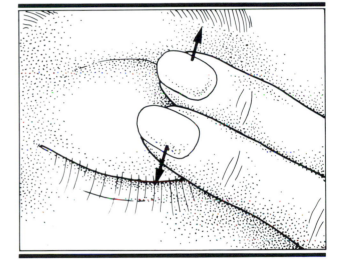

2. A. The wall of the lymphatic cyst is perforated with a sterile disposable needle to create a hole for drainage of the clear fluid. **B.** The collapsed cyst, seen following drainage.

3. Massage through the eyelids is used to collapse a punctured cyst.

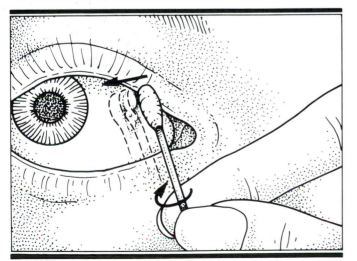

4. A cotton-tipped applicator is used to collapse cysts that do not spontaneously deflate.

42   Forced Duction Testing

Description/Indications. Forced duction testing investigates the passive movements of an extraocular muscle in its field of action and judges whether an ocular motility abnormality is due to mechanical myopathic resistance or paretic muscles, usually of neurogenic origin. Forced duction testing is one procedure not part of the routine ocular motility test battery. In certain situations, however, such as motility disturbances due to trauma, it can provide important diagnostic information. Forced duction testing is indicated when diplopia is of acute onset, a history of trauma precedes an ocular motor disturbance, or diplopia occurs in certain positions of gaze.

Instrumentation. Sterile cotton-tipped applicators, fixation "toothed" forceps, lid speculum, topical ophthalmic anesthetic solution.

Technique

Forceps: Instill topical 10% cocaine solution prepared by a pharmacist, using a cotton pledget (see p. 6). Place the pledget on the conjunctiva near the insertion of the recti muscle(s) to be tested, for 1 to 2 minutes (Fig. 1A).

With a toothed forceps, grasp the conjunctiva and Tenon's fascia at the insertion of the muscle to be tested, about 5 mm posterior to the limbus (Fig. 1B). This conjunctival area is grasped opposite to the quadrant where the globe will be rotated. Grasp the globe and gently rotate the eye in the indicated direction of movement. Have the patient hold a hand in the direction the eye will be moved and ask him or her to look at it. By having the patient look at the hand, innervation is controlled and cooperation ensured. Force is gently applied, slowly attempting to move the eye into the desired position (Fig. 1C). Uncooperative patients attempting to look in other positions of gaze may innervate antagonistic muscles, giving the false impression of mechanical resistance. If voluntary eye movements cannot be controlled then the test cannot be done under topical anesthesia. Once the eye is moved into the position of gaze or a restriction is felt, the forceps grasp is released from the conjunctiva, allowing the globe to return to its position of rest. The contralateral eye, if indicated, may then be tested in a similar manner comparing resistance between the two eyes. As the eye is rotated, do not press or push the globe back into the orbit since this may simulate ocular movement, leading to improper observations.

Cotton-tipped Applicator: The cotton-tipped applicator technique is a simpler and less traumatic method for doing the forced duction test (Fig. 2). Anesthetize the eye using a topical anesthetic solution and place a sterile cotton-tipped applicator tangential and just posterior to the limbus. Gently push the globe with the cotton-tipped applicator in a similar method as with the forceps. Move the involved eye into the affected positions of gaze, asking the patient to look at a target such as his or her hand to facilitate eye movement. Repeat the test on the contralateral eye. The disadvantage of using a cotton-tipped applicator is that it may slip from position because it does not grasp the eye securely. Cotton-tipped applicators do not provide the leverage and force that forceps do, but cotton-tipped applicators are easier to use, less traumatic, and work well in the majority of cases. With forceps the eye is pushed or pulled, looking for abnormal resistance, while with cotton-tipped applicators the eye is only pushed.

A lid speculum (see p. 90) may help in keeping the eyelids separated, especially in traumatic cases with eyelid edema. The lid speculum is also useful in uncooperative patients requiring assistance.

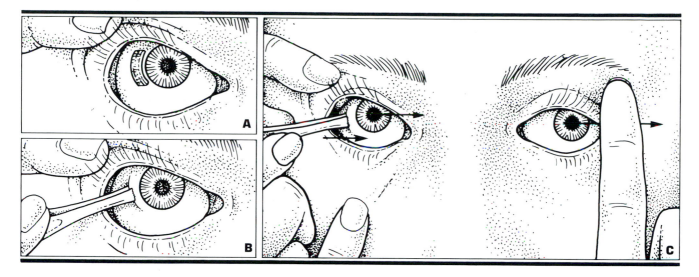

1. A. The pleget of cocaine is placed on the conjunctiva overlying the extraocular muscle insertions for 1 to 2 minutes for anesthesia. **B.** A toothed forceps is used to grasp the conjunctiva, about 3 to 5 mm posterior to the limbus. **C.** A gentle force is applied, attempting to manually rotate the globe.

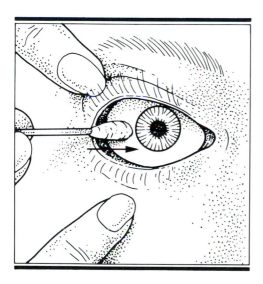

2. A cotton-tipped applicator is placed tangential to the globe and posterior to the limbus.

Interpretation. With forced rotation the globe should move freely in its excursions (negative test). If resistance is encountered (positive test), greater force is needed to move the eye. The opposite eye is used for comparisons, especially in subtle cases of fibrosis or contracture. To obtain the feel of a normal excursion, do the test on "normals" to sense what the expected minimal resistance is.

In motility disturbances due to mechanical restrictions, the globe will move only with increased force and at times not at all (Fig. 3). The increased resistance occurs in grades and not in an "all or none" fashion. In most cases of fibrosis, if enough force is applied, the eye can be made to move to some extent into any position of gaze.

In motility disturbances of neurogenic origin, whether secondary to trauma or ischemia, the globe will move easily with forced duction testing, giving a negative test. With traumatic damage, the orbital or intracranial nerves supplying the extraocular muscles may be contused, leading to the paretic muscles (Fig. 4). If the traumatic damage is severe, whereby the extraocular muscles are severed, a supranormal test will result where little if any resistance is sensed upon forced duction testing.

In cases of trauma, the forced duction test is used to determine if the muscle dysfunction is due to injury to the motor nerves supplying the muscles, extraocular muscle contusion, orbital edema, or entrapment of the inferior recti or inferior oblique muscles within a blow-out fracture site. If the test is positive and increased resistance is felt, suspect a muscle or soft tissue to be entrapped. The test is negative if the eye movements are smooth and a paretic muscle, probably secondary to neurologic injury, is suspected. A neurogenic injury, edema, or muscle contusion should resolve with time, while an entrapment injury will not and may require treatment; yet all may look identical upon preliminary examination.

If the force applied pushes the eye backward, the globe may be displaced posteriorly, giving the false impression of full motilities.

In individuals with a thyroid condition who present with diplopia, suspect a myopathy. The diplopia is usually on upgaze with an accompanying inferior heterotropia. The inferior rectus is frequently involved, becoming fibrotic, leading to the eye's inability to elevate. The superior rectus muscle is not abnormal, although it appears to be on first assessment. Differential diagnosis includes a paretic muscle versus a myopathy. If resistance is felt when the eye is elevated, a probable myopathy of the inferior rectus is present.

In Brown's tendon sheath syndrome, an apparent congenital paresis of the inferior oblique is noted. Upon forced duction testing, with the eye in the adducted position, a resistance is felt with elevation. This positive forced duction test differentiates Brown's syndrome from an inferior oblique paresis.

Contraindications/Complications. Forced duction testing is difficult to do on youngsters or other individuals not capable of controlling their fixation. In these cases false positives are possible, since resistance may be felt that does not truly exist. The test can be uncomfortable and in cases of inadequate anesthesia, painful if a forceps is used. A mild dull ache in and around the eye may occur for several hours after the procedure. Small subconjunctival hemorrhages are not uncommon. Cotton-tipped applicators must be carefully used since they may slip, causing a secondary corneal abrasion.

Forced duction testing is contraindicated during an acute hyphema where rebleeding is still a potential problem. The test is often uncomfortable and difficult to accomplish in acute cases of trauma with marked lid edema and pain. In such cases, a delay of several days may be needed.

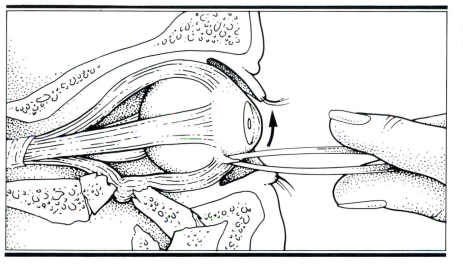

3. In a blowout fracture with entrapped muscles, the eye will not elevate with forced duction testing.

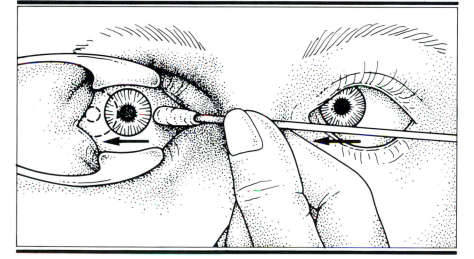

4. An ecchymotic right eye is seen with a sixth nerve paresis. With forced duction testing a full range of movements is seen. (*See also* Color Plate 42–4.)

43 Forced Generations Testing

Description/Indications. Forced generations testing is used to diagnose and grossly quantify ocular muscle abnormalities of neurogenic origin. It is indicated in the examination of suspected nerve paresis with extraocular muscle dysfunction, especially those secondary to trauma. A traumatic neurogenic etiology may be differentiated from muscle restriction. It is often used as a companion test with the forced duction test (see p. 138).

Forced generations testing is also used to follow and grossly quantify resolution of neurogenic muscle paresis, such as in a third or sixth nerve palsy. The test is done periodically over time, with the degree of resistance encountered recorded.

Instrumentation. Sterile cotton-tipped applicators, topical ophthalmic anesthetic solution, lid speculum.

Technique. Several drops of a topical ophthalmic anesthetic solution are instilled in each eye. A cotton-tipped applicator is placed at the limbus of the muscle of action to be tested, keeping it tangential to the eye (Fig. 1). The patient is given a target to look at such as a penlight or his or her hand and asked to look hard into the field of action of the muscle and nerve to be tested (Fig. 1). A slight force is applied to the applicator, attempting to push the eye in the opposite direction of gaze. The degree the eye can or cannot be made to move against its will is graded and recorded. Each quadrant of both eyes is tested in a similar fashion. Be careful not to push the eye into the orbit, causing the eye to retract and appear to move.

A lid speculum (see p. 90) may help in keeping the eyelids separated, especially in traumatic cases with eyelid edema. The lid speculum is also useful in uncooperative patients requiring assistance.

A suspected traumatic right sixth nerve paresis with impaired abduction would require a differential diagnosis between muscle entrapment or neurogenic paresis. The cotton-tipped applicator is first placed nasally, then inferiorly and superiorly at the limbus, asking the patient to look toward the applicator. An attempt is made to push the eye in the opposite direction. The applicator is finally placed at the temporal limbus of the right eye, asking the patient to look right (temporally) while the left eye is observed, making sure it turns directly into the nose. With the cotton-tipped applicator at the temporal limbus an attempt is made to push the right eye in toward the nose.

Interpretation. In normal extraocular motility function, it is difficult to move the eye against its will in any direction. A pull or tug will be felt on the cotton-tipped applicator with the eye refusing to budge, remaining firmly in its original position. This is a negative test (Fig. 2). In cases of partial or total paresis, with gentle force the eye can be moved against its will. This indicates a positive finding (Fig. 3). The degree of resistance depends upon the degree of neurogenic involvement. In the case discussed in the "Technique" section, if the right eye does not move nasally when force is applied at the temporal limbus with gaze to the right, then a negative test has occurred and sixth nerve function is intact. Some other cause of paresis must be found and additional testing, such as forced duction testing to rule out muscle restriction, is needed. If the eye can be moved nasally, then a right sixth nerve paresis is suspected with abduction weakness and no further testing is required.

To assess what normal muscle tone and resistance feels like, the test can be performed on normal patients, testing each quadrant of each eye.

The test can be quantified, noting the degree of resistance (mild, moderate, severe), and may be repeated at regular time intervals (biweekly for several months) to assess for change.

Contraindications/Complications. Care must be taken to anchor the cotton-tipped applicator at the limbus to prevent it from slipping, especially if it may roll across the cornea and lead to an abrasion. The test is contraindicated in any case of recent hyphema as further pressure may induce a rebleed.

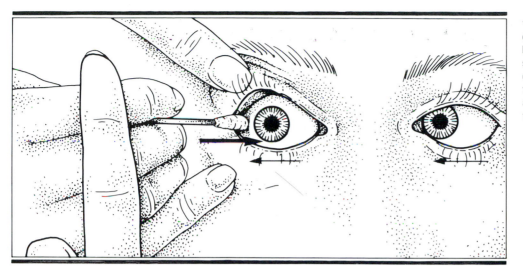

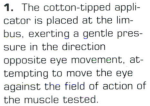

1. The cotton-tipped applicator is placed at the limbus, exerting a gentle pressure in the direction opposite eye movement, attempting to move the eye against the field of action of the muscle tested.

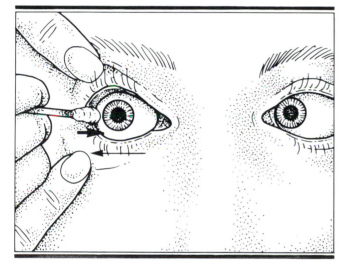

2. An example of a negative forced generations test.

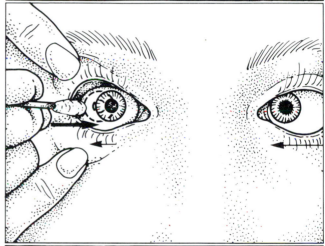

3. An example of a positive forced generations test.

V Suggested Readings

Casser L: Conjunctival abrasions and lacerations. *J Am Optom Assoc* 1987;**58**:488.

Catania LJ: *Primary Care of the Anterior Segment.* Norwalk: Appleton & Lange, 1988.

Duane DD, Jaeger EA (eds): *Clinical Ophthalmology.* Philadelphia, Harper & Row, 1987, vol 4.

Fedukowicz HB, Stenson S: *External Infections of the Eye.* Norwalk, CT, Appleton & Lange, 1985.

Grant WM: *Toxicology of the Eye,* ed 3. Springfield, IL, CC Thomas, 1986.

Norn MN: *External Eye Methods of Examination.* Copenhagen, Scriptor, 1974.

Rao NA: A laboratory approach to rapid diagnosis of ocular infections and prospects for the future. *Am J Ophthalmol* 1989;**107**:283.

Smith JL (ed): How to really do the forced ductions/generations test. *Neuro-Ophthalmology Audio Journal,* vol 11, no 4. Miami, Neuro-Ophthalmology Tapes, 1988.

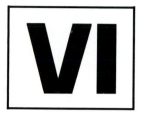

Corneal Procedures

44 Corneal Foreign Body Removal

Description/Indications. Foreign matter can become embedded in the cornea, leading to symptoms of varying intensity. Symptoms may include pain, foreign body sensation, lacrimation, blurred vision, and photophobia. A red eye frequently accompanies these symptoms.

Foreign body (FB) removal is indicated when an embedded, immovable object or particle is noted on the corneal epithelium. Rust or edema may be seen surrounding the FB. The ring of edema should disappear once the FB is removed, while the ring of rust needs to be eliminated (see p. 152) for the corneal epithelium to properly heal. A stromal FB penetrating the outer layer of the cornea, especially if centrally located, needs to be treated as a penetrating injury, with a surgical consultation obtained to remove the embedded particle(s) since scarring will occur and induced visual loss needs to be minimized.

The patient history is crucial to understanding how an FB got in the eye, when it did, how much, and what the material is. When the history indicates an injury from propelled debris (as from drilling, a grinder's wheel, or hammering metal on metal), a penetrating wound must be ruled out with a careful slit lamp examination, Seidel test (see p. 290), and dilated fundus examination (see p. 192).

There are several techniques for the removal of a corneal FB. The technique used will depend on the location, depth, and degree of embeddedness, with the goal being to remove the offending agent with as little tissue disruption as possible.

Superficial particles may be removed with an irrigating solution, whereas embedded particles require a needle, loop, or spud (Fig. 1). An object may appear to be loosely embedded, but if irrigation does not dislodge it (see p. 130), consider it embedded. Most particles left in the eye longer than 6 hours will have epithelial cell growth over the surface, requiring a more invasive technique.

A loop made from nylon or another semirigid material flexes and bends when placed under FBs. It is used to remove loosely embedded FBs. Because of its safety, the loop is useful for children with poor fixation, uncooperative patients, or for those practitioners uncomfortable with the use of a sharper instrument. A needle or spud is required for partially to deeply embedded FBs. A spud looks like a miniature spoon whose rounded curved edges are not as sharp as a needle's. Its shape allows for excavation and the flicking off of an FB from the surface. Because of its ease of use, it is the instrument of choice for removing most embedded corneal FBs. Needles come in different lengths and widths, varying from 18 gauge (thicker) to 25 gauge (thinner) in width and 5/8 to 2 inches in length (Fig. 1). The size used is up to examiner preference. The syringe is not used with the needle. Because of the sharp point of the needle, care must be taken to not snag or catch basement membrane fibers. An Algerbrush is used to remove the secondary rust. An Algerbrush should not be the primary instrument used for removing an FB. A cotton-tipped applicator is useful to sweep loosely embedded objects from the palpebral conjunctival surface but is not appropriate for removal of embedded objects in the cornea. The applicator tends to break or fragment the FB, removing the superficial material and leaving embedded particles behind (Fig. 2).

Corneal FBs rarely penetrate through Bowman's membrane since it has a consistency of a taut sheet of canvas and will usually trap FBs perforating the corneal epithelium (Fig. 3). Since Bowman's membrane is so strong, significant force is required for either an FB or an instrument to penetrate it. By working gently near the cornea and keeping the instrument tangential to the corneal plane, it will be difficult to inadvertently perforate the cornea.

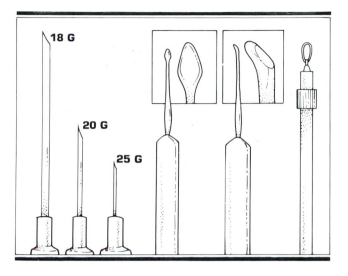

1. Needles, spuds, and a loop, the instruments used to remove corneal foreign bodies.

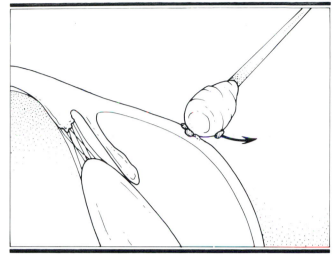

2. A cotton-tipped applicator is not a useful instrument to remove a foreign body since it may fragment the FB, leaving a disrupted corneal epithelium behind.

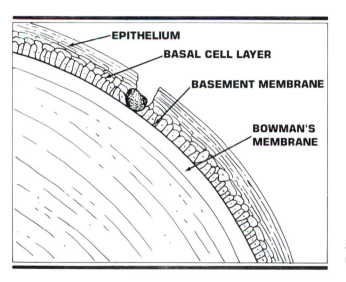

EPITHELIUM

BASAL CELL LAYER

BASEMENT MEMBRANE

BOWMAN'S MEMBRANE

3. A FB penetrating the corneal epithelium, lodged on Bowman's membrane.

Instrumentation. Spud, sterile disposable needle, loop, irrigating solution, topical ophthalmic anesthetic solution, lid speculum, cotton-tipped applicators.

Technique. Explain to the patient what will occur and how cooperation and good fixation will facilitate the procedure. Use a penlight and slit lamp to localize and assess the FB location, secondary inflammatory reaction, and any induced sequellae (rust ring, edema). Use a corneal optic section to determine the depth of the FB (see p. 22).

Loosely Embedded Foreign Bodies: Recline the patient in the examination chair, raise the upper lid with the thumb of one hand, and use the other hand to direct a stream of irrigating solution at the edge of the FB (see p. 130). If the fluid dislodges and floats the particle into the inferior cul-de-sac, use a moistened cotton-tipped applicator to sweep the object from the eye. If irrigation is not successful, a different technique is required.

Embedded Foreign Bodies: Instill 2 drops of a topical ophthalmic anesthetic solution into each eye.

Position the patient comfortably in the slit lamp with the forehead pressed forward against the headstrap (see p. 22). Set the magnification at medium power with a wide parallelepiped white light beam. Give the patient a fixation target that will be visible during the procedure. Move the fixation target so the eye is positioned for easy access to the FB. Secure the upper eyelid with the thumb of the non-instrument-holding hand. An assistant may be used to secure the upper lid. Use a lid speculum if cooperation or fixation are very poor or blepharospasm is a problem. Stabilize your arm on the instrument table or rest the fourth and fifth fingers of the instrument hand on the patient's cheek or bridge of the nose. Align the spud, needle, or loop by sighting outside the slit lamp, placing the instrument just in front of the corneal FB (Fig. 4). Once aligned, use the slit lamp for the remainder of the procedure.

Nylon Loop: Tease the perimeter of the FB so the surrounding tissue is loosened (Fig. 5A). Burrow the loop underneath the FB (Fig. 5B). Move the loop upward in a smooth, fluid, flicking-type motion (Fig. 5C), releasing the FB from the corneal surface.

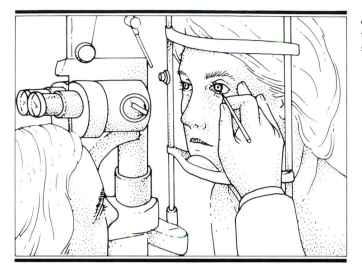

4. The spud is lined up with the FB by viewing outside of the instrument. Once aligned, use the magnification of the slit lamp to achieve the best results.

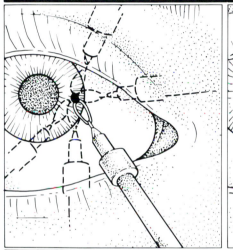

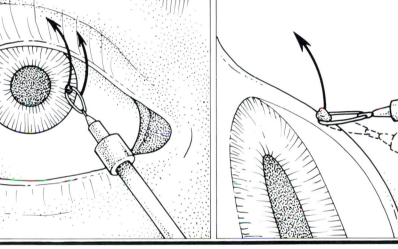

5. A. A loop is used to tease the edges to loosen the epithelium for subsequent removal.

5. B. The loop is seen buried underneath the FB.

5. C. The head is flicked upward so the FB will rise toward the surface.

Spud or Needle: Hold the spud or needle like a pencil, with the spud held by the shaft and a needle held either at the plastic base or also by the shaft. Approach the FB tangentially so that if the patient moves forward, the instrument will not penetrate the eye (Fig. 6). With small strokes, use the beveled edge of the spud or needle to loosen the edges of the FB (Fig. 7A). Bury the needle or spud under the FB. Flick the head of the instrument upward so the buried end raises towards the surface, bringing the FB with it (Fig. 7B, C). The spoonlike end of the spud can be used to scoop the FB from the cornea (Fig. 7D). Do not press on the FB with the instrument, impacting it further into the cornea.

Once the FB is removed, reassess the eye looking at the resultant corneal condition. Remove any residual rust with an Algerbrush (see p. 152). If a moderate to severe amount of corneal tissue disruption has occurred, it is likely a traumatic anterior uveitis will develop. Instill a cycloplegic, usually 2 drops of Homatropine 5%. Make sure the pupil is well-dilated and then apply a pressure patch. Place a broad-spectrum antibiotic ointment into the lower cul-de-sac and apply a pressure patch (see p. 156). Prescribe analgesics as necessary for the pain. Instruct the patient to leave the patch in place until the next visit in 24 hours. See the patient every 24 hours until patching is discontinued.

Interpretation. Once a FB is removed, the eye is reassessed looking for damage due to the injury and the removal process. Disruption of Bowman's membrane secondary to rust or a deep injury is noted since this may later cause a recurrent erosion. Corneal edema (Fig. 8) occurs when a FB remains in the cornea longer than 24 hours, and resolves once the FB is removed. Topical hypertonic agents (5% sodium chloride solution/ointment) may be used to hasten this recovery. The anterior chamber is evaluated looking for signs of secondary inflammation (see p. 36).

Contraindications/Complications. Infection or inflammation is possible after FB removal and is more likely with greater tissue disruption. Traumatic iridocyclitis is typically seen 24 to 36 hours after an injury and usually subsides when the cornea reepithelializes. Increasing inflammation or an eye that is not responding to therapy suggests the possibility of an intraocular FB with subsequent investigations required. Deeply embedded FBs at or below the stroma require surgical removal.

Corneal edema may occur due to the FB or the mechanical nature of the removal procedure and should disappear within a few days. Small linear scars at the level of Bowman's membrane may occur due to the sharp point of the needle snagging corneal fibrils as the FB is removed.

The patient needs to be counseled that symptoms of increasing severity can be serious, making it necessary to notify the doctor as soon as possible. Also recommend that patients use safety glasses in the future.

A certain amount of discomfort is expected after a FB is removed. The extent depends upon the nature of the FB, the amount of tissue disruption, and patient sensitivity. Analgesics may be used to decrease the discomfort. Never dispense a topical ophthalmic anesthetic solution for the pain. Once the eye is cyclopleged and patched, the level of pain usually diminishes dramatically.

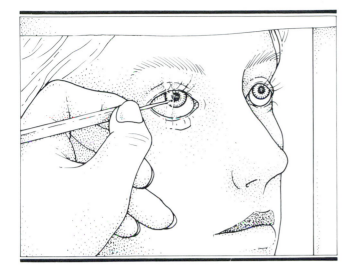

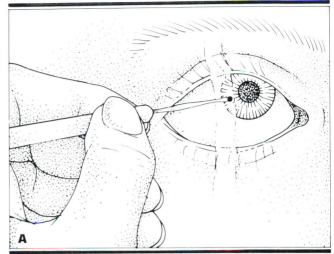

6. Always work tangentially to the cornea to avoid any mishaps with the needle or spud.

7. A. A spud is seen loosening the edges of a FB. (*Continued below*.)

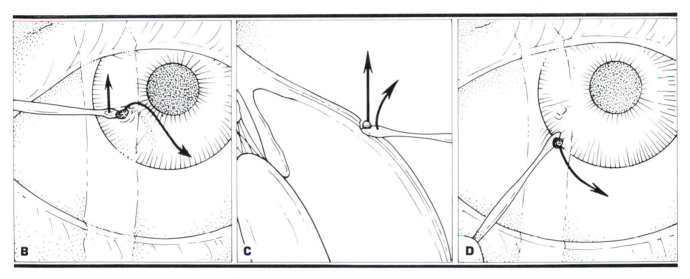

7. B. The spud is seen underneath the FB. (*See also* Color Plate 44–7.B.) **C.** A cross-section of the spud seen underneath a corneal FB. The head is flicked upward to dislodge the FB. **D.** The spud can be used to scoop away a FB.

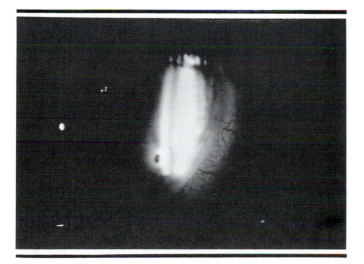

8. A ring of corneal edema seen surrounding a FB before removal.

45 Corneal Rust Ring Removal

Description/Indications. Corneal metallic foreign bodies begin to oxidize (rust) within 12 to 24 hours of lodging in the eye. The resulting siderosis will stain the corneal epithelial cells, basement membrane, and Bowman's membrane an orange-brown color. The rust usually forms a ringlike shape around the metallic foreign object. A ring of edema, appearing as a white band, may be seen around the band of rust (Fig. 1). The rust can affect the adherence of the epithelial cells to the basement membrane, leading to the potential development of a recurrent corneal erosion.

To avoid formation of a rust ring, metallic foreign bodies need to be removed as soon as possible (see p. 146). If a rust ring does develop, the stained epithelial cells and metallic particles should be removed after the metallic foreign body is eliminated.

The Algerbrush (Fig. 2) is commonly used to remove rust. It is a small, low speed, battery-operated drill with a tiny dental burr. The Algerbrush comes with several different size burrs. The smallest size (0.5 mm) is used most often. This burr will remove the rust particles cleanly with the least tissue disruption. The Algerbrush drill has a built-in clutch mechanism that will stop the instrument when a certain amount of resistance occurs. Bowman's membrane, being of canvas-like consistency, is very strong and requires a greater force to penetrate than the Algerbrush can produce. When the Algerbrush contacts Bowman's membrane, it shuts off. Thus, it is almost impossible to accidentally perforate the cornea when using this drill. The burrs can be removed from the drill for storage and sterilization after use. The epithelium is removed with the Algerbrush down to but not past the basement membrane. Going deeper will lead to scar formation.

A hand-held ophthalmic burr (Fig. 3) may also be used to mechanically remove rust particles. This method is useful when the whirring sounds made by the Algerbrush concern the patient. The drawback to using a mechanical burr is it tends to take longer to achieve the desired results. When an Algerbrush is not available or desired, a needle or an ophthalmic spud may be used. A jeweler's forceps may also be useful in removing a corneal rust ring.

Instrumentation. Algerbrush with burrs, ophthalmic burr, needle, spud, slit lamp, topical ophthalmic anesthetic solution.

Technique. Instill 2 drops of a topical ophthalmic anesthetic agent into each eye (see p. 2). Position the patient in the slit lamp and provide a suitable fixation target. Locate any rust ring and determine its density and corneal depth.

Ophthalmic Burr: Explain to the patient how the procedure is performed. Hold the burr between the thumb and index finger like a pencil. Locate the rust ring and align the burr tangentially to the cornea. Contact the rust area from the side and apply gentle pressure. Make a rolling motion and twirl the burr in your fingers so its head rotates on the cornea (Fig. 3). The rust is lifted off as the burr revolves in the cornea.

Spud or Needle: Locate the rust ring and align the needle or spud. Keep the instrument tangential to the cornea and make small sweeping motions in one direction as the corneal surface is touched. Scrape the epithelial surface lightly to remove any rust.

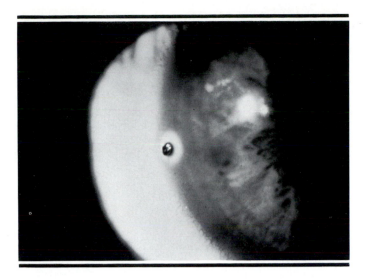

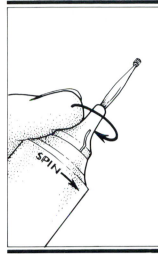

1. (far left) A metallic foreign body on the cornea, surrounded by a ring of rust and edema. (*See also* Color Plate 45–1.)

2. (left) The Algerbrush is turned on by rotating the base housing the burr.

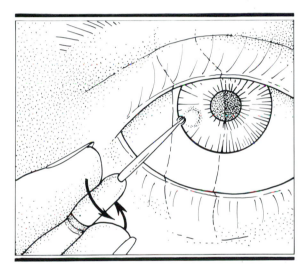

3. An ophthalmic burr is used to manually remove the rust. The burr is twirled to remove any rust particles.

Algerbrush: To alleviate patient apprehension with the Algerbrush, first describe what will occur. Explain that the drill's whirring-like noise in no way means it is "burrowing a hole" through the cornea. Encourage the patient to ignore the noise in order to reduce apprehension and improve cooperation and fixation.

Turn the Algerbrush on by rotating the base of the burr with your finger in the direction noted on the handle (Fig. 2). The burr will rotate and a whirring noise will be heard. Align the Algerbrush with the rust ring. This can be done by viewing through the slit lamp oculars or outside of the instrument. Rest your elbow on the slit lamp table or place your fourth and fifth fingers on the patient's nose or cheek to enhance stability of the Algerbrush. Viewing through the slit lamp, use a wide parallelepiped with white light and medium magnification, positioning the Algerbrush tangentially to the cornea. Lightly contact the rust ring and make small circular patterns (Fig. 4A). Try not to press down too firmly on the cornea. If the drill continually stops during the procedure, reduce the amount of pressure being applied. Continue drilling until all the rust is gone, if possible. A small excavation will be made as the rust is removed (Fig. 4B, C, D). Stop the burr by putting pressure with your finger on the burr housing.

Stop the procedure and reassess the cornea if rust is no longer being removed but the excavation is becoming larger. Further removal may be postponed for several days, watching for the rust to rise toward the surface and possibly lift off by itself.

Upon completion of the procedure, irrigate (see p. 130), instill an ophthalmic antibiotic ointment, and patch the eye (see p. 156). Ask the patient to return in 24 hours. Instill a cycloplegic agent if the cornea is significantly abraded to relieve pain and prevent posterior synechia formation associated with a secondary traumatic iridocyclitis.

Interpretation. A small craterlike depression will be visible after the rust is removed. This will begin to fill in with new epithelial cells over 24 to 48 hours. Any remaining ring of edema should disappear over 48 to 72 hours. Sodium chloride 5% solution and/or ointment may be used to hasten its removal.

At times the rust ring may break up or crumble as it is being removed, not allowing a clean excavation. This happens more often when the rust is deep. Some rust may stain Bowman's membrane and not be removable. If the rust does not remove cleanly, leave it in place and follow the patient. Rather than creating a large area of tissue disruption, patch the eye and have the patient return in 24 hours. Over the next several days the tissue around the rust will soften and the rust will work its way towards the corneal surface. The rust may dislodge by itself or the Algerbrush may again be needed to remove the remaining superficial rust. If a recurrent erosion occurs in the future around an old rust ring, a second attempt at removal may be considered.

Contraindications/Complications. Care must be taken whenever the cornea is scraped or manipulated in any way. The patient must be observed over several days after the procedure to watch for secondary infection or inflammation. Infection or inflammation is possible and more likely with greater tissue disruption. Traumatic iridocyclitis is typically seen 24 to 36 hours after the procedure and usually subsides when the cornea reepithelializes. Increasing inflammation or an eye that is not responding to therapy suggests the possibility of an intraocular foreign body with subsequent investigations required.

Explain to the patient there may be some discomfort after the topical anesthesia has worn off that should diminish within 24 hours. Analgesics are suggested when the patient is uncomfortable.

Small corneal scars are possible if Bowman's membrane is affected. The patient should be advised whenever a small scar occurs from a foreign body or rust ring.

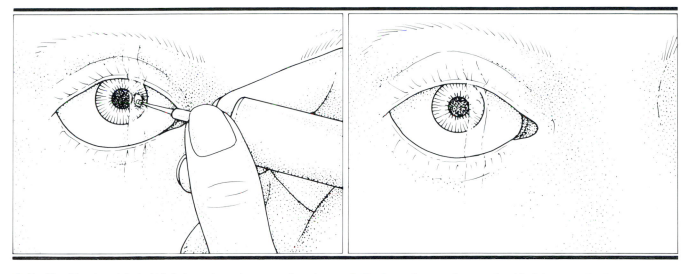

4. A. The Algerbrush is held lightly against the corneal surface as the burr revolves, removing any rust. (*See also* Color Plate 45–4.A.)

4. B. A small area of corneal epithelial excavation is present after the rust is removed.

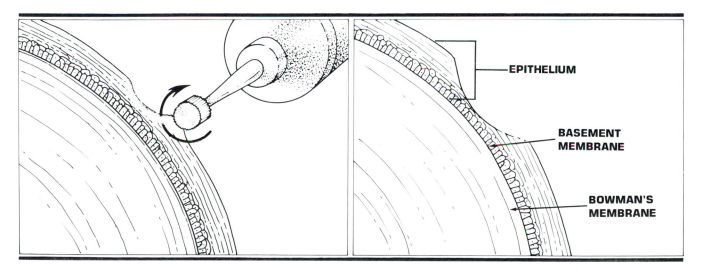

4. C. The burr removes epithelial cells as it rotates, leaving an excavated pit in the epithelium.

4. D. The corneal epithelium is removed down to, but not past Bowman's membrane.

46 Pressure Patching

Description/Indications. An injury to the corneal epithelium frequently requires a pressure patch to aid in the healing process and provide symptomatic relief. Small, superficial conjunctival or corneal abrasions, especially in youngsters, may resolve without patching, but in most cases patching is required to achieve swift resolution.

There are several ways to apply a pressure patch. No matter how the patch is applied or what material is used, its intention is to tightly close the eyelids to prevent blinking. The opening and closing of the eyelids will continually shear off new corneal cells, impairing the healing process and prolonging the foreign body sensation. The patch presses the basal layer of epithelial cells onto the basement membrane, increasing cellular adherence and decreasing cellular edema.

Instrumentation. Sterile gauze eyepatches, 1-inch hypoallergenic tape, topical ophthalmic antibiotic ointment, cycloplegic solution, sterile ophthalmic irrigating solution, topical ophthalmic anesthetic solution, alcohol swabs.

Technique. If the patient is photophobic, dim the exam room lights to improve patient comfort. Instill a topical anesthetic to improve patient comfort and cooperation.

Recline the patient in the examination chair. Inspect the patient's face, skin, size of nose, position of mouth, size and depth of orbit, and texture and oiliness of skin. Examine the orbit by viewing from both the front and side. These factors will effect how, where, and the number of patches used. Oil needs to be removed from the skin to ensure proper tape adherence. Use an alcohol swab to scrub the areas of the cheek and forehead where tape will be applied. Beards may interfere with adhesion of the tape; modify the tape's placement, and if needed, trim the beard.

Instill a cycloplegic solution, usually 5% Homatropine (see p. 2), if indicated, prior to patching. Make sure the pupil dilates fully before applying the patch. This is important in dark-eyed individuals who may dilate poorly. Maximum dilation will ensure patient comfort and limit the sequelae of traumatic iridocyclitis. Squeeze a small ribbon (¼ to ½ inch) of a broad-spectrum topical ophthalmic antibiotic ointment into the inferior cul-de-sac (see p. 10). Ask the patient to close both eyes for the remainder of the procedure.

Push any hair back away from the face. Fold one patch in half and place it over the closed eyelid (Fig. 1A). The initial pad may be dampened with water prior to its placement and laid flat to mold it to the eye. A second and third patch are placed over the initial patch, angling them so they point toward the junction at the nose and forehead (Fig. 1B). For shallow orbits two patches may suffice, while deep orbits may require a fourth patch to create pressure on the cornea. Keep the patches in place by asking the patient to place a finger on the patch. Tip the patient's head slightly backward to balance the patches on the eye, or apply a short piece of tape over the eyepads.

Cut a 6 to 7-inch piece of tape, placing one end at the midpoint of the forehead, and use the thumb of one hand to securely hold it in place. With the free hand lay the tape diagonally across the patches, pulling it taut as it runs toward the cheek and top of the mandible (Fig. 2A). Keep the tape away from the nasolabial fold and side of the mouth so that the patient may chew or talk comfortably without loosening the tape. Pinch the skin of the cheek upward where the end of the tape will fall. Release the pinched skin as the tape is placed on the skin (Fig. 2B). This increases the adherence of the patch. Ask the patient to attempt to open the eye; if he or she can't, the patch has been properly applied and the remaining pieces of tape can be applied.

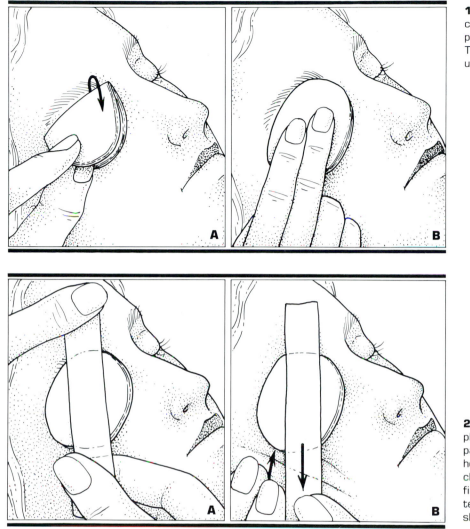

1. A. A folded patch is placed over the closed eye. **B.** Two or three additional patches are used to occlude the eye. The patient holds the patches in place until a strip of tape is applied.

2. A. The first strip of tape is placed down the center of the patch, being anchored at the forehead and on the cheek. **B.** The cheek is pinched upwards as the first strip of tape is placed. This tends to tighten the tape on the skin.

Cut a second piece of tape about 6 inches in length, starting it closer to the bridge of the nose and overlapping the first piece (Fig. 3A). Curve or contour this piece so it follows and covers the superior and lateral edges of the patch. Apply a third piece of tape, about 6 inches in length, starting temporally to the original piece of tape (Fig. 3B). Overlap the original strip of tape at the superior and inferior temporal edges. Apply a fourth piece of tape, 7 inches in length, in a downward direction along the route of the first strip. Pull this strip taut, making sure it overlaps the inner edges of strips two and three and covers all ends of the tape on the cheek (Fig. 3C). Use a fifth piece of tape, about 4 inches in length, to close off the lateral aspect of the patch, if still exposed.

Prescribe an analgesic if the patient is in considerable discomfort. Instruct the patient to leave the patch in place until reexamined in 24 hours, and to avoid taking a shower or getting the patch wet. Also explain that the eye may feel worse once the topical anesthestic has worn off.

Remove the patch by pulling down on the skin of the cheek and at the same time, with the other hand grasping the end of the first strip of tape, lift the end of the tape, starting from the bottom and advancing toward the forehead (Fig. 4). The eyepads will lift off as the tape is removed.

Interpretation/Management. After the patch is removed, wipe away any lid debris. Wait a few minutes before taking a visual acuity to allow the patient to become reacclimated. Use a penlight and slit lamp to assess the size and shape of the remaining corneal abrasion, corneal edema, discharge, hyperemia, and cells and flare (see pp. 20–39).

Mild to moderate abrasions usually heal in 24 to 36 hours, while larger abrasions may take 48 to 72 hours or more to resolve. If after 24 hours the abrasion has not totally healed, repatch with a cycloplegic and an antibiotic ointment, and ask the patient to return again in 24 hours. Infants and children heal extremely quickly while diabetics often heal slowly. Recurrent corneal erosions may require several days to resolve, especially in cases of anterior basement membrane dystrophy. Reepithelialization is indication that patching can be discontinued.

Contraindications/Complications. A pressure patch should never be applied whenever a penetrating injury is suspected. A protective shield should be applied and the patient referred promptly to an anterior segment specialist. An iridocyclitis may be part of the spectrum of sequelae due to the injury. Treatment with a steroid suspension is delayed until a patch is no longer required, since in most cases the inflammation is secondary to the epithelial loss and will resolve once reepithelialization occurs. Discharge, especially if increasing in severity, is a sign of ocular infection and must be dealt with promptly.

After removing the patch, several changes may be noted on the cornea due to the mechanical effects from patching and not due to the injury. Punctate staining secondary to the irritative effects of the ointment may be seen. This will resolve as the ointment is discontinued. Corneal edema or folds in the stroma and Descemet's membrane may be due to the pressure effects of the patch on the cornea. The folds and edema will disappear within 24 to 48 hours of discontinuation of the patch. Five percent Sodium chloride solution may hasten the recovery. Some individuals' skin may be sensitive to either the mechanical or allergic effects of the tape. A mild red erythematous area occurs on the skin where the tape was placed. This will disappear in several days after the patch is removed. A low-dose topical dermatologic steroid may hasten the recovery.

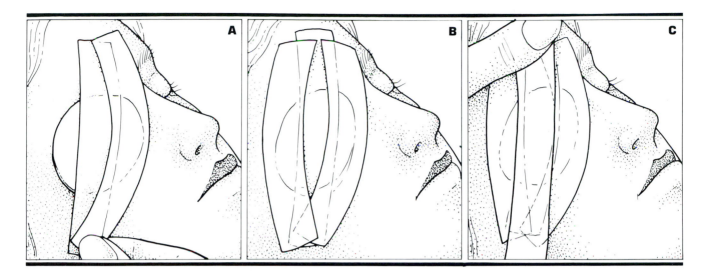

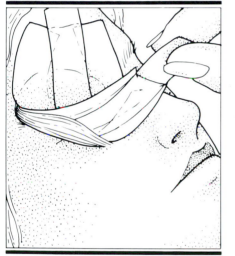

3. A. (above) The second strip of tape is placed inside the original strip. It follows the contour of the patch before ending on the cheek. **B.** The third strip of tape is placed to the outside of the original strip. **C.** The fourth strip of tape is centered over the patches. It overlaps the sides of the other pieces of tapes.

4. The bottom piece of tape is pulled upward to remove the tape and patch.

47   Corneal Debridement

Description/Indication. Loose, diseased, or damaged epithelial cells are frequently therapeutically removed to hasten corneal recovery. Debridement, usually performed with a cotton-tipped applicator, removes the damaged cells to allow healthy ones to grow in their place. The epithelial surface, having the consistency of a jello-like substance, will depress and furrow when pressure is applied, allowing the surface epithelial cells—especially those damaged—to be easily removed.

Debridement is used to remove necrotic tissue and loose cells surrounding a corneal abrasion, to remove a corneal dendrite, and to remove corneal filaments in filamentary keratitis. There are several methods of debridement. A "minimal wipe" form removes only the loose, damaged superficial tissue. For filaments or some corneal dendrites, a more extensive form of debridement is needed to remove the damaged epithelial cells and some small amount of surrounding tissue.

Instrumentation. Cotton-tipped applicators, topical ophthalmic anesthetic solution, slit lamp, sterile saline solution, Algerbrush.

Technique. Instill a topical ophthalmic anesthetic solution into both eyes. Using the slit lamp locate and inspect the area to be debrided. Give the patient a suitable fixation target.

Cotton-Tipped Applicator: Moisten the head of a cotton-tipped applicator with sterile saline solution. Approach the cornea with the applicator from the side where the lesion is located. Keep the applicator on a tangential plane to the cornea, lightly stroking the affected area in one direction (Fig. 1). For the minimal wipe form of debridement, remove the necrotic tissue surrounding the dendrite or abrasion, using gentle small strokes to lift the dead, damaged epithelial cells and tissue from the cornea.

For filaments or dendrites requiring further debridement, work the applicator in one direction, stroking the epithelium with a small amount of pressure to remove diseased cells (Fig. 2A, B). Take care not to roll the applicator or press directly on the cornea. Work from the side since this affords a better view of the lesion through the slit lamp and is less traumatic to the eye if the patient jerks forward unexpectedly. Repeat the procedure several times until all the cells in question, and a small amount of tissue surrounding the area, are removed.

Algerbrush: Keep the burr of the Algerbrush tangential to the corneal plane (Fig. 3) and allow it to skim across the epithelial surface. Watch the Algerbrush and cornea carefully, making sure to not remove too much tissue. The end-point for the procedure is when all possible damaged cells are removed and the tissue assumes a clean appearance.

Irrigate the eye (see p. 130), aiming a spray of sterile saline solution into the lower cul-de-sac to remove all remaining debris from the eye. For corneal filaments, instill a topical antibiotic solution into the eye prophylactically after the procedure. Use an antiviral solution in cases of "minimal wipe" debridement associated with herpes simplex keratitis. For a corneal abrasion, patch the eye and manage according to a corneal abrasion protocol (see p. 154). Follow the patient for several days after the procedure, monitoring for timely resolution of the lesion.

Contraindications/Complications. A cotton-tipped applicator can be cumbersome to work with and cause healthy tissue to be removed. If excessive tissue is removed, a corneal abrasion may result, necessitating patching. Debridement is contraindicated in any suspected case of penetrating injury or obvious ocular infection.

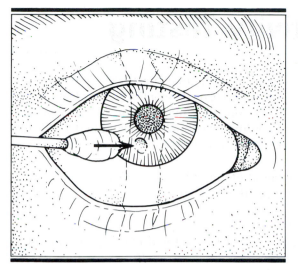

1. The lesion on the cornea is wiped with a cotton-tipped applicator in one direction only.

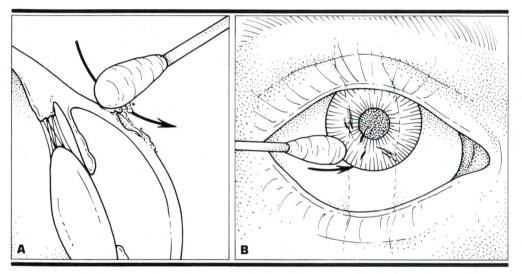

2. A. The loose necrotic cells are removed with a cotton-tipped applicator.
B. Several filaments are seen on the cornea as one is debrided.

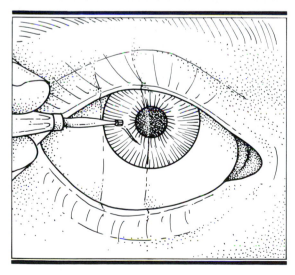

3. The Algerbrush being used to debride a corneal lesion.

48 Corneal Sensitivity Testing

Description/Indications. Corneal sensation may be reduced in pure ocular conditions and in neurological disorders affecting the nerves innervating the cornea. The assessment of corneal sensation can aid in the diagnosis of various conditions by ruling out those not associated with diminished sensation. In terms of management, the restoration of sensation may be one of several parameters used in assessing the resolution of a condition.

The cornea, conjunctiva, eyelid margins, and caruncle are all sensitive to touch and are innervated by the first branch of the fifth cranial (trigeminal) nerve. Of these structures the cornea is the most touch-sensitive. A cotton wisp is frequently used to assess corneal sensation. A gross qualification of the touch sense is made, comparing one eye to the other. A commercially available corneal sensation measuring device, Cochet and Bonnet's Aesthesiometer, is available to quantify corneal sensation. It uses a ballpoint-pen-like device with a nylon thread protruding from its front. The thread is changed in length to measure the minimum perceptible sensation. The shorter the thread used, the less the corneal sensation. Sensitivity is recorded as the length of filament.

Corneal sensation may be reduced in several ocular conditions including herpes simplex keratitis, herpes zoster keratitis, contact lens wear, trachoma, certain forms of corneal degeneration, types of vernal conjunctivitis, dense corneal scar formation, and glaucoma with elevated intraocular pressure. Corneal sensation may also be reduced for 3 to 5 months after ocular surgery. Central nervous system disorders, especially those secondary to brain tumors, may also effect corneal sensation. Certain conditions may permanently affect corneal sensation. For example, herpes simplex epithelial keratitis may reduce corneal sensation even after the acute condition has resolved.

A topical ophthalmic anesthetic cannot be used prior to testing corneal sensitivity. In addition, any other procedure that may irritate the cornea, eyelids, or conjunctiva must be postponed until after corneal sensation is tested.

Instrumentation. Sterile cotton wisp, sterile cotton-tipped applicator.

Technique. Before the procedure, demonstrate to the patient how the test is done. Explain that he or she may feel a sensation as the eye is touched but that it should not be painful. Ask the patient to signal as soon as a sensation is felt.

Prepare the cotton wisp by drawing out a small tuft of cotton from a cotton ball or cotton-tipped applicator (Fig. 1A). Twirl and twist the ends of the cotton strands to form a point (Fig. 1B). Inspect the cornea with the slit lamp to ensure no corneal irritation is present that may affect the results or be misinterpreted after the procedure as due to the cotton wisp.

Seat the patient and ask him or her to look up. Move the cotton wisp carefully toward the center of the cornea, trying to avoid its being seen by the patient. Gently touch the cornea, keeping the wisp perpendicular to the corneal plane (Fig. 2A). Be careful to touch the center of the cornea rather than the periphery. Continue to touch the wisp to the cornea until the patient signals the wisp is felt (Fig. 2B) or the wisp, contacting the cornea, bends slightly (Fig. 2C). If the patient indicates that he or she senses the touch, ask the patient to grade the sensation on a numeric scale. Observe the patient to see if he or she blinks or begins tearing when the wisp contacts the cornea. Test the other eye in a similar fashion, asking the patient to compare the sensation to the other eye. Do one stroke at a time, repeating the test 30 seconds later. Do not repeat strokes continuously since summation will occur, negating any results.

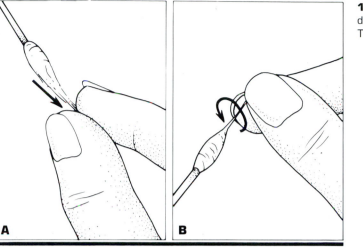

1. A. (far left) To prepare the cotton-tipped applicator, draw a small piece of material from the head. **B.** (left) The cotton is twirled and twisted to form a point.

2. A. The patient looks up as the cotton-wisp is advanced toward the center of the cornea, trying to avoid being seen by the patient.

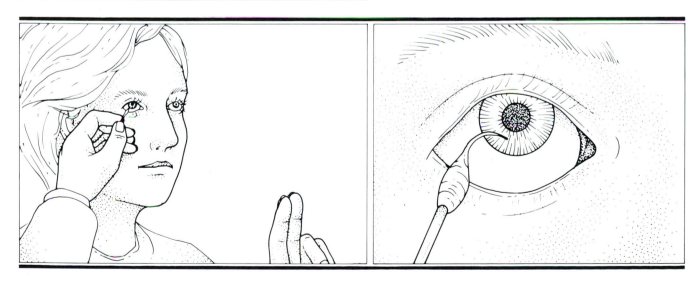

2. B. One end-point for the test is when the patient signals that the cotton wisp is felt. The signal may be raising a hand or verbalizing when the sensation is perceived.

2. C. Another end-point for the test is when the cotton-wisp contacts the cornea with enough force that the wisp bends. The test stops at this point, even if a signal has not been made.

Do the test several times for each eye; intermittently, do not touch the cornea but continue to ask the patient to respond as if the cornea was being touched. This will allow the assessment of the reliability of patient responses.

After the test, reevaluate the cornea using fluorescein dye to assess corneal integrity and what, if any, irritation is due to the test. If the cornea is compromised, explain to the patient that he or she may feel a foreign body sensation for a few hours.

Interpretation. The patient is asked two questions: Do you feel the cotton wisp touching the eye, and, if so, can you quantify the sensation on a subjective numeric scale? The corneal sensation can be graded with the least sensitive level occurring when the cotton wisp is laid on the cornea for several seconds without response. The patient is also asked to compare the sensation between the two eyes, since one eye is usually either disease-free or less involved than the other.

Most individuals will demonstrate a blink reflex when the cornea is touched. Unfortunately, blinking cannot be used as a sign of sensation, since patients may blink as a protective reflex if they see the wisp advancing.

Reduced corneal sensitivity without a history of past corneal disease, trigeminal nerve disease, contact lens wear, or other ocular condition, may be indicative of a cerebral tumor. Visual field analysis along with a referral to a neurologist may be indicated.

Although the test is subjective and prone to several variables, it is still worthwhile, especially when used with other diagnostic tests.

Contraindications/Complications. Care must be taken whenever the test is done on a diseased cornea; the examiner should wash the hands prior to manipulating the cotton wisp and always use a clean, sterile cotton wisp. While not usually painful, it is briefly irritating. The procedure may cause a mild amount of corneal punctate staining so corneal evaluation after the procedure is in order. In the rare event that excessive staining is seen, a topical antibiotic may be instilled either in-office or for several days depending on the amount of corneal irritation noted. Explain to the patient that after the procedure he or she may experience a mild foreign body sensation for a few hours.

VI Suggested Readings

Abrahamson IA Jr: Management of ocular foreign bodies. *Am Fam Physician* 1976;**14**:80–87.

Bartlett JD, Jaanus SD (eds): *Clinical Ocular Pharmacology.* Boston, Butterworth, 1989.

Catania LJ: *Primary Care of the Anterior Segment.* Norwalk, CT, Appleton & Lange, 1988.

Clompus RJ: How to find and remove corneal foreign bodies. *Rev Optometry* 1983; Sept:53–58.

Clompus RJ: How to manage corneal abrasions. *Rev Optometry* 1985; Nov:75–84.

Duane DD, Jaeger EA (eds): *Clinical Ophthalmology.* Philadelphia, Lippincott, 1988, vol 4.

Gombos G: *Handbook of Ophthalmological Emergencies.* Garden City, New York Medical Examination Publishing Co, 1977.

Grayson M: *Diseases of the Cornea.* St. Louis, Mosby, 1983.

Leibowitz HM (ed): *Corneal Disorders: Clinical Diagnosis and Management.* Philadelphia, Saunders, 1984.

Mandell RB, Polse KA, Bonanno J: Reassessment of optical pachometry, in Cavanagh HD (ed): *The Cornea. Transactions of the World Congress on the Cornea III.* New York, Raven, 1988, chapter 35.

Paton D, Goldberg MF: *Management of Ocular Injuries.* Philadelphia, Saunders, 1976.

Pavan-Langston D: *Manual of Ocular Diagnosis and Therapy.* Boston, Little, Brown, 1985.

Vinger PF: How I manage corneal abrasions and lacerations. *Physician Sports Med* 1986;**14**:170–179.

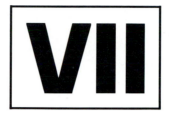

Ocular Laboratory Procedures

49 Cultures

Description/Indications. Certain external infections that threaten the integrity of the eye require laboratory analysis to identify the microorganism(s) involved. Ocular laboratory studies center on two areas: cytology and microbiology. Whereas cytological studies (see p. 177) help identify bacteria, viruses, fungi, and allergens, microbiological culture techniques are mainly used for bacterial identification. Viral cultures are also available and becoming more common as laboratories acquire the necessary instrumentation.

Culture studies involve the growth of colonies of microorganisms onto suitable media. A small amount of material from the eye containing microorganisms is spread onto solid media plates. The plates are incubated and evaluated for the development of distinct colonies. The characteristics of growth are specific for each microorganism and aid in identification. After each microorganism is grown and isolated, the characteristics of each pathogen are described. Culture results are also used to study the sensitivity of microorganisms to specific antibiotics. The patterns of resistance each organism has to specific antibiotics are studied, leading to more effective antibiotic usage. Sensitivity studies should be requested whenever cultures are taken. It takes 24 to 48 hours before culture results are available, so treatment is usually instituted with broad-spectrum agents. The treatment is modified if the culture and sensitivity results indicate other antibiotics might be more effective.

Cultures are indicated when clinical findings are insufficient to arrive at a diagnosis, when the tissue reaction is severe, or when the infection has not responded in a suitable time course to treatment. Specific indications for culture include hyperacute conjunctivitis, neonatal conjunctivitis, postoperative infections, chronic conjunctivitis, and central corneal ulcers not of viral origin.

Agar plates are the solid medium used to grow microorganisms for isolation and identification. Blood agar is the most commonly used plate. It is a general, all-purpose medium that will grow most bacterial organisms. Neisseria and Haemophilus do not grow well on blood agar; therefore chocolate agar (a polypeptone agar enriched with hemoglobin) is also used. Blood and chocolate agar plates are requested for all eye cultures. Other media such as Sabouraud's agar (fungi isolation) and Thayer-Martin agar (gonococcal identification) might be required, depending on the case presentation. The media plates are refrigerated prior to use and are brought to room temperature prior to inoculation. Thioglycolate broth (liquid media) is useful as a transportation medium and will grow facultative anaerobic organisms.

When results reveal a sparse growth of an organism known to be part of the normal eye flora, the noninvolved eye is cultured for comparison. There are common pathogens in all eyes and by comparing the normal to pathogenic flora, misinterpretation can be avoided.

When possible, specimens should be directly inoculated onto the solid media plates and promptly delivered to a laboratory. When not feasible, transport media are available. Amies, Stuart, Cary-Blair, Transgrow, and liquid thioglycolate broth are examples of some transport media used to keep bacteria viable until the sample is plated by the lab. The laboratory used will often supply a preferred choice of transport and growth media with specific directions.

Sterile conditions are required for any microbiological test so that extraneous microorganisms do not contaminate the findings. Wear gloves, be meticulous and clean with each step of the procedure, and obey all rules for universal precautions.

Because anesthetics decrease the number of organisms available for recovery, lid and conjunctival cultures need to be taken before their instillation. Proparacaine is the anesthetic of choice when needed because it inhibits bacterial growth the least of all the topical anesthetics. Cultures are therefore taken before scrapings and smears for which an anesthetic is required. Antibiotics also limit the number of organisms available for culture. It is necessary to discontinue the antibiotic at least 1 and usually 2 days before culturing.

Applicators used to collect material from the lids and conjunctiva may be made from cotton, calcium alginate, or Dacron polyester. Calcium alginate swabs are preferred, being soft, inert, and soluble.

Instrumentation. Sterile cotton-tipped applicators, calcium alginate swab, Kimura platinum spatula, alcohol lamp, topical ophthalmic anesthetic, blood agar plates, chocolate agar plates, Sabouraud's agar plate, specialty agar plates, trypticase soy broth, thioglycolate broth (transport medium), biomicroscope, lid speculum.

Technique

Eyelids: Before culturing lid margins, clean away any crusts or debris. Moisten an applicator with nonpreserved saline solution to scrub the lid margins. Moisten a separate applicator with trypticase soy broth (if available) or unpreserved sterile saline solution. Pull the lid away from the eye and wipe along the margin of the eyelid (Fig. 1). Roll the applicator along the lid margin three or four times so that it absorbs some material. Do not rub the lid margins. Immediately inoculate the solid media plates.

To streak an agar plate using a sample from an eyelid from the right eye, place the applicator in the lower part of the plate and slowly streak a capital ''R'' (Fig. 2). This is the designated symbol for a culture specimen taken from the right eyelid. A capital ''L'' is the symbol for material from the left lid margin. Material from the eyelids is placed on the bottom part of a plate and material from the conjunctiva on the top.

Roll the applicator along the surface of the plate (Fig. 3A), avoiding the edges. Do not let the applicator dig into the medium and break the surface (Fig. 3B). Use a separate plate for each eye to prevent crowding of the growth, thus avoiding interpretation difficulties. Routinely inoculate both blood and chocolate agar plates as well as any other media indicated.

It is preferable to inoculate the solid medium plates immediately after obtaining the sample. When solid medium plates are unavailable, use a transport medium. The preferred transportation medium is a glass tube of thioglycolate broth. Remove the cap and flame the rim of the tube, allowing the tube to heat for a few seconds (Fig. 4A). Place the applicator tip first into the tube of thioglycolate broth, breaking off any part of the wooden stick that has been touched (Fig. 4B). Reflame the top of the tube and cap tightly. It is important that the wooden stick remaining in the tube be untouched. Therefore, try to touch only the peripheral end of the applicator.

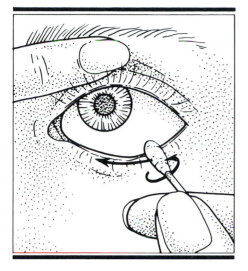

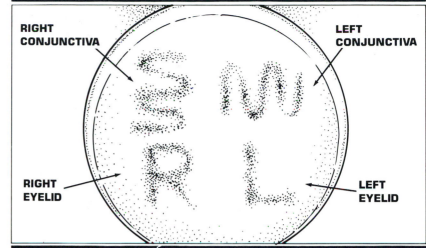

1. Wiping the eyelid margin with a pre-moistened applicator to obtain a sample for culture.

2. The symbols are made on the medium plates to designate where the material plated is from.

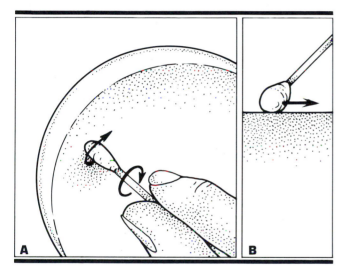

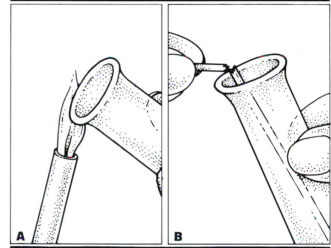

3. A. Using a cotton-tipped applicator to inoculate a plate. **B.** The cotton-tipped applicator should not break the surface as the plate is streaked.

4. A. Flaming the top of a tube of thioglycolate broth. **B.** The wooden end of a cotton-tipped applicator is broken off, removing all material that has been touched.

Label the sample with patient's name, doctor's name, time and date of sample, eye, and medications used and if they have been discontinued (Fig. 5). Fill out the laboratory forms and request the antibiotics to be tested in the sensitivity studies.

A Culturette is a commercially prepared transport container used for cultures. It is readily available and consists of a rayon-tipped applicator packaged in a cylindrical container containing modified Stuart's medium. Use the applicator to obtain the culture and slide it back into the container so the top of the applicator fits flush at the end of the tube. Squeeze the ampule at the bottom of the tube, breaking the seal and allowing the liquid medium to surround the applicator tip (Fig. 6). Recap, place the container back in the envelope from which it came, label, and ship to a laboratory.

Lacrimal Sac/Meibomian Glands: Samples from the lacrimal sac or meibomian glands can also be plated and are placed in the position on medium plates as any sample would be from the eyelids. To obtain meibomian secretions, express the meibomian glands (see p. 94). Using a moistened applicator, collect the secretions by rolling an applicator along the lid margins. Plate the collected material or place in a suitable transport medium. To obtain secretions from the lacrimal sac, gently palpate the sac (see p. 114), watching for discharge to regurgitate from the punctum. Collect the discharge with a moistened applicator, plate, and transport. Label each sample, noting where the material is from.

Conjunctiva: The inferior palpebral conjunctiva is the usual site for obtaining conjunctival specimens. Evert the lower lid, pulling it down and away from the eye. Gently roll a moistened applicator along the entire inferior palpebral conjunctiva (Fig. 7). Allow the applicator to absorb as much material as possible.

Roll the applicator several times to collect as much material as possible. Do not rub the conjunctiva and avoid touching the applicator to the lashes, lid margins, or your hand. Plate immediately or place the material in a transportation medium. A vertical zig-zag or helical pattern, placed on the top part of the media plate, is the symbol for material from the right conjunctiva, and a horizontal zig-zag pattern is the symbol for material from the left conjunctiva (Fig. 2).

Cornea: Use a Kimura platinum spatula to obtain specimens for cultures from a corneal ulcer. Instill a topical ophthalmic anesthetic in each eye. Using an alcohol lamp, flame a Kimura spatula for sterilization, heating it for several seconds and allowing to air cool. Focus on the ulcer using a slit lamp and place the spatula temporally and tangentially to the corneal lesion. Provide a suitable fixation object and explain to the patient what the procedure entails. Use the edge of the blade rather than the belly, gently scraping away and discarding any necrotic tissue and debris surrounding the ulcer. Gently scrape the advancing edge and then the central ulcer bed (Fig. 8), only removing the surface cells. The advancing edge and the ulcer bed are each a separate sample, being plated on their own media. Always move the spatula in a downward motion away from the eye, taking care to not use excessive force. A downward motion allows greater control and if the patient moves, with the spatula moving away from the eye, little danger of penetration exists. The spatula must not contact anything but the ulcer. When blepharospasm or fixation are problems, a lid speculum may be of help. Eyelid and conjunctival cultures are obtained routinely before scrapping a corneal ulcer, and if a lid speculum is required, it is inserted after obtaining lid and conjunctival specimens.

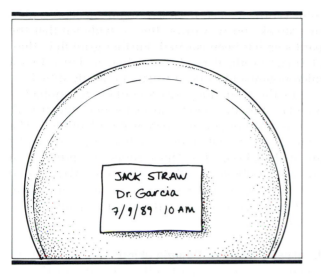

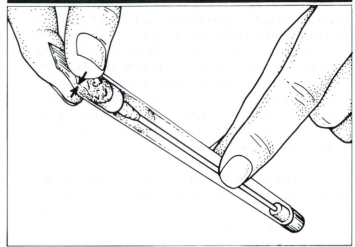

5. An example of a completed label, attached to a solid medium plate to be sent to the lab.

6. The ampule of a Culturette is squeezed, breaking the seal and providing a transport medium for the specimen still in place on the cotton-tipped applicator.

7. Using a moistened cotton-tipped applicator, the inferior palpebral conjunctiva is rolled to obtain a specimen.

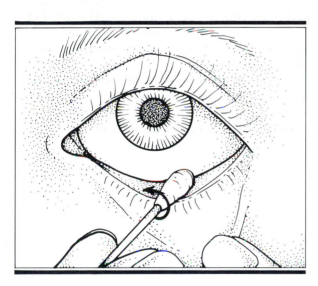

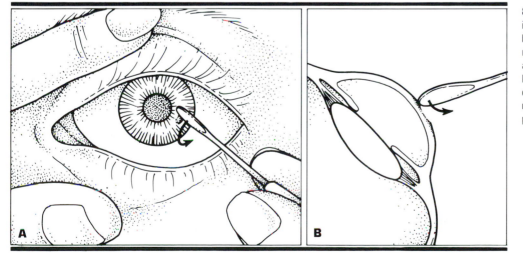

8. A. (far left) The spatula is used to scrape the ulcer bed to obtain a sample. The movement is always down and away from the eye.
B. (left) Both the leading edge and central ulcer bed need to be scraped and plated independently.

Take multiple samples of both areas of the ulcer, flaming the spatula after each sampling. Place the first samples retrieved on slides for Giemsa and Gram staining. Next inoculate blood, chocolate, and Sabouraud's agar plates by lightly streaking the spatula over the surface. Make a minimum of two rows of "C's" (Fig. 9) with each "C" representing a separate sample. Label the plates. Because of reduced growth, transport media are not utilized for cultures from corneal ulcers.

Interpretation. When growth is seen, the density, shape, and description of the colonies is important. Colonies are described looking at the size, pigmentation, shape, surfaces, odor, transparency, and consistency (Fig. 10). Any of these characteristics can be quantified from 1+ to 4+. The growth can also be quantified in a 1 to 4+ fashion or in colony-forming units (CFU). If changes to the medium occur, such as hemolysis, these need to be noted. From the description of the culture growth, a microorganism may be identified. Any growth away from a streak is viewed as a contamination and not microorganism growth. Preliminary results are usually available in 24 hours, with the final results in 48 to 72 hours. In a conjunctival infection, if streaks from both the lids and the conjunctiva are plated, the greatest growth should be observed in the conjunctival streak. In evaluating the rows of streaks from a corneal ulcer, if a microorganism is present in two streaks on two rows, this is evidence that the pathogen has been isolated. Further growth in thioglycolate broth, if used, is further evidence that a microorganism has been isolated and identified.

In the laboratory, discs containing antibiotics are placed on the blood agar plates once the growth of the microorganisms has been identified. The zones in the inhibition of growth around each tablet are analyzed (Fig. 11). These zones are indicators if specific antibiotics will be effective. Drugs that should be requested for testing include ampicillin, bacitracin, cefazolin, erythromycin, gentamycin, and sulfonamides.

Contraindications/Complications. Care must be taken whenever any part of the lids, conjunctiva, or cornea is cultured. Create as little trauma as possible, especially when corneal scrapings are done because an infected cornea is weakened and prone to perforate with excessive pressure. The number of samples may need to be limited in severe corneal ulcers extensively thinned by inflammation and in danger of perforation.

The collected ocular material may be infectious and even dangerous. Obey all rules for universal precautions, using gloves, washing hands, and cleaning and sterilizing all equipment.

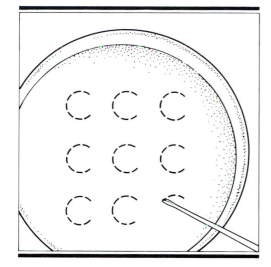

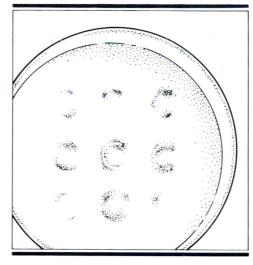

9. (far left) The spatula is used to directly inoculate the media plates, forming rows of "C's."

10. (left) A culture at 48 hours of growth.

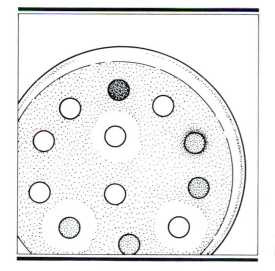

11. A plate showing sensitivity studies, using discs impregnated with antibiotics to inhibit microorganism growth and quantify the level of resistance.

50 Cytology (Smears and Scrapings)

Description/Indications. Ocular cytological studies (smears and scrapings) are indicated when an ocular infection or inflammation presents whose ominous appearance and questionable assessment suggest the need to identify or exclude certain organisms to arrive at a diagnosis. Smears and scrapings provide information regarding the morphology of the microorganism(s), inflammatory cellular response, and epithelial cell composition. This information is used to better understand possible etiologies and to formulate a treatment regimen.

Specific indications for obtaining cytological studies include any central corneal ulcer not of viral origin, hyperacute purulent conjunctivitis, neonatal conjunctivitis, postoperative infections, and chronic or recurrent conjunctivitis.

Smears and scrapings are taken after culturing (see p. 169), since a topical anesthetic is usually required to obtain samples and due to its bacteriostatic effect, can decrease the number of viable organisms available for culture. Samples are also preferably obtained before antibiotics are used.

A cotton-tipped or calcium alginate applicator and Kimura platinum spatula are used to lightly scrape off epithelial cells from the surface of the eyelids and conjunctiva. A spatula can collect more material than an applicator; if upon microscopic examination insufficient cells are present after using an applicator to obtain the conjunctival sample, retake the sample using a spatula. Only a Kimura or Lindner platinum spatula is used to scrape corneal ulcers. Once obtained, the sample is placed on a glass slide, fixed, stained, and examined under a microscope. The practitioner may read the slide or utilize a community laboratory for this purpose. Smears results are usually available the same day, which is one advantage they have over cultures.

The stain(s) used for reading the slides depend upon the presentation and clinical suspicions. The two most common stains are the Gram and Giemsa stains. The Gram stain is used to differentiate bacterial microorganisms into two groups, Gram positive and Gram negative, and to provide information regarding the morphology of the organism. This division of organisms into smaller, more specific groups helps in their identification and diagnosis. The Giemsa stain or a modified variation (Wright's stain) is used when the etiology is unknown and information is needed regarding the cytological response. The Giemsa stain does not provide a great deal of information for bacteria since, whether gram positive or negative, all will stain alike. The Giemsa stain is useful to differentiate a viral from allergic from bacterial response, especially for conjunctivitis, by determining the type of inflammatory cells, condition of the epithelial cells, and presence of cytoplasmic inclusion bodies. The Giemsa stain also identifies fungi (hyphae), yeast forms, and the bacterial morphology, though the Gram stain may better accomplish the latter. In general, both the Gram and Giemsa stains are used for each case, since they tend to complement each other.

The monoclonal antibody test is used to diagnose chlamydial infections. A smear is stained with the monoclonal antibody, and read using a fluorescent microscope. Other special stains are available to evaluate fungal, atypical bacterial responses, and Acanthamoeba. A lab can be of help in deciding which stains to choose.

Instrumentation. Sterile cotton-tipped applicator, calcium alginate applicator, Kimura-type platinum spatula, topical ophthalmic anesthetic solution, alcohol lamp, glass slides, 95% methyl alcohol, slit lamp.

Technique

Eyelids: If scales or crusts cover the lid margin, use a moistened applicator to gently scrub the margins prior to obtaining a smear. Then pull the lid taut and using a dry sterile cotton-tipped or calcium alginate applicator, rub the margin of the eyelid in one direction, rubbing at or near the base of the lashes alongside the lid margin (Fig. 1). The applicator should not be rolled. Transfer the material to a glass slide by gently rocking the applicator at the center, depositing the contents onto the slide (Fig. 2). The material is spread firmly and evenly in a thin layer over a small area in the center of a clean glass slide. If the material is dry, several drops of unpreserved saline solution may be added to allow the specimen to spread evenly. The slide needs to be promptly fixed. The preferred method, especially for Giemsa stain, is to place the slide in a 95% methyl alcohol solution for at least 5 minutes (Fig. 3). After 5 minutes remove the slide, allow to air dry, label, and prepare for transport to a local laboratory. Alternate methods for fixing the slide include air-drying or placing the slide over a flame for a few seconds. When a flame is used, the slide is held above it so the bottom is gently heated without being touched (Fig. 4). Throughout the procedure, be careful not to touch any part of the eye other than the eyelids.

Meibomian/Lacrimal: Meibomian secretions may be obtained by expressing the meibomian glands (see p. 94) and collecting the material with a dry applicator, smearing the material onto the center of a glass slide, and fixing. Collect secretions from the lacrimal canaliculus and lacrimal sac in suspected cases of dacryocystitis. The lacrimal sac is palpated (see p. 114) until material regurgitates from the punctum. The material is collected with a sterile dry applicator, wiped onto a clean glass slide, and promptly fixed. Care must be taken to not touch the eyelids as this sample is retrieved.

Conjunctiva: Conjunctival specimens are obtained using a dry applicator or spatula. Usually the sample is taken from the inferior palpebral conjunctiva, but the superior palpebral conjunctiva is used when it is the predominant tissue affected. To obtain a sample from the inferior cul-de-sac, have the patient look up, and evert the lower eyelid. Move the applicator over the inflamed area or blindly rub the conjunctiva if a specific pathology is not seen. Start at one point and advance the applicator several times, moving approximately one-quarter inch in length for each turn in one direction only (Fig. 5). Do not roll the applicator. Place the material on a clean glass slide and promptly fix.

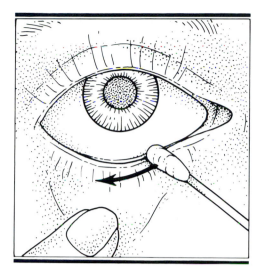

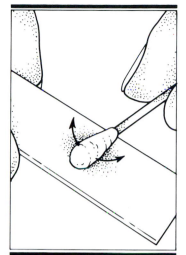

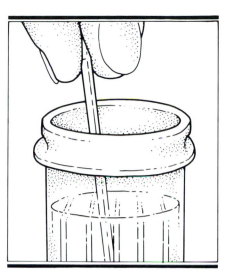

1. A dry applicator is used to obtain a smear from the lid margin. Note that the applicator is moved in one direction only.

2. Using gentle pressure, rock the applicator gently onto the center of the glass slide to transfer its contents.

3. The glass slide is placed in a bath of 95% methyl alcohol for 5 minutes for fixation.

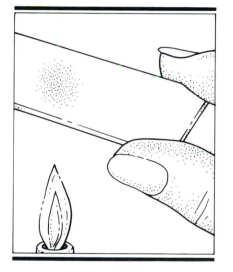

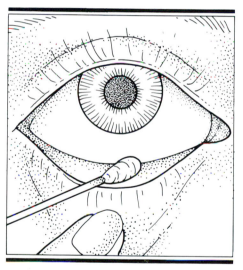

4. The slide may be held above a flame to fix the specimen.

5. A dry applicator is used to obtain a sample from the inferior palpebral conjunctiva.

A platinum spatula may also be used to obtain samples from the conjunctiva. Place a drop of a topical anesthetic agent in the eye. The spatula is sterilized, placing the blade into the flame of an alcohol lamp for several seconds. Remove and allow to cool to room temperature, not letting it touch anything that may effect its sterility. Remove any excess secretions with a moistened cotton-tipped applicator. Evert the lower eyelid, and anesthetize the eye. The spatula should gently scrape the conjunctiva, holding the blade perpendicular to the surface so its edge collects cells as it grazes along (Fig. 6). Move in one direction only for several passes, having the patient look away as the procedure is done. As it is scraped, the conjunctiva will blanche mildly, but should not bleed. Press firmly, but if bleeding occurs, lighten up on the force applied. Gently tap the side of the spatula blade on the edge of the glass slide to remove excess fluid (Fig. 7A). Turn the spatula over and while holding it flat, gently tap it to the center of the glass slide, transferring the material in a smooth, even fashion (Fig. 7B). Fixate the slides.

Cornea: Corneal ulcers need to be scraped, using a Kimura or Lindner platinum spatula. Instill several drops of a topical ophthalmic anesthetic solution. Pass a Kimura spatula through a flame for sterilization and allow to cool. Use a slit lamp to better visualize the ulcer and with a moist applicator, gently remove any necrotic tissue or discharge from the ulcerated area. This material may be used for culture (see p. 169). Using the side of the spatula blade, gently scrape the base and advancing edge of the ulcer (Fig. 8), avoiding excessive force to the cornea. The corneal surface and crevice are lightly grazed, picking up superficial cells as the spatula blade moves along. The material is spread onto glass slides, fixed, and prepared for transport to the laboratory. Gram and Giemsa stains are indicated on any specimen collected from a corneal ulcer.

Label any slide being prepared for transport to a laboratory. Include the name of the patient and doctor, date and time of sample, and the eye the specimen was taken from. If antibiotics have been used, this needs to be noted. A form is completed for each test required and the slide is placed in the container or envelope provided by the laboratory for transportation.

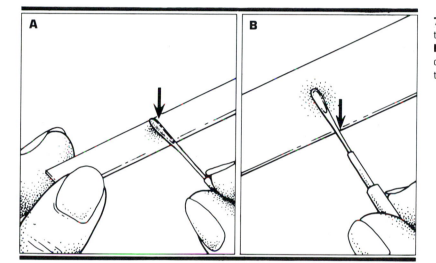

6. A spatula can also be used to collect a sample from the inferior palpebral conjunctiva.

7. A. (far left) The spatula is lightly tapped on the edge of the slide to release excess fluid. **B.** (left) The spatula is then tapped over the center of the glass slide to release its contents.

8. The spatula being used to scrape a corneal ulcer, making sure to get samples from both the advancing edge and ulcer base.

Interpretation. All material, whether from the eyelids, conjunctiva, or cornea, will be stained and evaluated. The Gram stain is used to divide bacteria into two groups: those retaining (Gram positive) or losing (Gram negative) the primary crystal violet stain when treated with 95% methanol. Gram-negative organisms do not retain the primary stain and are subsequently counterstained with safranin, appearing red under the microscope. The makeup of the cell wall determines if the stain is preserved. The Gram stain is also useful in describing the morphologic appearance of the microorganisms. Three shapes (cocci, rods, bacilli) and four organizational patterns (single, pairs, clusters, chains) can be identified (Figs. 9 and 10). Not all shapes occur for all organized patterns. Gram-positive cocci may be observed as single units, in pairs, in clusters (Staphylococci), or in chains (Streptococci). Gram-positive rods or diplococci (Pneumococci) may be seen, and Gram-negative organisms may appear as diplococci (Neisseria), diplobacilli (Moraxella), and rods (*Pseudomonas aeruginosa*, Haemophilus). Organisms having a similar morphologic appearance with Gram's stain may be definitively diagnosed with a culture (see p. 169). The Gram stain will also identify hyphae from fungal infections, seen as large filaments under a microscope. While hyphae usually pick up the Gram stain, this is not absolute, and on occasion filaments may be noted on a smear not picking up the stain. The Gram stain is especially useful in evaluating bacterial corneal ulcers and providing guidance on the microorganism involved and the choice of therapeutic agents.

The Giemsa stain provides information regarding the inflammatory cell response, condition of the epithelial cells, and presence of cytoplasmic inclusion bodies within the epithelial cells. When polymorphonuclear leukocytes (PMN) are the predominant cell, a bacterial infection is suspected. Fungal infections and conjunctivitis associated with membrane formation may also give a predominant PMN response. Mononuclear cells (lymphocytes) are associated with adenoviral infections, viral infections, and toxic reactions. A predominant response of eosinophils is found in allergic and hypersensitivity conditions. Epithelial cell changes include intracytoplasmic inclusion bodies, seen in neonatal chlamydial infections, and keratinization associated with keratitis sicca. Intracytoplasmic inclusion bodies are less commonly seen in adult forms of Chlamydia. The Giemsa stain can also give information like the Gram stain on cell morphology.

On occasion the number of cells available for interpretation may be small, leading to a negative report. This is more common when a dry applicator is used to obtain the sample. The specimen may be retaken, using a spatula to generate a larger representation.

Contraindications/Complications. Care must be taken when using a spatula or applicator to obtain samples from the eye. Bleeding, while not uncommon since cells are being removed from the superficial layers of the eyelids and conjunctiva, is an indication that excessive force is being applied. Corneal ulcers can be particularly problematic to test since the cornea may already be thinned and any additional force may lead to perforation.

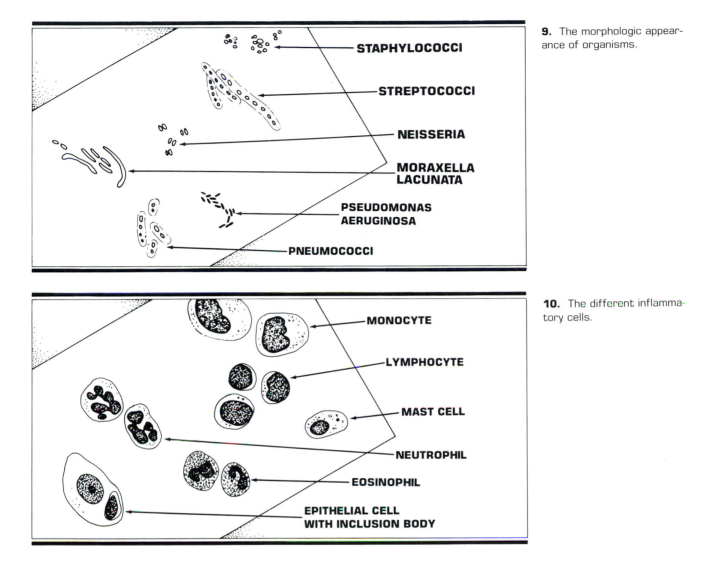

9. The morphologic appearance of organisms.

STAPHYLOCOCCI

STREPTOCOCCI

NEISSERIA

MORAXELLA LACUNATA

PSEUDOMONAS AERUGINOSA

PNEUMOCOCCI

10. The different inflammatory cells.

MONOCYTE

LYMPHOCYTE

MAST CELL

NEUTROPHIL

EOSINOPHIL

EPITHELIAL CELL WITH INCLUSION BODY

VII   Suggested Readings

Fedukowicz HB, Stenson S: *External Infections of the Eye.* Norwalk, CT, Appleton & Lange, 1985.

Finegold SM, Baron EJ: *Bailey and Scott's Diagnostic Micro-* *biology.* St. Louis, Mosby, 1986.

Leibowitz HM: *Corneal Disorders: Clinical Diagnosis and Management.* Philadelphia, Saunders, 1984.

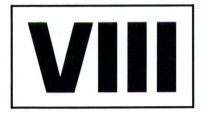

Posterior Segment Procedures

51   Direct Ophthalmoscopy

Description/Indications. Direct ophthalmoscopy allows for the visual examination of the retina and ocular media. The hand-held direct ophthalmoscope utilizes the patient's eye as a simple magnifier by aligning its viewing and illuminating beams (Fig. 1). This produces an erect, magnified, well-detailed real image of the retina. Compared to other fundus-viewing instruments, it is the easiest to master, provides for greatest patient comfort, can be used through smaller pupils, and provides the most accurate estimate of the patient's visual compromise due to media opacification. Disadvantages of the direct ophthalmoscope include its limited illumination, lack of stereopsis, close working distance, dependence on refractive errors for clarity and magnification, and small field of view (approximately two disc diameters). Although acceptable screening views are obtained through an undilated pupil, routine pupillary dilation enhances the field of view. The examined eye's pupillary margin and crystalline lens peripheral optical distortions limit the extent and quality of off-axis and peripheral fundus views.

Direct ophthalmoscopy is indicated for posterior fundus screening, evaluation of an eye's media, and evaluation of a patient's fixation pattern.

The ophthalmoscope head (Fig. 2) connects to a handle that serves as the power source. The head contains a variable range of plus and minus lenses used to compensate for refractive errors. The light is projected through a variably sized aperture and correcting lens to illuminate the fundus. Adjusting the aperture changes the beam size, which helps control reflections. A red-free filter is available to more easily identify hemorrhages and the nerve fiber layer. A bull's-eye fixation target is included in many ophthalmoscopes to test the fixation pattern (visuoscopy).

Magnification is determined by the patient and examiner's refractive powers, axial lengths of their globes, and compensating lenses used. A myopic person's inherent uncorrected plus power, along with the correcting minus ophthalmoscope lens, yield a magnified image (Galilean telescope design) for the emmetropic examiner. The hyperopic eye minifies (reversed telescopic design) the usual 15X magnified image created when both the examiner and the patient are emmetropic. High astigmatic or spherical refractive errors require that spectacle correction be worn by the examiner and/or patient to improve the clarity of the image, avoid distortion, and/or avoid unacceptable image size.

Instrumentation. Direct ophthalmoscope, topical ophthalmic mydriatic solution(s).

Technique. Dilate the pupils whenever possible with a topical mydriatic solution. Position the patient's eyes at a similar level to yours. Ask the patient to fixate a nonaccommodative distance target. Dim the room lights to maximize pupil dilation and reduce glare. Holding the ophthalmoscope in your right hand, align your right eye with the ophthalmoscope's aperture and brace it against your cheekbone. Attempt to keep your opposite eye open to minimize accommodative spasm and eyelid discomfort. Place the right index finger along the right side of the lens dial wheel. Dial in a +10 lens. Push down and rotate the rheostat illumination dial, usually located toward the top of the handle. Set the illumination in the mid-range of beam intensity, varying it as needed to improve the clarity of the image. To examine for media opacities, direct the ophthalmoscope's light beam into the patient's right pupil at a distance of 10 to 12 inches, angled from a slight temporal position (Fig. 3). Move forward until the reflex is in focus and examine for opacities. If an opacity is present, ask the patient to look in a certain position while you keep the ophthalmoscope stable, or move the ophthalmoscope beam keeping the patient's eye stable. Determine if the opacity moves in the same or opposite direction as your movement. Same-direction movement indicates that an opacity is in front of the posterior crystalline lens area (geometric center of eye), while against movement indicates an opacity posterior to the lens. Use the slit lamp to confirm any findings.

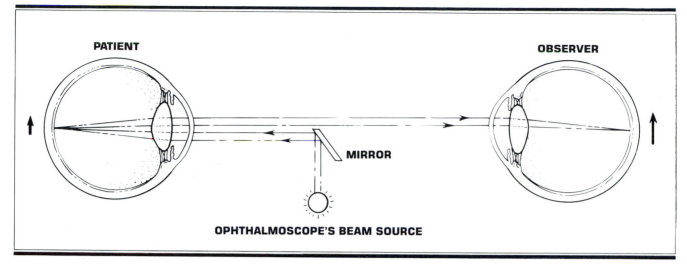

1. Basic optical principle of direct ophthalmoscopy.

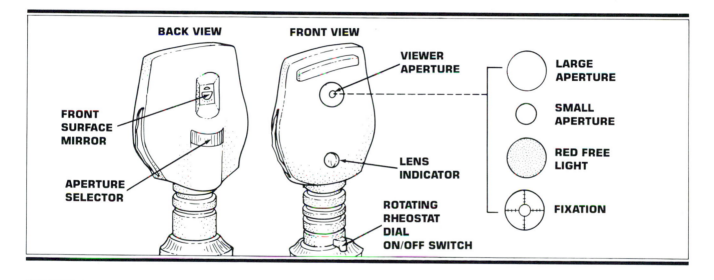

2. (above) Ophthalmoscope head components and aperture selections.

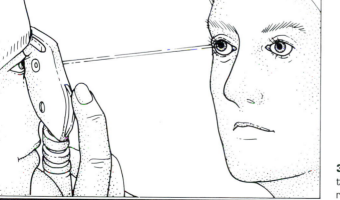

3. (left) Positioned at 10 to 12 inches in front of the patient, the examiner moves forward and observes the red reflex for opacities, judging their location.

Reduce the plus power as the patient's eye is approached. Attempt to keep your head position vertical so as to not block the patient's fixation with his or her opposite eye. Stop when your knuckles lightly touch the patient's cheek (Fig. 4A). This area of contact can act as a rotational point for examination movements, insuring a close working distance and resultant optimal field of view (Fig. 4B). Slowly continue with plus reduction until the retina is in focus, noting any anomalies along the way. Approximately a circular area two disc diameters in size is visualized when emmetropia (Fig. 5) is present. Direct your fixation slightly nasally and inferiorly to locate the optic disc. Note its color, margins, shape, peripapillary retinal changes, presence or absence of spontaneous venous pulsation, and the horizontal and vertical cup/disc ratios. Observe disc tissue for sloping margins of the cup and/or pallor. Estimate the depth of the cup by focusing at the anterior-most cup edge and then reducing plus power until the bottom is clear (1 diopter = ⅓ mm).

Follow the retinal blood vessels outward from the disc into the posterior pole in a systematic quadrantal fashion (Fig. 6). Go as far as possible, noting the A/V ratio, crossing appearances, vessel caliber, arterial light reflex, and the surrounding retinal tissue for blood, fluid, exudate, elevation, or pigment alteration. Make small dioptric power adjustments if needed to compensate for ocular movements, unsteadiness, and changes in tissue area observed. Increase the range of the retinal area visualized by asking the patient to look in the same direction as the quadrant being examined. To examine the retinal periphery, view from 180 degrees away and angle your head to go out as far as possible (nasally for temporal retinal exam, inferiorly for superior retinal exam).

Examine the macula area. Ask the patient to look directly at the ophthalmoscope beam for the exact localization of the foveal area. Note the presence or absence of the foveal reflex. To determine the patient's fixation pattern, change the ophthalmoscope's aperture to the bull's-eye target, instruct the patient to occlude the opposite eye with his or her hand and to fixate on the center of the target.

Gently hold the patient's upper lid against the superior orbital rim with your opposite thumb for viewing the inferior fundus, for photophobic patients, or for patients with small palpebral apertures. It may also be necessary to secure the sensitive patient's lower lid downward against the inferior orbital rim with the ring finger of the hand holding the ophthalmoscope to keep the eyelids open. Record all pertinent data in the patient's record.

Repeat the entire procedure on the opposite eye by moving to the patient's opposite side and using your left hand and eye.

Interpretation. The optic disc should be evaluated for its color, margins, shape, peripapillary retinal changes, presence or absence of spontaneous venous pulsation, and the horizontal and vertical cup/disc ratio, noting any accompanying disc tissue sloping and/or pallor. Fundus vasculature, pigment changes, and clarity of ocular media should all be noted. Although with a dilated pupil the examiner is capable of visualizing the far peripheral retina, the ophthalmoscope's magnification and limited field of view do not lend themselves to an efficient examination of the periphery.

Contraindications/Complications. Aside from some discomfort due to glare, this noncontact procedure should present no risk to the patient. Patient and examiner health may be better protected by the examiner wearing a surgical mask.

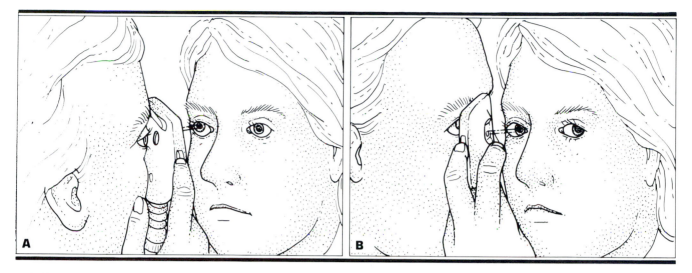

4. A. Proper examiner–patient alignment using the knuckles as a point of rotation during examination. **B.** The examiner should rotate in the opposite direction of the fundus area being examined.

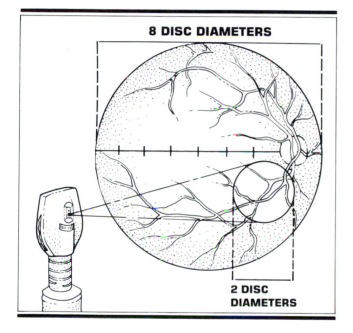

5. Direct ophthalmoscopy yields a two-disc-diameter field of view with emmetropic eyes, while indirect ophthalmoscopy with a 20-diopter lens yields an eight-disc diameter field of view.

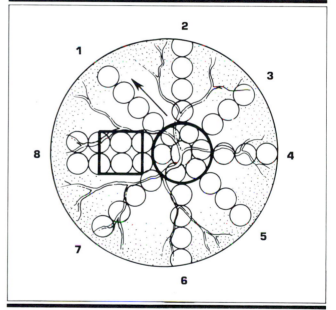

6. In the systematic evaluation of the fundus, after viewing the optic disc (large dark circle), follow the retinal blood vessels in an organized pattern outward from the disc (as shown in steps 1 through 8), finishing with an examination of the macula (large square).

52 Monocular Indirect Ophthalmoscopy

Description/Indications. Monocular indirect ophthalmoscopy combines the advantages of increased field of view (indirect ophthalmoscopy) with erect real imaging (direct ophthalmoscopy) to produce a viewing system for ocular fundoscopy. By collecting and redirecting peripheral fundus-reflected illumination rays, which cannot be accomplished with the direct ophthalmoscope (see p. 186), the indirect ophthalmoscope extends the observer's field of view approximately four to five times. An internal relay lens system reinverts the initially inverted image to a real erect one, which is then magnified. This image is focusable using the focusing lever/eyepiece system (Fig. 1). The end result is an ophthalmoscope with a 40 to 45-degree (eight disc diameters) field of view and approximately 5X magnification.

The instrument itself has an illumination rheostat at its base, a focusing lever for image refinement, a filter dial with red-free and yellow filters, a forehead rest for steady proper observer head positioning, and an iris diaphragm lever to adjust the illumination beam diameter (Fig. 2). Its disadvantages include lack of stereopsis, limited illumination, fixed magnification, and fair to good resolution.

Indications for use of monocular indirect ophthalmoscopy include the need for an increased field of view of the retina, small pupils, uncooperative children, patient's intolerance of the brighter light from the binocular indirect ophthalmoscope, basic fundus screening, one-handed examination technique, and a monocular examiner unable to appreciate the advantages of a binocular instrument. Binocular indirect ophthalmoscopy (see p. 192), however, with its superior stereoscopic viewing system, still remains the technique of choice whenever possible.

Instrumentation. Monocular indirect ophthalmoscope, topical mydriatic solutions.

Technique. Dilate the patient's pupils with topical mydriatic solutions. To examine the right eye, stand to the patient's right side, remove any spectacle correction the patient is wearing, and have him or her fixate straight ahead and level with the left eye. Keep your habitual refractive correction in place, turn on the instrument rheostat, dim the room lighting, push the iris diaphragm lever fully to the left to maximally increase the aperture size, and center the red dot on the filter dial to position the open aperture for normal viewing. Slide the front dust shield button fully downward to prevent illumination and viewing obstruction.

Place the forehead rest against your forehead and align your right eye through the instrument eyepiece with the patient's right eye, holding the handle with your right hand. Position yourself several inches in front of the patient and focus through the patient's pupil onto the fundus using your thumb and focusing lever (Fig. 3). As you approach, stop approximately 4 to 5 inches (18 mm) from the patient's eye. Adjust the focusing and iris diaphragm levers to produce a clear maximally illuminated fundus view. Continue to approach the patient until your knuckle lightly touches the patient's cheek. As your working distances decreases, fundus magnification will increase. Angle the light slightly nasally to illuminate the optic disc.

After scanning the tissue surrounding the optic disc, ask the patient to look upward and scan the superior posterior pole, pivoting around the pupil as a rotational center. Direct the patient to look superior temporally, then superiorly, and finally, superior nasally. With each position of gaze direct the ophthalmoscope light beam from the opposite direction (Fig. 4), focus on the central posterior pole, and track anteriorly as far as possible to examine as much retinal tissue as can be visualized. Repeat the same procedure nasally, temporally, and then inferiorly in a similar fashion. Use the opposite hand to control obstructive eyelids. Make fine adjustments with the focusing lever as your vertex distance varies.

Repeat the same procedure on the left eye, using your left eye, left hand, and positioning yourself at the patient's left side.

Interpretation. As with direct ophthalmoscopy, observe any media opacities as you focus through the eye onto the fundus. The optic nerve, retinal vasculature, and retinal tissue should be examined for anomalies. Use of the red-free filter will enhance the contrast of the retinal vasculature and any hemorrhages.

Although vitreous base views are possible with the monocular indirect ophthalmoscopy, its greatest effectiveness extends anteriorly to the peripheral equatorial region. The 40+ degree field of view of the monocular indirect is approximately the same as that of the binocular indirect ophthalmoscope.

Contraindication/Complications. This noncontact, moderate illumination procedure, when performed properly, presents no potential for light damage to the patient.

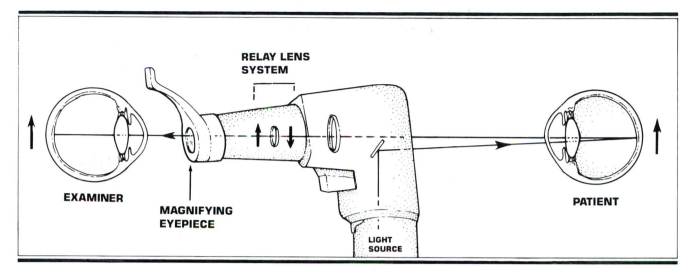

1. The optical principle of monocular indirect ophthalmoscopy, demonstrating the resultant erect, magnified image.

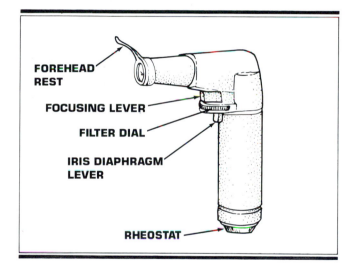

2. The monocular indirect ophthalmoscope.

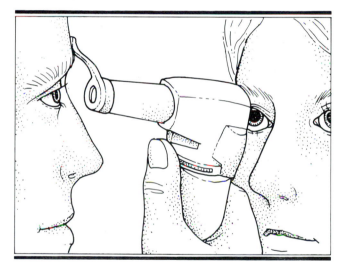

3. The examiner is properly positioned with thumb on the focusing lever.

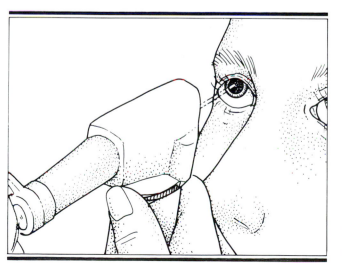

4. The patient is asked to look in the same direction as the fundus area being examined, while the light beam is directed from the opposite direction.

53 Binocular Indirect Ophthalmoscopy

Description/Indications. Binocular indirect ophthalmoscopy (BIO) is a technique used to evaluate the entire ocular fundus. It provides for stereoscopic, wide-angled, high-resolution views of the entire retina and overlying vitreous. Its optical principles and illumination options allow for visualization of the fundus regardless of high ametropia, hazy ocular media, or central opacities. The examiner's use of different powered condensing lenses, variable illumination intensity, scleral indentation (see p. 200), and multiple viewing angles, allow for total fundus inspection. A more detailed inspection of certain retinal areas may require the complementary use of fundus biomicroscopy techniques: 90-diopter lens (see p. 210), fundus contact lens (see p. 204) or Hruby lens (see p. 208).

The optics of BIO (Fig. 1) consist of light beams directed into the patient's eye that produce reflected observation beams from the retina. These beams are focused to a viewable, aerial image following placement of a high plus-powered condensing lens at its focal distance in front of the patient's eye. The resultant image is real, magnified 1.5X to 3.5X, reversed left to right, inverted top to bottom, and located between the examiner and the condensing lens (Fig. 2). The examiner views this image through the oculars of the head-borne indirect ophthalmoscope.

The BIO (Fig. 3) consists of a headband apparatus, optical viewing system, and rheostatically controlled illumination source. The headbands provide proper and comfortable instrument placement, with adjustment controls located at the crown of the head and occipital notch area. The light source's variable-intensity illumination beams are directed downward and reflected laterally by an adjustable mirrored surface located in the instrument's main housing. These optics allow the fundus-directed illumination beams to pass off-axis to the returning reflected observation beams, minimizing corneal light reflexes. The ocular lens system has knobs or sliding track adjustments to horizontally align the low plus-powered eyepieces (+2.00 to +2.50 D) with the examiner's interpupillary distance (IPD). Prisms incorporated into the instrument optically reduce the examiner's IPD, allowing it to be imaged along with the illumination beam within the patient's pupil. Stereoscopic viewing is thus produced. Therefore, the two images of the examiner's pupils and that of the light source are located inside the patient's dilated pupil for binocular viewing. The small-pupil BIO has the ability to further condense these three points to allow passage through undilated pupils.

Condensing lenses are double aspheric with a multilayered antireflective coating available in various powers, diameters, tints, and designs. During examination the more convex lens surface faces toward the examiner, while the less convex surface faces the patient's eye (noted by a white line encircling the lens). The standard +20-D lens produces approximately 2.5X magnification and a 35-degree or eight-disc diameter field of view. This is in contrast to a direct ophthalmoscope, which produces approximately 15X magnification and a two-disc diameter fundus view (Fig. 4). As the condensing lens power is decreased, the resultant visual field decreases and magnification increases; therefore, compared to the standard +20-D lens, a +14.00-D lens yields 3.5X magnification and smaller field, while a +28-D yields 1.5X magnification and larger field. Clear and amber lenses are available. Amber or yellow lenses appear to increase patient comfort by reducing scattered light, thereby reducing irritating glare. They produce an image as sharp as a clear lens. Examiners have their own preferences relative to fundus color perception with a clear versus a yellow lens.

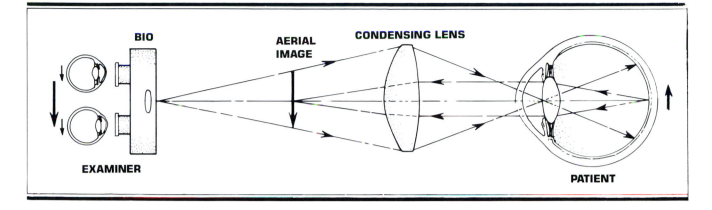

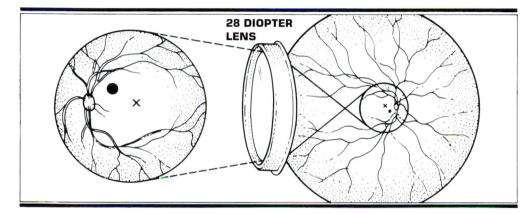

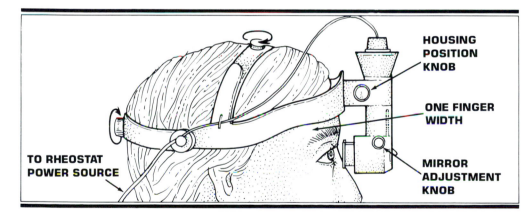

1. (above) BIO optical principles: a magnified, reversed, inverted fundus image is formed and viewed at a point between the examiner and the condensing lens.

2. (left) BIO with a condensing lens produces a magnified, reversed, inverted aerial fundus image for examiner inspection.

3. (left) BIO is balanced and secured on your head. The crown top strap is initially adjusted to absorb most of instrument's weight, and then the occipital strap is tightened. The front headband is positioned approximately one index finger width above the eyebrows. The oculars are placed close to your eyes or lightly abutting any spectacles.

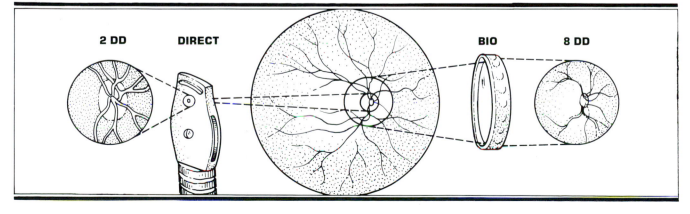

4. Visual field comparison between the BIO (8 DD) and direct ophthalmoscope (2 DD).

Advantages of BIO include stereopsis, large field of view, bright illumination, minimal peripheral view distortion, and complete peripheral tissue access when used with scleral indentation. Other advantages include a comfortable working distance and relative independence from patient refractive error or moderate media opacification. Disadvantages include initial cost, the need for pupil dilation, patient's moderate glare discomfort, initial examiner adjustment to the inverted/reversed image, low magnification with loss of fine detail, and the initial learning time needed to become comfortable and proficient with its use.

Indications for BIO examination include thoroughness of routine ocular health assessment; patient symptoms of flashes, floaters, spots, or other visual symptoms consistent with vitreous detachment, syneresis, inflammation or hemorrhage, or retinal tear or detachment; and patient history of peripheral vision loss, blunt ocular trauma, previous retinal detachment or peripheral retinal disease, diabetes, significant vascular disease, metastatic carcinoma, posterior vitreous detachment, or parasympathomimetic therapeutic drug treatment (pilocarpine therapy). Airborne communicable disease that might be passed with a closer working distance unless a mask is worn, or uncooperative patient behavior most commonly found in children, are also indicators.

BIO teaching mirrors are available that allow another observer to simultaneously view the same fundus with the examiner (Fig. 5).

Recognition of fundus anatomical landmarks (Fig. 6) assist the novice BIO practitioner as he or she develops proficiency and confidence with the instrument. These same landmarks are helpful to the more experienced practitioner for specific localization and recording of significant fundus findings. Posterior pole reference points include the optic disc; central retinal artery and vein; fovea; and the anatomical macula, which includes the area between the major superior and inferior temporal vascular arcades. The actual posterior pole anterior limit is identified by connecting the vortex vein ampullae with an imaginary line. Approximately 60 to 70% of the entire fundus is considered posterior pole. These prominent, thicker ampullae, numbering 4 to 15 per eye, represent the merging of multiple swirling choroidal venous tributaries as they exit posteriorly from the choroid through the scleral canal. The equatorial region is immediately anterior to these large collecting vessels, which are most commonly found in each oblique quadrant and best seen in lightly pigmented patients.

The peripheral retina comprises the remaining 30 to 40% of the fundus and is divided into superior and inferior regions by the long posterior ciliary arteries and nerves. This artery and nerve emerge at the retinal equator and traverse anteriorly to the ora serrata in a characteristic "ribbonlike" hyper and hypopigmented pattern. The short ciliary arteries of the choriocapillaris and their accompanying nerves, numbering 10 to 20, are found perpendicular to the ora serrata. These pigment-mottled lines are most commonly seen in the vertical meridians (6 and 12 o'clock). The ora serrata represents the end of the choroid and the retina. The choroid continues on as the pigmented pars plana while the retina becomes the nonpigmented single epithelial layer on the pars plana surface. The temporal ora serrata border is characteristically smooth while the nasal border has a scalloped surface. Just posterior to the ora serrata is an age-related, circumferentially oriented, wide band of mottled pigment that represents the vitreous base or posterior firm attachment of the posterior vitreous to the retina.

Instrumentation. Binocular indirect ophthalmoscope, condensing lens(es), topical mydriatic solution(s), reclinable examination chair or table.

Technique

BIO Adjustment: Loosen both the crown and occipital headstraps. Place the loosened BIO onto your head and position the bottom of the front headband approximately one index finger width above your eyebrows (*see* Fig. 3). Tighten the crown strap until this headband position begins to stabilize as most of the instrument's weight begins to rest on the top of your head. Position the back headstrap on or below the occipital notch and tighten until the instrument appears to be securely positioned. Make fine adjustments as needed. Loosen the knob(s) that control the instrument's main housing (oculars and light tower). Fixating straight ahead and level, vertically position the oculars to within eyelash distance from your uncorrected eyes aligned tangential to or slightly angled downward from the ocular surface. This should maximize your visual field and minimize horizontal diplopia. If you wear distance spectacles, lightly abut the oculars up against their front surface.

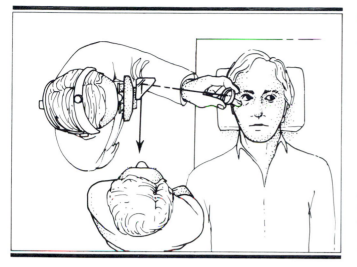

5. (left) A teaching mirror is attached to the BIO for simultaneous fundus viewing by two people. The observer should be positioned at twelve inches or less from the mirror.

6. (below) Ocular fundus with anatomical landmarks. (a) Long posterior ciliary artery and nerve. (b) Short posterior ciliary artery. (c) Vortex vein. (d) Vitreous base (nasal). (e) Vitreous base (temporal). (f) 20 D lens view. (*See also* Color Plate 53-6.) (Courtesy of Anthony Cavallerano, OD.)

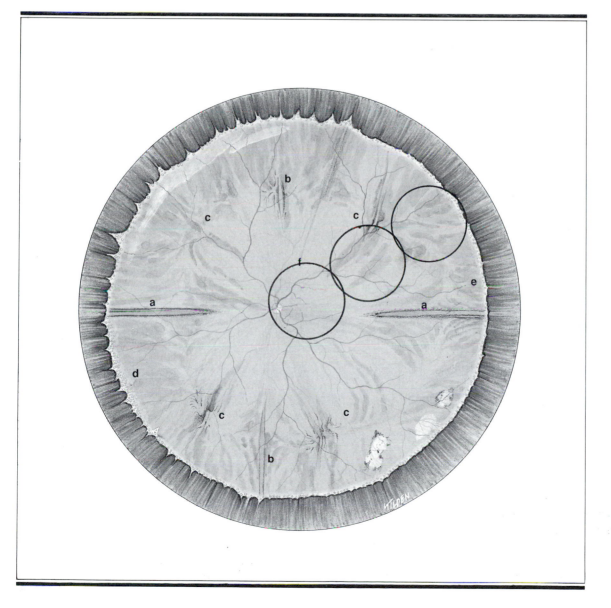

Horizontally align each ocular by closing one eye and fixating your centrally positioned thumb at 16 to 20 inches. Adjust the ocular alignment knob or slide the oculars to place an identical centrally positioned thumb in each ocular's field of view (Fig. 7). After individual alignment, view the thumb binocularly as a single clear object, thus creating an optimal setting for stereoscopic viewing. Make fine vertical and horizontal adjustments as needed to maximize the optics. Turn on the BIO power source and fixate straight ahead on a wall or your hand at 16 to 20 inches looking at the projected light source. Use the mirror knob to vertically place the light source at the upper one-half to one-third of the field. The illumination beam will then pass superior to the reflected observation beam. In a darkened room, this step would precede centration of the oculars. Observe the location of the light filament in each ocular's field of view to ensure that it is horizontally centered or displaced slightly nasally. Refer to the manufacturer's guide if it is not. These light filaments should be defocused at the 18 to 20-inch working distance.

The only required major adjustment to a BIO personally used by one practitioner is the occipital headstrap adjustments. A brief review of all adjustments and alignments should be made with each BIO use, however.

BIO Technique: Dilate both of the patient's pupils with topical mydriatic solution(s), preferably using both a parasympatholytic and sympathomimetic agent to maximize dilation and patient comfort. Seat the patient in a reclinable examination chair which, when reclined, will give the examiner 270 degrees access at the patient's head. Carefully recline the patient using good neck support until his or her facial plane is parallel to the floor and approximately at the level of your hips to allow for extension of your arms with a slight bend (Fig. 8). Direct the patient to fixate straight upward at the ceiling. Dim the room lighting to eliminate any overhead glare sources. With the BIO headset in place and with the voltage set to mid-range, stand to the right shoulder side of the reclined patient at his or her 8 o'clock position. Gently secure the patient's right upper lid against the superior orbital rim with your left thumb and rest your remaining fingers on the patient's forehead for self-support and for future condensing lens support (Fig. 9). Hold a clean +20-D condensing lens with the thumb, index, and middle fingers of your right hand, positioning the more convex surface toward you or the lens' white-ringed edge closest to the patient. Place your thumb between the knurled rings of the lens and place your index and middle fingers on the upper and lower knurled rings, respectively, for maximum lens control. Lightly secure the right lower lid against the inferior orbital rim with the ring and/or smallest finger of the same hand completing palpebral aperture separation and establishing a pivot position for adjustments of the condensing lens.

From a working distance of 18 to 20 inches (arm's length) and positioned almost above the patient, direct the light beam into the pupil, producing a complete red pupillary reflex. Pivot the condensing lens laterally and place it close to the ocular surface between you and the patient, noting an erect image of the patient's eye through the lens. Pull backward on the lens, maintaining the central position of the pupil reflex, until the entire lens fills with a fundus image. This "tromboning" movement of the lens is used continuously during BIO. Make fine adjustments in the lens tilt and vertex distance to produce a distortion-free, full lens view. Increase the illumination when poor visualization occurs secondary to media opacification. At this point an "optical viewing system" has been created consisting of your fixation line through the BIO oculars to the focused aerial image, through the condensing lens' optical center, through the center of the pupil, to the fundus area of regard (Fig. 10). An imaginary rod through these points reminds the examiner to bend the torso in unison with the lens in order to maintain this identical alignment as the condensing lens is tilted to view other fundus areas.

If a single, stereoscopic, clear image is seen, initiate a systematic examination of the fundus, beginning with the less photosensitive peripheral retina. Direct the patient to look back toward the 12 o'clock position at his or her forehead. Tap the forehead with your fingertips if fixation assistance is needed. From a position 180 degrees opposite to the patient's direction of gaze, in this instance inferiorly, direct the illumination beam into the right eye, using the just discussed "optical system" design. Begin posteriorly near the equator and track superiorly toward the ora serrata, attempting to maintain a full condensing lens view and an intact "optical system." This will require you to lean slightly over the patient and then tip your torso at the hip backward and to the right, as fixation is directed more and more superiorly. With the pupil as the rotation point, illuminate and view any specific retinal area by rotating yourself and the light source opposite in direction to the area of regard thus directing the beam onto the retina from 180 degrees away.

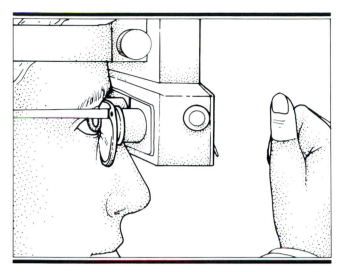

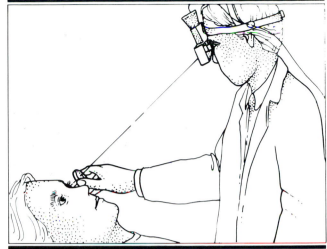

7. Eyepiece alignment: alternately close each eye and view the centrally placed thumb at 16 to 18 inches. Slide the oculars until each eye is seeing identical, centered images with resultant stereopsis.

8. The patient is reclined backward at the level of your hips, positioning the plane of his or her face parallel to the floor.

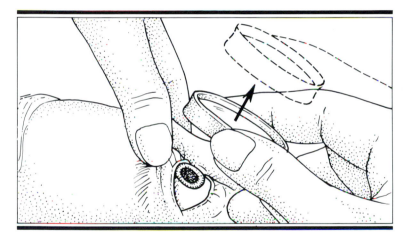

9. The patient's upper and lower lids are gently retracted while centering the condensing lens over the red reflex; lens movement in a "tromboning" motion will yield a fundus view.

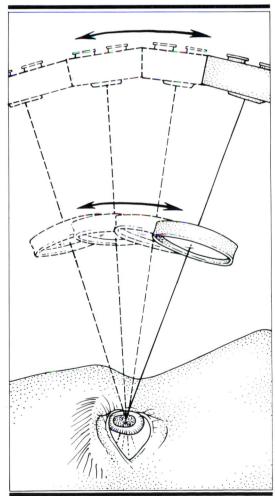

10. All examiner movement during examination is performed maintaining the patient's pupil as the center of rotation as the examiner's visual axis and condensing lens are changed in unison.

Note that the far peripheral retina is viewed through an optically oval or elliptical pupil opening, reducing the lens image quantity or lens filling and your stereopsis (Fig. 11A, B). Frequently tilt your head to reposition the illumination beam and ocular alignments in the pupil (Fig. 11C). After reaching the superior retina's peripheral limit, direct the light source out of the patient's pupil, ask him or her to blink and then to look superior nasally. Reposition the light back into the "optical system," begin equatorially and again smoothly track the retina anteriorly. Repeat this procedure in a clockwise direction for all eight cardinal meridians. View and review overlapping areas. Ask the patient to look in the direction of the quadrant to be examined. Circle the patient's head as you examine downward toward the inferior retina. To prevent patient distress and light intolerance, remove the light source and allow the patient to blink briefly following changes in fixation.

Having completed the peripheral retina inspection, reposition yourself at the patient's 8 o'clock position and ask him or her to fixate the ceiling. With minimal torso and "optical system" movements, scan the superior and lateral posterior pole meridians beginning near the disc and moving anteriorly to the vortex areas. Ask the patient to look toward each of your shoulders as you examine the inferior posterior pole meridians with similar movements. Overlapping areas are viewed and reviewed.

Repeat the same examination on the left eye either by carefully leaning over the patient or by positioning yourself on the opposite side of the patient at his or her 4 o'clock position. Rotate the head of the chair away from the standard instrument stand to create the needed 270 degrees of access area. Ambidextrous examination is encouraged but not required as it will be needed for scleral indentation. After examining the left eye's periphery and posterior pole, ask the patient to look directly at the light source with each eye for better macular examination. Use a lower-powered condensing lens than the standard +20 D if greater magnification is needed.

Interpretation. The initial work with the smaller, inverted, reversed, condensing lens image can be quite trying. It is important to remember that it is only the lens view that is different. If you are directing light into the superior aspect of the fundus, you are indeed looking at superior retina. As you scan more anteriorly, the newly illuminated retinal tissue image appears in the condensing lens at its opposite edge closest to you. Much of the initial concern with image reversal and inversion can be reduced by performing most of the posterior fundus examination standing at the head of the reclined chair facing the patient's face. When looking straight down at the patient from this position you have changed your viewing relationship, such that your face is now inverted and reversed relative to the patient's. This nullifies the image change and the orientation of what you see is now a "normal" fundus view. Fundus drawing (see p. 214) will also help to overcome this hurdle.

If only a red reflex is seen or if the lens is only partially filled with fundus details, trombone the condensing lens off the pivot finger. If no details are seen, place the condensing lens at 2 inches and move your headset light source closer or further away. If no fundus details are still seen, suspect media obstruction. Poor fundus visualization due to patient blepharospasm may be decreased by reducing the light intensity or by possibly holding the eyelids more gently.

Complications/Contraindications. Maximal dilation may be contraindicated in certain patients. Physical or vascular conditions may prevent reclining of the patient. In this case, examination can be done in the sitting position, which requires additional repositioning of both the patient and examiner during examination.

The examiner's inability to hold the condensing lens stable can reduce viewing quality. Consider bracing the edge of the condensing lens against the thumb of the hand holding the upper lid and also against the patient's nose in certain positions.

Significant corneal disruption or opacification hinders fundus visualization with indirect ophthalmoscopy. Therefore, do not perform fundus contact lens examination prior to BIO.

Vertical diplopia is frequently the result of a tilted BIO housing, which can be corrected by gross tilting of the headset. Horizontal diplopia is commonly caused by incorrect IPD settings or a working distance too close to the patient. Too close a working distance with a smaller pupil will not allow fundus visualization. A tight headband adjustment will induce unnecessary examiner discomfort.

American National Standards Institute (ANSI) modified findings recommend that with voltage set at half power, continuous viewing of a single fundus area should not exceed 40 seconds duration.

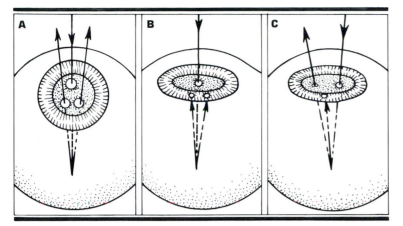

11. A. A normal round pupil area contains the illumination beam and the examiner's visual axes. **B.** Oval pupil can obstruct the examiner's visual axis. **C.** Examiner's head tilting can reposition the three beams for better viewing.

54   Scleral Indentation

Description/Indications. Views of the anterior fundus are limited by the iris, edge of the crystalline lens, and the patient's globe–orbit configuration. Even with maximum pupillary dilation, these factors make viewing the pars plana, ora serrata, and some areas of the peripheral retina difficult when solely using the binocular indirect ophthalmoscope (BIO) (Fig. 1A). Scleral indentation is a technique used to inwardly displace optically inaccessible or poorly defined areas of the peripheral fundus, aligning them with the examiner's axis of observation (Fig. 1B). Scleral indentation not only allows for the simple inward displacement of tissue, but also allows it to be viewed stereoscopically from multiple angles by elevating and rolling the tissue with a scleral depressor. Lesions that might otherwise go undetected or misdiagnosed can be identified by employing this technique. The practitioner must master the BIO technique (see p. 192) before learning scleral indentation.

Indications for scleral indentation include symptoms of flashes, floaters, spots, or hazy or decreased vision; history of blunt trauma; high axial myopia; aphakia; or any previously diagnosed peripheral retinal anomaly.

One purpose of peripheral fundus examination is to identify retinal breaks or areas with rhegmatogenous potential. Proper indentation technique attempts not only to place the area of concern on the observation axis, but also to produce a change in viewing perspective to assist in diagnosis. Placement of the area along the sloping edge of the indentation (Fig. 1C) produces a darkened subretinal appearance with resultant enhanced contrast between the intact retina and any retinal break. Indentation also produces oblique viewing, which increases apparent tissue layer density, thus reducing retinal translucency, again increasing the contrast between a retinal break and the retina. Indentation allows for greater ease in viewing tissue layer separation and surface irregularities by creating multiple viewing angles along and between tissue layers.

There are several types of scleral depressors available, with the choice depending mostly upon personal preference. The thimble type (open or closed tip), double-ended flat, and cotton-tipped applicators are commonly employed (Fig. 2). Ambidexterity with both the condensing lens and the depressor greatly facilitates the technique. The anatomic configuration of the patient's face usually determines whether the right or left hand is used. A gentle touch during indentation yields the best results.

Instrumentation. Binocular indirect ophthalmoscope, condensing lens (20 D and 30 D), scleral depressor (indentor), topical ophthalmic mydriatic solutions.

Technique. Maximally dilate each eye with topical mydriatic solutions. Recline the well-dilated patient, being sure to allow for enough room at the patient's head for unrestricted examiner movement around it. Perform BIO before scleral indentation to identify fundus areas warranting further study.

In preparation for superior retinal examination, stand at the patient's right side. Hold the depressor between the left thumb and index finger, with the middle finger placed along its shaft, and ask the patient to look downward. Locate the superior lid fold, which corresponds to the top of the tarsal plate, and place the depressor tip at this point with its curve directed toward the globe (Fig. 3A). Ask the patient to slowly look backward just beyond the straight up position, allowing the depressor to maintain its lid position as it follows the eye back into the orbit (Fig. 3B, C). The depressor is now positioned perpendicular to with its tip tangential to the globe. Place the depressor between 7 (ora) and 14 mm (equator) from the limbus along the side of the globe corresponding to the area of regard and apply gentle pressure. If the patient is uncomfortable, too much pressure is probably being applied, the depressor is not tangential, or you are indenting too far anteriorly.

With the depressor in position, tilt your torso to the right. Shine the indirect beam into the pupil, directing it superiorly, attempting to place the depressor tip and the light on the same observation axis. Standing 180 degrees away, observe the overall red reflex and note the presence of a darkened alteration to the reflex corresponding to the depressor position. Practice finding this reflex change using only the BIO and the depressor. Place the condensing lens in front of the eye's darkened reflex area, follow the depressor shaft into the eye, and look for an elevation of the retina at the opposite side of the lens. If not present, do not add any additional pressure. First, scan the adjacent fundus, adding a little movement to the depressor for easier recognition. If still unsuccessful, reposition the light or the depressor, making sure that gentle pressure is being applied tangentially, not perpendicularly, to the globe.

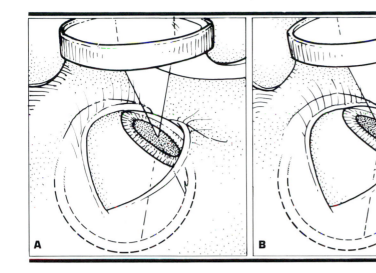
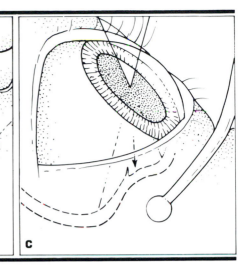

1. (above) **A.** Even with extreme gaze and maximum dilation, some anterior fundus tissue cannot be seen with the BIO alone. **B.** Scleral indentation displaces tissue inwardly to place it onto the examiner's axis of observation. **C.** The area of regard is placed along the sloping edge of the indented tissue for different viewing perspectives.

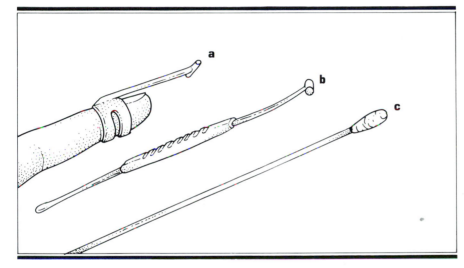

2. (left) Three common designs for scleral depressors are the (a) thimble-design, (b) double-ended flat and (c) cotton-tipped applicator.

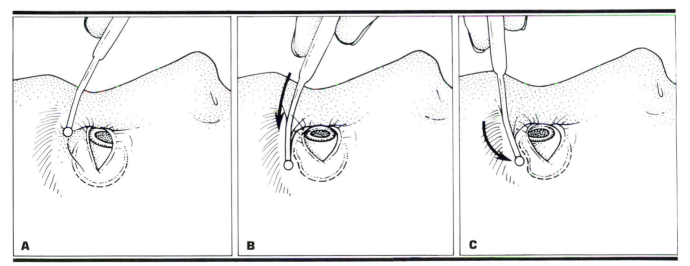

3. A, B, C. The depressor is placed at the upper lid's superior tarsal plate margin and follows the globe backward, remaining in this position.

Attempt to maintain a common axis between the BIO, condensing lens, pupillary center of rotation, and the depressor (Fig. 4). If the elevation is seen, but not in the proper position, move the depressor opposite to the direction you want the visualized elevated area to move, or ask the patient to look into that position of gaze. To see the ora serrata have the patient look further backward toward his or her forehead and your depressor. To view more posteriorly, instruct the patient to partially lower the eyes. During the learning process, make correcting movements with the depressor horizontally and vertically, eventually progressing to oblique corrective movements. Reposition the plane of the patient's face to assist in bypassing anatomical obstructions. For example, a patient with a prominent frontal bone will require the chin elevated to tip the frontal bone out of the way for inferior fundus viewing (Fig. 5).

Each circumferential placement of the depressor usually allows for the visualization of 1½ clock hours of the fundus. The need for repositioning of the depressor with each clock hour to be examined depends upon the age of the patient and his or her accompanying tissue flaccidity. With an older patient with flacid lids, attempt to move the depressor one additional clock hour by sliding the depressor without the patient's refixation. For additional circumferential examination, reposition the depressor at the desired position(s). With younger patients having firmer orbital texture, reposition the depressor for each clock position.

To perform inferior fundus indentation, ask the patient to initially look upward toward his or her forehead. Place the depressor at the inferior-most edge of the lower tarsal plate, and then ask the patient to look straight ahead or downward keeping the chin level or tilted slightly upwards (Fig. 6A). As the eye returns downward to the straight ahead or inferior gaze position, allow the depressor to follow the globe back into the orbit (Fig. 6B). Examine the inferior fundus by clock hours in the same manner as the superior fundus.

Difficulty will arise when the 3 and 9 o'clock areas are indented. Begin as if you were going to examine the 10 or 2 o'clock position. After placement of the depressor at the edge of the superior tarsal plate, "drag" the lid around to the 9 or 3 o'clock position exerting gentle pressure (Fig. 7). If poor results occur, anesthetize the globe with a topical solution and depress directly on the scleral tissue.

Interpretation. Contrast enhancement of a retinal defect is produced because part of the incident light beam from the indirect ophthalmoscope is reflected obliquely away from the examiner's view, yielding a darker choroidal/retinal pigment epithelial background against the inner translucent retina. In addition, angular displacement may place another structure optically behind a defect, also enhancing tissue contrast. Whenever a translucent tissue is viewed obliquely, its apparent tissue density is increased resulting in increased contrast. Retinal surface irregularities leading to retinal holes, tears, or other peripheral anomalies are more easily detected when viewed from different angles produced with indentation.

Complications/Contraindication. Incomplete pupillary dilation will frequently be the cause of unsuccessful scleral indentation. Placement of the condensing lens prior to the visualization of the darkened reflex will often lead to poor depressor localization. The gentle depression of the globe must be tangential rather than perpendicular to attain the desired results. Slight discomfort may be reported by some patients during testing. Depression on the tarsal plate or too close to the limbus and ciliary body will also produce patient discomfort. Extreme gaze toward the quadrant of regard is not always needed for good anterior retina visualization. Inadequate examiner torso tilting can limit fundus views.

Proper scleral indentation is not believed to enlarge retinal holes or cause retinal detachment. Do not perform indentation on eyes that have undergone recent intraocular surgery. Use caution when depressing glaucoma patients, as IOP does increase during this technique. Do not perform depression on eyes that may have a penetrating injury, hyphema, or ruptured globe.

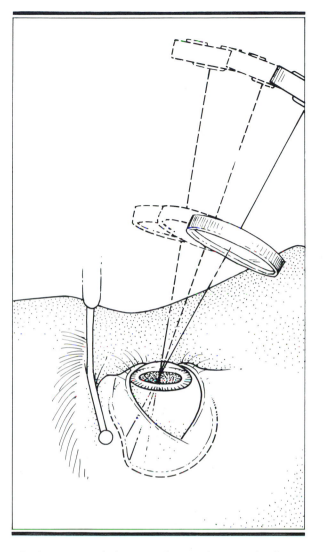

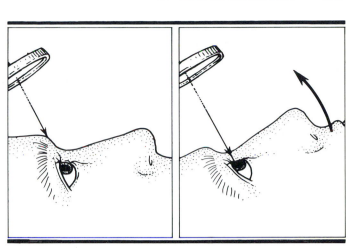

5. To avoid anatomical restrictions during examination, tilt the patient's face away from the obstructive tissue.

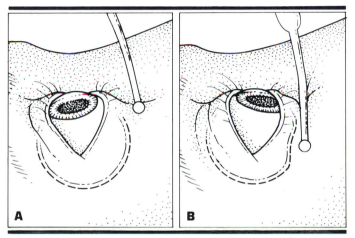

4. A common axis between the examiner, condensing lens, pupillary center, and area of indentation should be maintained during examination.

6. A, B. The depressor is placed at the lower lid's inferior tarsal plate margin and maintains this position as it follows the globe downward.

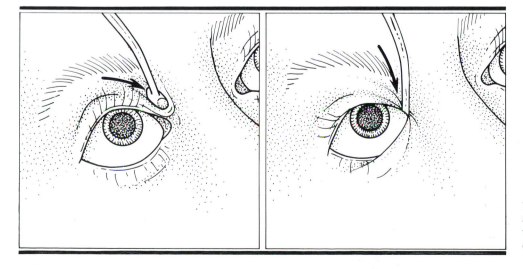

7. The horizontal meridians are examined by "dragging" the edge of the superior lid downward and then indenting.

55 Retinal Evaluation: Three-Mirror Lens

Description/Indications. The three-mirror fundus contact lens, used with the biomicroscope, allows for stereoscopic examination of the retina extending from the optic disc to the ora serrata including the vitreoretinal interface. The entire vitreous cavity can also be visualized and studied. It is helpful to have performed binocular indirect ophthalmoscopy (see p. 192) prior to three-mirror lens examination so that specific areas requiring further scrutiny can be identified.

The fundus lens' inner concave surface is placed centrally in contact with the anesthetized cornea, similar to the positioning of a gonioscopic lens (see p. 72). A viscous ophthalmic solution or gel is used as a cushioning and bonding agent. The direct contact bonds the lens and ocular surfaces, producing an optical continuity that yields a view with few distortions or reflections. The lens neutralizes the corneal refractive power, extending the biomicroscope's range of focus posteriorly to the retina (Fig. 1). Lateral and axial biomicroscopic views with this lens, through a maximally dilated pupil, are relatively independent of the patient's refractive error.

The lens' name is somewhat of a misnomer because not only does it have three mirrors for fundus viewing, but also a central viewing lens. Lens design (Fig. 2A) consists of a 64-diopter central lens power with an inner surface 7.6 mm radius of curvature, capable of displaying the central fundus 30 degrees from the axis. The optic disc and macula can be examined with this centrally positioned lens for subtle changes. The three enclosed reflecting mirrors are spaced 120 degrees apart with varying angles of inclination (73, 67, and 59 degrees) corresponding to the equatorial fundus, anterior equator to posterior ora serrata, and ora serrata/pars plana regions, respectively (Figs. 2B and C). The latter lens is also used in gonioscopy for viewing of the anterior chamber angle (see p. 72). The 73 and 67-degree mirrors are frequently used with the differential diagnosis of peripheral retinal holes, tears, or other anomalies. Selection of the desired mirror depends upon the fundus area to be examined. The resultant views are reversed in an antero-posterior direction (inverted) only, not laterally as in binocular indirect ophthalmoscopy. For example, the inferior retina is seen inverted and directly in a superiorly positioned mirror. The fundus lens–biomicroscope combination allows for a variety of magnified views using different slit widths and illumination options. The additional magnification with the three-mirror lens is a clear advantage over the binocular indirect ophthalmoscope when a detailed examination is required.

Instrumentation. Three-mirror lens, slit lamp, topical ophthalmic anesthetic, topical mydriatic solutions, cushioning solution or gel.

Technique. Maximally dilate the pupil with topical mydriatic solution(s). Anesthetize the cornea with topical 0.5% proparacaine hydrochloride solution. Place 2 or 3 bubbleless drops of methylcellulose into the clean, concave surface of the lens. Position the patient in the slit lamp, encouraging him or her to maintain contact with the slit lamp forehead rest and to not squeeze the eyes shut during testing.

Pull the slit lamp away to allow adequate room for lens placement. Instruct the patient to look upward and open the eyes widely. Hold the lens with your thumb, index and middle finger, tilting it slightly backward to retain the fluid (Fig. 3A). Depending upon the palpebral aperture size, tightness of the lids, and patient cooperation, the thumb of the opposite hand may be needed to secure the upper lid against the superior orbital rim. Place the lens on the eye with either hand; however, since the outside hand (left for the right eye, and vice versa) usually holds the lens in position during the procedure, it might be easier to perform the insertion procedure with the same hand.

Steady your hand by placing your ring finger on the inferior orbital rim while pulling the lower lid down to widen the cul-de-sac. Tuck the inferior edge of the lens into the inferior cul-de-sac (Fig. 3B) placing it in contact with the bulbar conjunctiva to assist with continued control of the inferior lid margin. Bring the top of the lens forward and ask the patient to look straight ahead (Fig. 3C). Look for a central cornea image which indicates proper alignment, and release the upper lid (Fig. 3D). Keep mild pressure on the lens during testing; however, if its placement is insecure, apply additional pressure. Watch for corneal folds or striae or induced arterial pulsation, which are indicators of excessive lens pressure. Utilize an elbow rest if additional stability is needed and secure the lens by placing your remaining fingers on the patient's cheek or on the biomicroscope's upright bar.

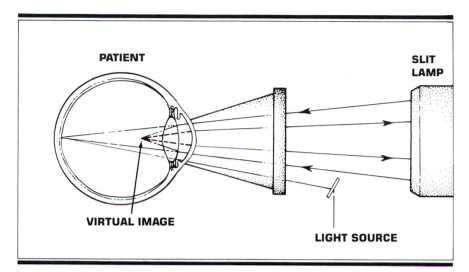

1. (left) Optical principle of the three-mirror contact lens

2. (below) **A.** Frontal view of the lens with its four optical surfaces. (1 = central posterior pole; 2 = equatorial area; 3 = anterior peripheral fundus; 4 = ora serrata, pars plana). **B.** Diagramatic projections of viewing range for each lens component. **C.** Panoramic diagram of specific viewing areas associated with each lens surface.

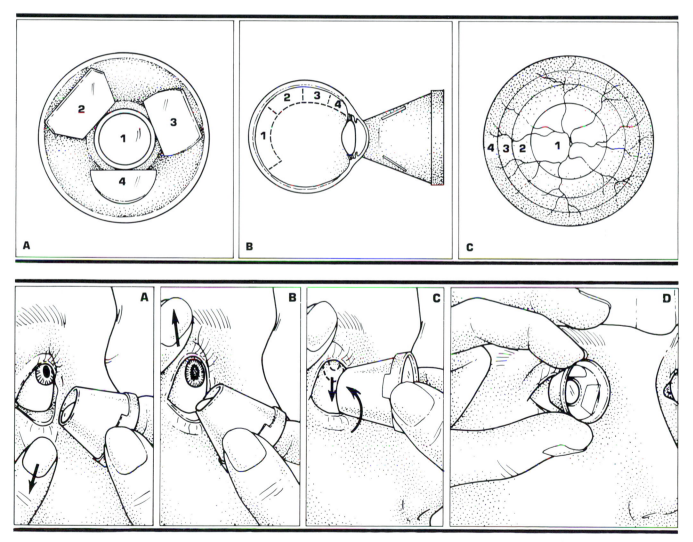

3. A. The fluid-filled lens is tilted slightly backward as the eye is approached. **B.** The lens is tucked into the inferior cul-de-sac. **C.** The top of the lens is brought up against the eye as the patient lowers his eye to look straight ahead. **D.** The thumb and index finger hold the lens securely against the eye.

Set the slit lamp magnification initially at 10X and the beam width at 3 to 4 mm with the light beam and microscope placed coaxially (Fig. 4). Instruct the patient to look straight ahead at a fixation target placed directly in front of the opposite eye. Move the slit lamp forward, keeping the beam centered in the middle of the lens. Continue moving forward through the pupillary red reflex until the posterior pole is in focus. Stop the axial movement behind the crystalline lens if central vitreous inspection is needed. Position the joystick vertically to allow for fine fingertip focusing. Examine any desired area of the central 30 degrees of the fundus, making small horizontal and vertical beam movements. Adjust magnification, beam width, light intensity and illumination angle (0 to 20 degrees), and beam rotation as needed. Ask the patient to look directly at the beam for central macular examination.

Examine the remaining posterior pole and equatorial regions by directing the light beam into the rectangular peripheral mirror. Rotate the lens on the eye using the thumb and middle or index finger to position this mirror directly opposite (180 degrees) to the retinal area to be examined (Fig. 5A). Rotate the light beam parallel to the meridian of regard (Fig. 5B). Place the illuminating column (light beam) on the same side as the mirror being used when obliquely examining the inferior retina with a superiorly positioned mirror. Place the illuminating column to the opposite side of the mirror being used when obliquely examining the superior retina with an inferiorly positioned mirror. Maintain adequate pressure on the lens with rotation movements to prevent air bubbles from entering and disrupting the view, or to keep an eyelid from sliding under the lens and squeezing it out from the eye. Attempt to eliminate acquired bubbles with lens rotation, tilting, and gentle pressure. Remove and reinsert the lens if obstructive bubbles persist. Use the same procedure with the square mirror when examining the peripheral retina from the equator to the vitreous base. Use the small semicircular mirror with wide dilation to expose the vitreous base, ora serrata/pars plana, and lens zonular areas, as well the anterior chamber angle when used for gonioscopy. Tilt the lens in the same direction as the specific

examining mirror to extend its peripheral range of view (Fig. 6A), or ask the patient to look in the opposite direction as the mirror to also extend the range (Fig. 6B). Pull back on the joystick slightly to examine the overlying vitreous.

Remove the fundus lens by asking the patient to look upward and blink firmly; or alternatively, ask the patient to continue to fixate straight ahead as you grasp the lens, while with the opposite hand's thumb you press on the globe at the lens' inferotemporal edge. Press through the patient's lower lid to ensure cleanliness (Fig. 7). Lightly irrigate the cul-de-sac areas with sterile ophthalmic saline solution after lens removal (see p. 130) to remove the residual cushioning solution. Clean the lens' concave surface with mild soap and water and dry gently with a soft tissue or cloth. Do not immerse the entire lens underwater. Inform the patient that he or she may experience some temporary blur and mild irritation during the remainder of the day. No prophylactic treatment is needed.

Interpretation. The three peripheral mirrors yield an image that is reversed in an anterior–posterior direction (Fig. 5B). As you move peripherally on the mirrored surface or "climb the mirror," new fundus tissue will appear on the inner edge of the lens.

Contraindications/Complications. Apprehensive, young, or poorly fixating patients may make this procedure difficult to perform. Inadequate pupil dilation or significant media opacities can all hinder success. Patients with surgical wounds, pathologic epithelial keratopathies, possible perforating injuries, or recent significant blunt trauma injury, should not be examined with this contact technique. The cushioning solution frequently causes punctate staining or haze, affecting corneal transparency; therefore, photography or other noncontact procedures should be completed prior to three-mirror evaluation. IOP is temporarily decreased following fundus lens use, also necessitating that IOP measurement be performed first. Minor corneal abrasions are possible with poor technique. A vasovagal reflex is possible with compressive procedure of the globe.

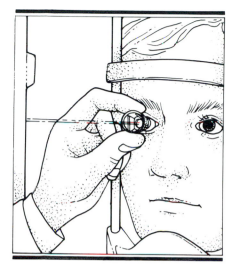

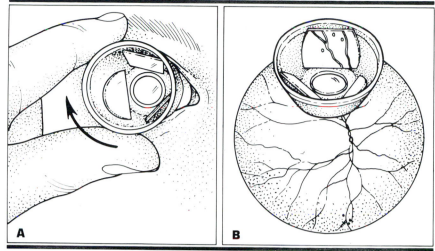

4. The light beam is directed centrally into the lens and focused on the retina.

5. A. Fingertip rotation of lens is done while maintaining adequate pressure against the eye. **B.** The biomicroscope's beam is directed into the lens mirror positioned at 12 o'clock to produce an inverted image of a 6 o'clock fundus lesion.

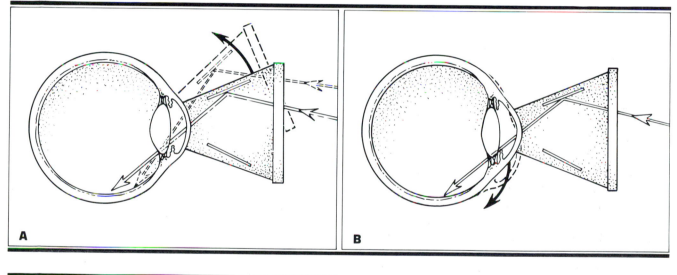

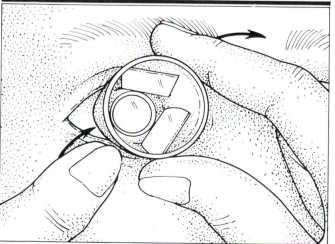

6. (above) **A.** The lens is tilted opposite in direction to the area being examined in order to extend the view anteriorly. **B.** Alternate method: The patient is asked to look slightly opposite in direction to the employed mirror to extend the anterior range of view.

7. (left) Lens suction can be broken by indenting the globe at the lens' inferotemporal edge.

56 Hruby Lens Examination

Description/Indications. The Hruby lens is a −58.6 diopter plano/concave lens mounted on the slit lamp that extends the microscope's focal range posteriorly to the retinal plane. By effectively neutralizing the eye's refractive power, this system results in an erect, stereoscopic, virtual image located in the anterior segment near the posterior lenticular surface (Fig. 1). The iris, located anterior to the lens image, acts as a diaphragm or field stop limiting or extending the stereoscopic field of view.

The major function of the Hruby lens is the noncontact examination of the optic disc, macula, posterior pole, and central vitreous. Prefocused or focusable Hruby lenses are available on specific slit lamps. The easily accessible, noncontact features of this lens make it useful in many situations. Reflections off the lens and the eye's anterior surface can produce bothersome aberrations.

Instrumentation. Hruby lens, slit lamp, topical mydriatic solutions.

Technique. Dilate the patient's pupils with mydriatic solution(s). Position the patient comfortably at the slit lamp with instructions to always keep the forehead in contact with the headstrap. Insert the post of the Hruby lens into the slotted sliding track with the concave lens surface facing the patient (Fig. 2). The Zeiss slit lamp has a self-adjusting Hruby lens that swings down into place and is operational after pushing a small release button on the mechanism arm (Fig. 3). Instruct the patient to fixate straight ahead with the nontested eye, while positioning the lens as close to the tested eye as possible (approximately 10 to 20 mm). Make initial adjustments with the gross movements of the slit lamp, and refinements with subtle movements of the Hruby lens handle (Fig. 4). Position the slit lamp joystick in the vertical position, allowing for fine focus adjustments during the examination with your fingertips. Adjust the slit beam to a 2 to 3-mm width, in direct alignment with the center of the Hruby lens; set magnification at 6X or 10X; and set illumination intensity to a moderate level. Move the slit lamp forward, maintaining lens focus and centration of the pupillary red reflex. Pass through the crystalline lens making note of any opacities seen with the induced retroillumination. Continue the movement forward through the vitreous until retinal tissue and blood vessels are clearly in focus.

Make fine adjustments by varying the beam width and height, magnification, illumination intensity, and the angle of illumination (0 to 10 degrees) to improve the image. Make fine adjustments also with the Hruby lens focusing handle. Control fixation with the slit lamp fixation light or with another fixation light or target. Position the latter target beside your ear on the nontested eye's side. Move the fixation target to centrally position the desired area for examination, noting that the ocular tissue in view will move in the opposite direction as the target movement. Continue to make fine joystick focusing adjustments during the exam, remembering that the more centrally positioned the red reflex and the smaller the lens distance to the cornea, the better the stereoscopic view.

Pull back on the joy stick to place the vitreous in focus when examination is desired.

Interpretation. The resultant Hruby lens image is erect, stereoscopic, and magnified. This provides for an adequate examination of the optic disc, macula, and central retinal tissue and lesions.

Complications/Contraindications. Patient's poor fixation, slit lamp positioning difficulties, poor glare tolerance, limited dilation, and significant media opacities all can yield poor results or limited success. The multiple optical interfaces of this system allow for fair to good views due to induced reflections and aberrations. Consider using a fundus contact lens or 90-D lens if the Hruby lens views are unacceptable.

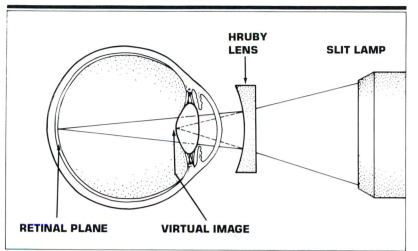

1. Optical principles of Hruby lens.

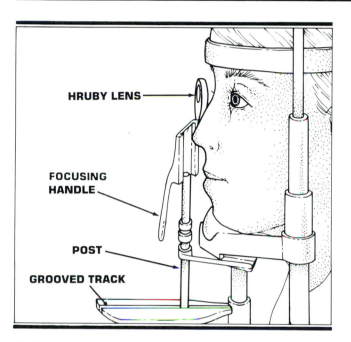

2. The focusable Hruby lens is placed in slide track and then adjusted for proper positioning.

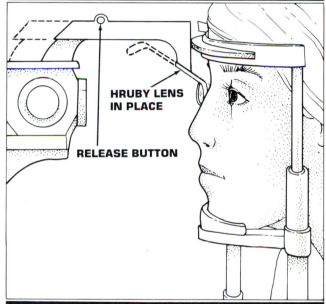

3. The self-focusing, slit-lamp-mounted Hruby Lens (Zeiss model) requires the button be pushed to release the lens bar, followed by downward rotation of the lens.

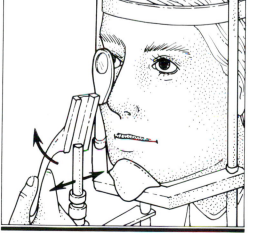

4. To decrease the lens vertex distance, pull backward on the handle; to increase vertex distance, push inward.

57 90-Diopter Lens Examination

Description/Indications. 90-diopter lens evaluation provides for a noncontact, stereoscopic, well-illuminated view of the retinal posterior pole and corresponding vitreous. It is an alternative procedure to the Hruby lens (see p. 208) and the retinal three-mirror lens (see p. 204). As with binocular indirect ophthalmoscopy (see p. 192), a high plus-powered ophthalmic condensing lens is used to focus diverging illuminated posterior segment light rays to form an aerial image. This image is located between the lens and the biomicroscope oculars. The resultant optical system (Fig. 1) provides the examiner with a magnified, real, inverted, reversed image. The image's small size requires the variable magnification capabilities of the biomicroscope for detailed examination. The auxillary condensing lens used is double aspheric, optically coated, and most frequently hand-held. The asphericity produces fewer optical aberrations and more uniform illumination.

Clear and yellow-coated lenses are available in powers of +60, +78, and +90 D, with the +90 D presently the most popular. The yellow tint eliminates ultraviolet and shortwave (blue and violet) visible wavelengths. Recent studies demonstrate that this reduces patient glare sensitivity as well as the potential for retinal photochemical damage. The resultant field of view of the 90 D lens, which is theoretically 70 degrees but in clinical practice approximates 30 to 40 degrees, depends upon the biomicroscope beam width, magnification, and the patient's pupil diameter. Successful lens alignment requires visual axis centration, proper and stable vertex distancing and lens tilting, along with continuous minor readjustment of the lens throughout the procedure. Pupil dilation is required, with the patient experiencing a moderate amount of glare during the procedure.

The hand-held, noncontact aspect of this technique allows for ease of performance, as well as a simple procedure for interruption or discontinuation. A steady lens holder is available as an alternative lens positioning technique. The 90-D lens can be used for routine posterior pole examination with cooperative patients, apprehensive patients, young individuals, recent postoperative patients, infected or inflamed eyes, and/or acute posttraumatized globes, which may all disallow the use of other more involved contact-type examination techniques.

Aside from its noncontact advantage, it also provides for a field of view three to four times larger than that of the Hruby lens, and also for easier lens adjustment to reduce induced glare and reflection. High-quality stereoscopic disc evaluation and posterior pole disease examination are both possible with this technique.

Instrumentation. Biomicroscope, condensing lens (60, 78, or 90 D), topical mydriatic solutions, optional steady lens holder.

Technique. Maximally dilate the patient's pupils. Comfortably position the patient at the biomicroscope with instructions to keep the forehead pressed up against the forehead rest. Adjust the slit beam to a 2 to 3-mm width, moderate illumination, and at either 6X or 10X magnification. Reduce the beam width and height if patient discomfort is a problem. Align the biomicroscope directly in front of the eye to be examined. Aim the light source at the cornea perpendicularly or up to 10 degrees off-axis, and move it to within a few inches of the eye. This should produce a large retroilluminated red pupillary reflex. Instruct the patient to fixate straight ahead with the opposite eye looking past your ear, or to fixate the properly positioned biomicroscope fixation light. Grasp the lens perimeter with your thumb and index finger. Viewing from outside the biomicroscope, introduce and center either surface of the double aspheric +90-D lens directly in front of the patient's eye at a distance of approximately 1 to 2 cm (½ inch). Stabilize the lens holding your hand against the patient's cheek (Fig. 2A), the slit lamp upright bar, or the headstrap with the remaining fingers. Use your middle finger to secure the top eyelid and the ring finger for the bottom lid against the orbital rim (Fig. 2B) if an adequate palpebral aperture width cannot be maintained by the patient.

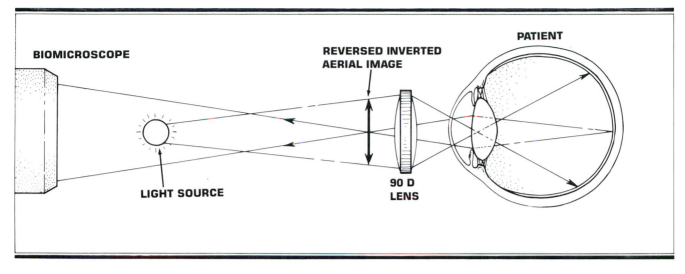

1. 90-Diopter lens optical principles

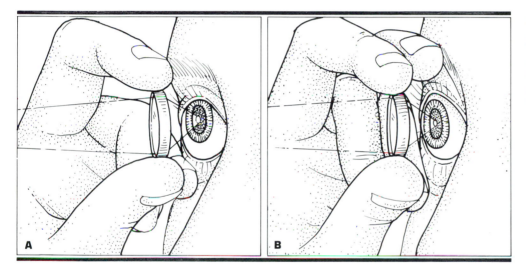

2. A. The lens is positioned and stabilized by resting the fingertips on the patient's cheek. **B.** The lens is stabilized and the eyelids are secured open with the finger tips.

While viewing through the oculars, pull back on the slit lamp joystick until the narrowed red reflex beam is focused on the retina. As with the BIO, make minor lens adjustments in the centration, tilt, and vertex distance of the condensing lens to improve the image. Gradually widen the slit beam as much as the patient will tolerate without creating added problems with reflection or discomfort. Place the joystick in the upright position to allow for fine focusing. Scan the fundus with lateral and vertical movements of the joystick. Do this in a systematic manner for all nine cardinal meridians. One suggested technique (Fig. 3) is to begin at the optic disc, move the beam inferiorly with the joystick or vertical knob, and track the superior vascular arcade and surrounding retina around temporally. After reaching the lens' temporal limit without patient eye movements, move the light beam superiorly and then track the inferior arcade back toward the disc. Examine the nasal retina next, and then finally direct the beam toward the macular area. To extend your views more anteriorly, ask the patient to look in each direction of the remaining posterior retina to be viewed, tilting the lens as fixation changes.

Tilt the lens to the left with left gaze and to the right with right gaze. Tilt the inferior edge inward and closer to the globe with upgaze (Fig. 4A). Tilt the superior edge inward and closer to the eyebrow with downward gaze, retracting the upper lid as needed (Fig. 4B). Pull back on the joystick for examination of the overlying vitreous. Angle the light beam for better viewing if needed.

Interpretation. As with binocular indirect ophthalmoscopy the resultant reversed, inverted lens image takes some time to adapt to. It is only the lens view itself that is different, as the quadrant that you are illuminating and examining is the quadrant being seen.

Complications/Contraindications.   Photophobic patients greatly restrict the quality and length of examination time. Proper placement of the condensing lens and a reasonable exposure time to the illuminating light source produces no danger to the ocular tissue. Unsteadiness may be resolved by using the available steady mount lens holder.

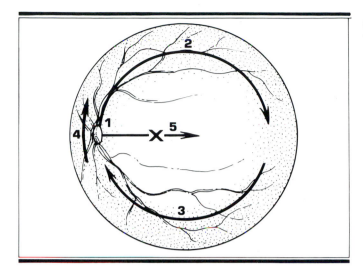

3. After examining the optic disc, scan the fundus in a systematic manner as illustrated.

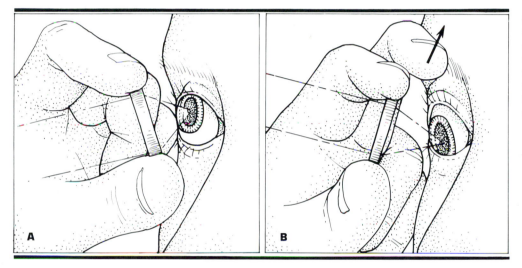

4. A. The lens is tilted backward with upgaze to view superior retina more anteriorly. **B.** The lens is tilted downward and the upper lid secured against the superior orbital rim to view inferior retina more anteriorly.

58 Fundus Drawing

Description/Indications. A fundus diagram or drawing is used to illustrate and record retinal conditions and associated vitreous anomalies. It is especially useful in illustrating conditions such as large retinal detachments that occupy areas too large in size to be documented by a single photograph. The technique of fine detailed fundus drawing or retinal diagramming is developed with practice, patience, and being a "stickler for detail." Mapping out a complete fundus appearance requires sound binocular indirect ophthalmoscopy (see p. 192) and scleral indentation (see p. 200).

Fundus drawings assist the novice practitioner in mastering the concept of the inverted, reversed, and smaller image created with binocular indirect ophthalmoscopy (BIO). An accurate drawing is the result of a systematic and thorough fundus examination utilizing good spatial orientation skills. It requires that the examiner be precise in his or her descriptions and use the universal color code for fundus drawings that allows other practitioners to understand them. These detailed geographic recordings are excellent for publication or for future review, and may prove invaluable in situations where media opacification occurs between the office visit and scheduled surgery.

The standard fundus drawing chart (Fig. 1A) provides a graphic, anatomic skeleton upon which normal and abnormal ocular tissue conditions are located and recorded. Projection of the eye's spherical surface onto this flat plane recording sheet produces a disproportionate amount of area alloted for the peripheral ocular tissue (Fig. 1B), yielding lateral and circumferential distortion. Since fundus drawing is commonly performed with peripheral retinal anomalies, this works in the examiner's favor for additional drawing space, but actual dimensions must be kept in perspective when reviewing the total picture. Three concentric circles on the standard chart circumferentially designate subdivisions of the fundus. The inner or equatorial circle, which in a three-dimensional drawing would actually have the largest diameter, encloses the posterior pole (disc, macula, and major vasculature). The middle circle represents the posterior border of the ora serrata and the termination of retinal photorecep-

tors. Between the inner and middle circle is the peripheral retina, which in actuality makes up 30 to 40% of the entire retina. The outer circle represents the anterior limit of the fundus (pars plana) visible to the examiner with scleral indentation. This area is not routinely examined by the general practitioner.

The recording chart has other helpful subdivisions, increasing the accuracy of the fundus representation. Roman numerials (I to XII) or numbers (1 to 12) are positioned to designate the clock hours around the perimeter of the drawing, with accompanying radial lines directed toward the posterior pole running through the concentric circles. Lesions can thus be described by clock hour and anterior–posterior fundus position. These radial lines also allow for superior and inferior fundus delineation (above and below the 3 and 9 o'clock positions) as well as temporal and nasal (left or right of the 12 and 6 o'clock positions). The point at which the 12 to 6 and 3 to 9 o'clock lines would cross if extended designates the fovea or center of the diagram. In the upper-right-hand corner of the chart (the XII end) is the designation of OD or OS. In a corner at the opposite end of the chart (the VI end) are the inverted and reversed words "inverted image." When the recording chart is positioned for use, these words can be read normally when standing at the patient's feet and looking toward his or her head. There is additional space designated on the chart for the patient's name and date.

Regardless of which eye is being examined on a reclined patient, the chart is always positioned with the XII (12) closest to the patient's feet and the VI (6) closest to the head (Fig. 2). To gain a better perspective as to actual in vivo fundus dimensions and orientation, the examiner should designate retinal distances using the common nonlinear measurement of the disc diameter (DD). An 18 to 20-diopter condensing lens provides an 8-DD view (Fig. 3). The equator is 6 DD from the fovea and also 2 DD anterior to the vortex vein ampullae. Between the equator and the ora serrata, enclosing the peripheral retina, is a 4-DD distance. Comparing the eye to the chart, the distance between each clock hour at the equator is approximately 6 DD, whereas, at the ora it is approximately 3 DD.

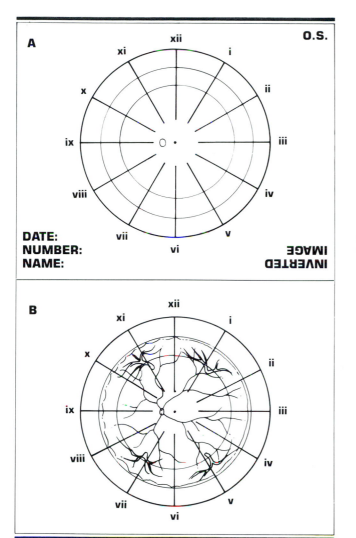

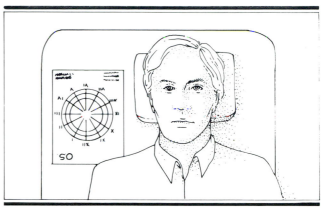

2. The fundus chart is positioned at the patient's right shoulder with the XII designated position closest to his or her feet.

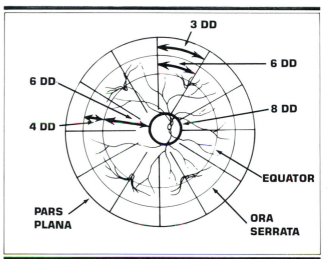

1. A. An example of standard fundus drawing chart. **B.** The peripheral fundus has a disproportionate amount of space allotted to it, requiring the examiner to place it in proper overall perspective.

3. Disc diameter (DD) measurements provide for a more realistic overview of actual fundus distances. A 20-diopter condensing lens has a field of view of approximately 8 DD.

Instrumentation. Binocular indirect ophthalmoscope (BIO), condensing lenses, scleral depressor, BIO recording charts, clipboard, common lead pencil, colored pencils or markers (red, black, blue, green, yellow, brown), topical ophthalmic mydriatic solutions.

Technique. Perform a complete fundus examination with the BIO and any other fundus viewing technique required for detailed assessment. Use a higher-powered condensing lens with its larger field of view when extensive retinal tissue involvement exists.

To prepare for fundus drawing, recline the well-dilated patient in the examination chair or on a retinal examination table. Secure the recording sheet to a clipboard with the Roman numeral XII facing the patient's feet and VI closest to the head, which is effectively inverting and reversing the chart. Place the clipboard beside the patient's right ear on the examination table or on a separate table. Left-handed examiners may choose to place the board to the left side of the patient's head.

First, document any significant posterior pole findings. Stand at the head of the chair or table looking down at the patient (Fig. 4) placing yourself in an inverted and reversed position relative to the patient. Begin with the right eye if both eyes are to be diagrammed. Ask the patient to fixate straight up at the ceiling. Lean slightly over the patient and using the BIO, observe the fovea seen to your left and the optic disc to your right in the condensing lens. Direct the patient's fixation to your left ear, examining the nasal disc area and beyond, and record directly on the chart just as seen. Direct his or her fixation to your right ear, examining the temporal disc and macula areas, and record. Direct fixation to your chin for superomacular viewing, and to your forehead for inferomacular viewing. This technique should provide a view of the central posterior pole region. Record your findings directly onto the chart, drawing them exactly as seen in your condensing lens view. Place a red dot or cross in the foveal area, inferotemporal to the disc, if this area is normal. Do not attempt to draw C/D ratios or other disc anatomy from BIO viewing as there are other more accurate instruments for this.

Examine the equatorial and oral areas using the following technique for each clock hour of the fundus. Stand 180 degrees away from the area to be examined and ask the patient to look toward the same area under examination. Record your findings on the area of the chart closest to you and corresponding to 180 degrees away from the quadrant examined (Fig. 5). For example, to examine the patient's right eye at the 2 o'clock position, stand on the patient's right side at his or her 8 o'clock position, ask the patient to look up and to the left toward 2 o'clock, and examine this area. Record your findings at the Roman numerial II chart area (8 o'clock position) on the chart exactly as seen in the lens. Remember that as you scan peripherally toward the ora, new retinal tissue will appear in the condensing lens closest to you at the near side of the lens. With each view, concentrate not only on retinal tissue, but also on any overlying vitreous changes. Continue in a systematic fashion to scan and examine each clock hour starting posteriorly and moving toward the ora serrata, viewing from 180 degrees opposite to the examined area. Complete examination will require you to circle the patient's head. Repeat the oral region examination with the scleral depressor for any areas with incomplete views. Record all initial findings in regular lead pencil for ease of correction. Draw and color all necessary findings (Fig. 6) using the universal color code (*see* Color Plate 58–6). Draw only the retinal vessels that are specifically helpful to the fundus description. It is usually easier to draw the required vasculature from the far periphery posteriorly.

Repeat the entire procedure for the left eye if indicated.

Interpretation. The composite drawing can illustrate any normal and abnormal finding seen in the fundus. An example of fundus drawing is presented (Fig. 7).

Complications/Contraindication. Prolonged fundus viewing of a single area to study detail should be avoided. The ANSI standard states that no continuous view of one area is to exceed 40 seconds using a setting of ½ voltage. Scleral indentation should be performed gently and avoided when contraindicated (see p. 202).

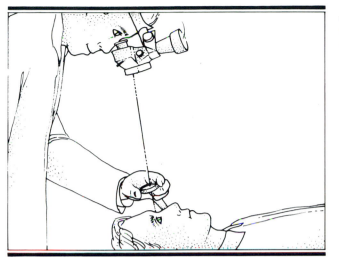

4. By standing at the patient's head and changing spatial orientation, the condensing lens' reversed and inverted image can effectively be nullified for simpler viewing.

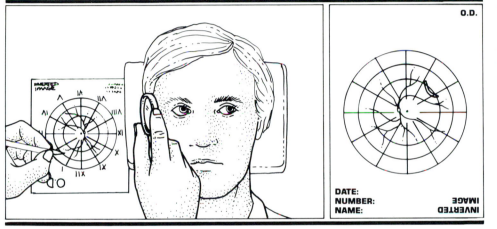

5. Direct the BIO light beam from 180 degrees away from the retinal quadrant under examination (here, the patient's right eye), and ask the patient to look toward the same examined quadrant.

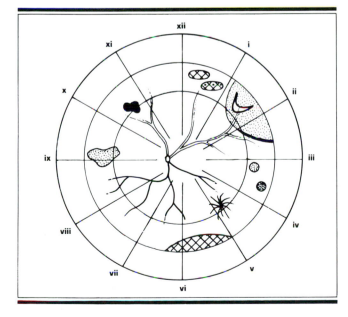

6. The fundus drawing color coding system. (*See* Color Plate 58–6 for the universal color chart.)

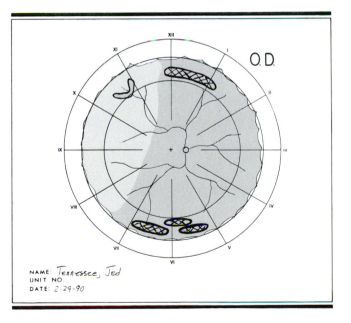

7. A fundus drawing example: retinal tear with detachment. (*See also* Color Plate 58–7.)

59 Amsler Grid Test

Description/Indications. Amsler grid testing is used to examine for and monitor functional disturbance(s) to the central visual field, 10 degrees on all sides of fixation. It is useful in detecting central and paracentral scotomas and distortion. The standard Amsler chart consists of a perfectly squared, white-lined grid pattern superimposed on a dull black background with a central white fixation dot (Fig. 1). The squared edges, straight lines, and good contrast provide a geometric design in which the eye can best identify pattern "errors" or disturbances. When the target grid is held at 28 to 30 cm (approximately 12 inches) and viewed by a patient wearing his or her habitual near corrective lens, each 5-mm square subtends a visual angle of 1 degree. The overall chart is 20 by 20 degrees square, projecting itself over the macular area (Fig. 2).

The standard Amsler grid is used the majority of the time, but a set of seven different grids (Amsler grid book) is available for use in specific circumstances. For example, chart 3 (red grid on a black background) may be used to test for a small central scotoma associated with optic neuritis. A central field weakness (relative scotoma) may manifest better with this chart due to red desaturation related to optic nerve disease (see p. 226).

A patient with unexplained visual acuity loss, despite a healthy macular appearance, requires detailed central field inspection with an Amsler grid. This test should be performed prior to pharmacologic mydriasis. The standard Amsler grid charts and instructions are frequently sent home with patients with macular disease for daily or frequent self-monitoring of inactive, active, or potential maculopathies.

Instrumentation. Amsler grid chart or book, patient's reading Rx, recording sheets.

Technique. Seat the patient comfortably and instruct him or her to wear his habitual near Rx. If the patient's near correction is not available, put the appropriate near Rx in a trial frame. Ask the patient to hold the uniformly illuminated chart in front of the testing eye at 28 to 30 cm (approximately 12 inches) (Fig. 3). Occlude the opposite eye, avoiding globe compression.

Ask the patient if he or she sees the chart's central white spot and make note of the answer. If "yes," remind the patient that central fixation must continue throughout the entire test. Continually remind the patient of central fixation during testing.

Ask the patient the following standard questions and note the responses:

1. Do you see the white spot in the center of the squared chart?
2. While you are looking only at the spot, do you also see all four corners of the chart at the same time?
3. While you are still looking at the spot, do you see an uninterrupted, even network of lines and squares; or do you see spots, holes, or any blurry or missing lines?
4. While you continue to look at the spot, are all the vertical and horizontal lines straight and parallel or are they distorted or wavy? Are all the small squares equal in size and perfectly regular?
5. Still looking at the white spot, do you see anything else; like vibrations, shining, colors, tint, or wavering lines?
6. Still looking at the white spot, at what distance from this center point do you see the blur or distortion(s)? How many boxes away is it and how many boxes are involved?

Record all significant data. Switch the occluder to the other eye and repeat the questions. In the case of subtle grid changes, alternately cover each eye and ask the patient to compare.

If the patient calls the office reporting any changes on his or her Amsler grid, schedule an examination within the next 24 to 48 hours.

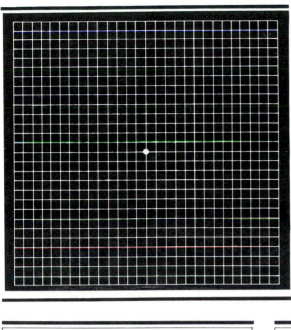

1. Standard Amsler grid testing chart (Chart 1).

2. Amsler grid tests the majority of the macular area.

3. Patient holds uniformly illuminated Amsler chart at 28 to 30 cm wearing habitual near corrective lens while occluding the opposite eye.

Interpretation. If the patient answers yes to question 1, then there is no central scotoma; move on to question 2. If the answer is "yes, but it's blurred," then there may be a relative central scotoma. Ask the patient to describe the extent of central grid involvement and move to question 2. If the answer is no, then there probably is a dense central scotoma. Switch to Chart 2 (Fig. 4) for the last five questions, since it has two diagonal white lines that cross in the center of the chart where the white spot would be. This should allow the patient to estimate where the center of the grid is for fixation purposes as the other questions are asked. The validity of the grid test decreases when poor central fixation is present.

If the answer to question 2 is yes, then continue on to 3. If the answer is no, then other visual field testing is indicated.

If the answer to question 3 is no, then continue on to 4. If the answer is yes, then relative or absolute juxta-central and paracentral scotoma(s) exist (Fig. 5). Have the patient point to and describe the defect(s). The patient may use the black on white recording grid sheets to better demonstrate them. Chart 4 has spots with no lines, which may be helpful in localizing scotomas.

If the answer to question 4 is yes, then continue to 5. If the answer is no, metamorphopsia is present.

Ask the patient to localize the area(s) of metamorphopsia. Use the patient recording grid sheets for documentation or ease of reporting. Chart 5, which has one-directional lines capable of being oriented horizontally or vertically, may assist in identifying the involved areas. Chart 6, which has doubling of the Amsler grid lines horizontally along the reading axis, may also be helpful with metamorphopsia testing.

If the answer to question 5 is no, then continue on to 6. If the answer is yes, then entopic phenomena may be present as an early indicator of maculopathy.

Question 6 has probably been answered by this stage. The goal is to localize the retinal problem. Chart 7 may help with fine central changes as it has duplication and finer subdivision of the central Amsler grid.

Record all desired information.

Complication/Contraindications. This is a noninvasive test that presents no risk to the patient. Poor central fixation or reduced near-point acuity will markedly decrease the test's reliability. The patient's understanding of the test and his or her ability to relate subjective findings to the examiner also determine the test's success.

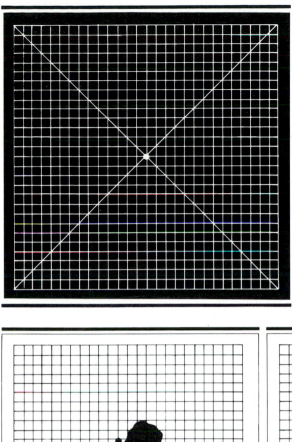

4. Chart 2: Amsler grid with diagonal lines used to aid fixation when central scotoma is present.

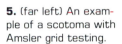

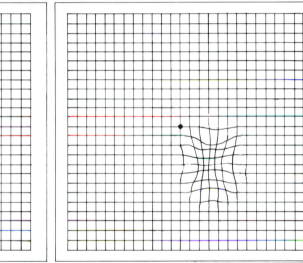

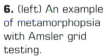

5. (far left) An example of a scotoma with Amsler grid testing.

6. (left) An example of metamorphopsia with Amsler grid testing.

60 Photostress Recovery Test

Description/Indications. The photostress recovery test, humorously dubbed the "poor man's ERG," measures the return of visual function to the macula after a timed exposure to a bright light stimulus. A test light bleaches the visual pigments to produce a subsequent decrease in visual acuity. The time of recovery to within one line of the entering visual acuity is measured, being dependent upon the resynthesis of the photoreceptor visual pigments. This process is dependent upon the metabolic ability of the involved photoreceptors, the juxtapositioned retinal pigment epithelium (RPE), and the photoreceptor–RPE complex interactions. Any disease process that disrupts photopigment resynthesis or separates the receptors and RPE could lead to an increased photostress recovery time.

The photostress recovery test is indicated when a patient presents with decreased vision and equivocal ocular findings, requiring the differential diagnosis between early optic nerve and macular disease.

Instrumentation. Penlight or transilluminator, acuity chart, watch with second hand.

Technique. Do not dilate the patient's pupils prior to the test. Determine and record the patient's best corrected visual acuities. Remove any spectacle correction. Totally occlude the involved poorer-seeing eye. Place a strong penlight or transilluminator 3 to 5 cm (1½ to 2 inches) in front of the "normal" eye (Fig. 1). Ask the patient to stare at this light for 10 seconds. Remove the light, continue to occlude the opposite eye, replace any spectacle Rx, and ask the patient to look at the distance acuity chart (Fig. 2). Have the acuity chart already set up displaying the patient's previously recorded best acuity and one line less in resolution (for example, 20/20 BVA and 20/25). Ask the patient to begin to read the letters as soon as focus returns. Time and record how long it takes for acuity to return in order to read one line less than the original best correctable visual acuity.

Occlude the previously tested eye, and repeat the same test on the opposite eye. Record your results.

Interpretation. The relative difference between recovery times in each eye is the best criterion for analyzing results. Normal recovery time is 50 to 60 seconds. Abnormal recovery time can range from 90 to 180 seconds or greater. Recovery time is age related, and therefore patients over 40 years of age will probably show some symmetric increase in "normal" recovery times.

Optic nerve disease is a conduction deficit unrelated to bleaching and regeneration of photopigments. Therefore, optic nerve disease should yield a negative photostress recovery test result. Macular disease, such as central serous choroidopathy, will show a positive photostress recovery test. A positive test may indicate the need for more advanced testing such as intravenous fluorescein angiography (see p. 228).

Validity of this test markedly decreases with acuity less than 20/80. Also, significant media opacification may yield a relative asymmetry in recovery time caused by decreased light stimulation rather than retinal disease.

Contraindications/Complications. There are no contraindications or complications with the photostress recovery test.

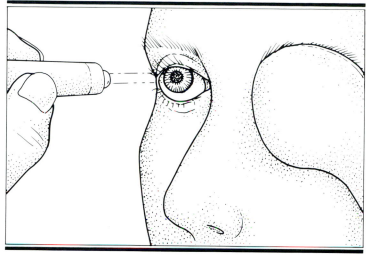

1. The nontested eye in question is occluded and a steady bright light source is presented to the opposite eye for 10 seconds.

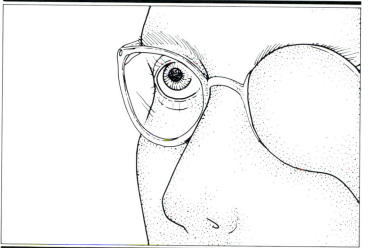

2. After replacing any spectacle correction and keeping the nontested eye occluded, the recovery time is measured for return of acuity to one line less than the original best visual acuity. The same procedure is repeated on the opposite eye.

61 Brightness Comparison Test

Description/Indications. The confirmation of optic nerve disease can be aided by a few basic in-office tests. The brightness comparison test involves the alternate presentation of a bright light stimulus to each eye followed by a series of questions on the subjective quantification of the "brightness" difference for each eye. A strong penlight, transilluminator, or binocular indirect ophthalmoscope (moderate setting) is used as the light source. A clean white, evenly illuminated card may also be used as a target. This test aids in the differential diagnosis between fundus disease and optic nerve disease when the ocular health appearance is equivocal. Optic nerve lesions usually produce a generalized depression in light sensitivity, perceived by the patient as objects appearing dimmer. Fundus disease, however, even with extensive pathology, tends not to be reported as dimmer, provided the testing light diffusely illuminates the interior of the eye.

This test is considered the subjective parallel to the swinging flashlight test for an afferent pupillary defect.

Instrumentation. Penlight, transilluminator or binocular indirect ophthalmoscope.

Technique. Occlude the patient's left eye and direct the bright light stimulus toward the right eye (Fig. 1). Ask the patient to look directly at the light with the right eye. Quickly occlude the right eye and present the identical stimulus at the same viewing distance and angle toward the left eye (Fig. 2), again asking the patient to look directly at the light. Alternately cover each eye (Fig. 3) and ask the patient if a brightness difference exists between the light stimulus as seen with each eye. Shine the light at each eye for about 1 to 3 seconds.

If the patient notices a difference in brightness, ask him or her to place a value on the level seen as the test is repeated. Present the light stimulus again, first to the healthier, better-seeing eye. Ask that if this light were worth one dollar in brightness value, then how much is the other eye's image worth? Ninety cents? Fifty cents? Present the same light stimulus to the suspicious eye and record the patient's subjective response. Record the response as RE and LE (for example, RE 100 and LE 50).

Interpretation. A definite brightness difference between the two eyes supports the suspicion that optic nerve dysfunction may be present. In the example recording of RE 100 and LE 50, this would be interpreted that the perceived brightness in the left eye is only half that of the right, lending support to the diagnosis of optic nerve disease in the left eye.

Complications/Contraindications. A marked difference in ocular media clarity between each eye could produce a false positive result. Incorrect results are possible if the light source is not strong enough to maintain stable, identical intensity during testing. Nonidentical angles of stimulus presentation or unequal testing distances may also induce error. The patient's ability to describe any difference seen can limit the test's value.

The amount or duration of the light stimulus during testing presents no danger to the patient.

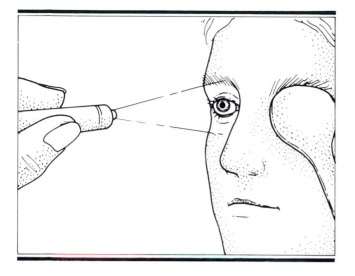

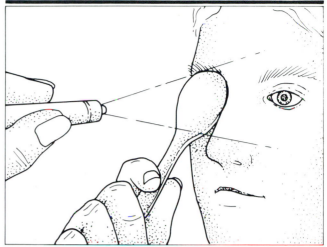

1. A bright white stimulus is presented to the patient's right eye while the left is well occluded, asking the patient to note the level of perceived brightness.

2. The patient's right eye is occluded and the identical stimulus is presented to the left eye, again asking the patient to note the level of brightness.

3. The light source is alternately presented to each eye and the patient is asked if a difference in brightness exists.

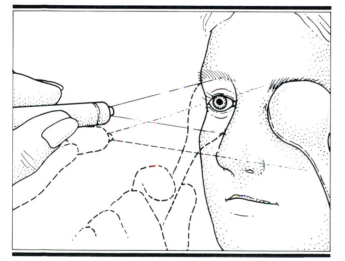

62 Red Desaturation Test

Description/Indications. The perception of certain colors frequently decreases or appears desaturated in the presence of optic nerve dysfunction. In contrast, macular disease does not usually affect gross color recognition. Red desaturation testing, along with other basic screening tests such as the brightness comparison test (see p. 224) and photo-stress recovery test (see p. 222), is performed when any unexplained loss or dysfunction of vision occurs.

The in-office screening for differences in red color perception between the patient's two eyes or in the different fields of view of one eye, may be diagnostic for optic nerve disease. The presence of optic nerve dysfunction and its accompanying diminished conduction may elevate pure cone threshold, thus acting as a filter barrier to the more sensitive cones, with a resultant decrease in color perception. An afferent pupillary defect frequently accompanies an eye that exhibits red desaturation. The level of color desaturation does not always correlate with the degree of visual impairment. Red desaturation in different areas of the visual field may be diagnostic for suspected chiasmal disease. Simultaneous field comparison of red stimuli may assist in the diagnosis.

Instrumentation. Red mydriatic solution caps or comparable red targets.

Technique

Alternating Red Comparison: Do not perform any bright light testing prior to red desaturation testing so each eye will be at an equal state of light adaption. Place the instrument stand's overhead light behind the patient and direct it forward to evenly illuminate yourself and the patient's visual field (Fig. 1). Occlude the eye in question and ask the patient to look at a red mydriatic solution cap with the "normal" eye (Fig. 2A). After a few seconds, switch the occluder (Fig. 2B) to the opposite eye, asking if there is any difference between the targets. If no definite response is given, repeat the test, asking the patient if each cap is equally as red, one is dimmer or brighter than the other, or one appears washed-out in color. Record the answer in relative value terms such as "slightly dimmer, much dimmer" and so on.

Simultaneous Testing—Foveal Versus Parafoveal Areas: An alternative method to test for central red desaturation is by unilateral presentation. Ask the patient to fixate a centrally positioned red cap with the eye in question. Hold the targets at your chest level, allowing your white lab coat to act as an even background. Present another red cap simultaneously several inches to one side of center (Fig. 3). Ask the patient to look directly at the central red cap and tell you if either the central or the peripheral cap's color is equal to or brighter than the other. Be sure that both caps are evenly illuminated and the opposite "normal" eye is occluded.

Monocular Visual Field Color Comparison: Another method of red desaturation testing is monocular visual field color perception comparisons. This is used most commonly with suspected early temporal field weakness in pituitary tumors, looking for possible quadrantic or hemispheric defects. Occlude one of the patient's eyes. Evenly illuminate yourself and the patient's field with the overhead lamp. Place two red caps approximately 8 to 12 inches apart, arm's length in front of the patient, and instruct him or her to fixate a target in between the two caps, such as your lab coat button or a properly positioned pin (Fig. 4). Ask the patient to look at the central fixation target and the decide if either red cap seem brighter or dimmer than the other. To more closely examine the superior quadrant, especially the superior temporal quadrant, keep the fixation point the same but elevate both targets to the superior quadrants (Fig. 5). Record the answers, occlude the opposite eye, and repeat the testing.

Interpretation. A positive response of a dimmer or desaturated red stimulus between eyes, especially with any subjective report of visual dysfunction, may necessitate further neurologic workup (such as meticulous pupillary, visual field, or visual evoked response testing, neurology consultation, CAT scan, or MRI).

While looking at the central red fixation cap and comparing it to the peripheral red cap, the central cap should be as red or redder than the other. If the central cap is reported as a dimmer or duller red, a central scotoma and optic nerve disease should be suspected.

In cases of pituitary tumor the temporal fields—more specifically the superior temporal fields—may exhibit characteristic weakness to red stimuli. If a positive response is given, visual field testing should be initiated.

Contraindications/Complications. As with any subjective test, the examiner's interpretation of the responses and the patient's reliability can lead to false positive or negative results. Uneven illumination of the testing objects can also introduce error.

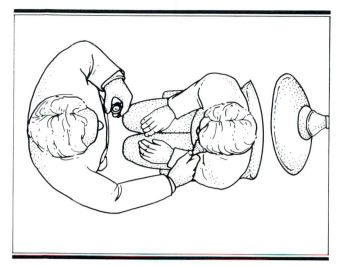

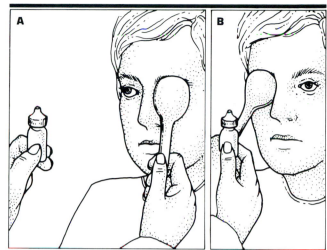

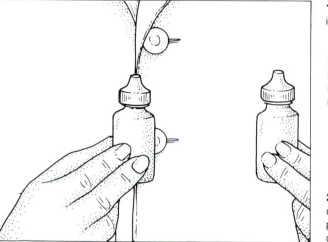

1. (above left) The examiner is centrally positioned with even illumination directed from behind the patient onto the targets.

2. A. (above right) The patient's involved eye is occluded as a red stimulus is presented to the opposite eye. **B.** The occluder is switched to the opposite eye and the identical red stimulus is presented to the involved eye.

3. (left) The nontesting eye is occluded while one red target is centrally positioned and another is placed off-center. Ask the patient to fixate centrally and state whether the center or off-center red target is brighter.

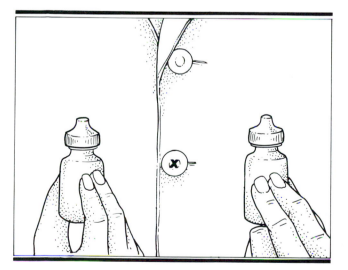

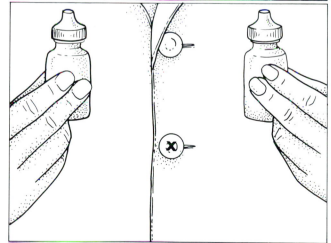

4. The patient fixates a centrally positioned fixation target between the two red caps. He or she is asked if there is a difference in redness between the caps.

5. The patient is asked to fixate centrally and to compare the brightness of the elevated red caps.

63 Fluorescein Angiography

Description/Indications. Fluorescein angiography (FA) is a diagnostic photography procedure used to detect vascular compromise to the retina and choroid and optic nerve. It may also be used to identify areas of the fundus amenable to laser treatment, and to evaluate and monitor postlaser success. FA studies the presence and extent of intra, extra, and subretinal vasculature alterations that may not be observable ophthalmoscopically or detected with other examination techniques. Many vision-threatening conditions require FA for differential diagnosis and treatment.

Fluorescein is a stable, pharmacologically inert vegetable dye. Following intravenous injection, 80% of it binds to plasma proteins, mostly albumin. The remaining 20% is free and unbound within the bloodstream and is responsible for actual fluorescence during testing. When light energy of 465 to 490 nanometers (blue light) is directed at these fluorescein molecules, they fluoresce yellow-green with a peak emission of 520 to 530 nm. A fluorescein camera (Fig. 1) has a blue excitation filter (such as the Kodak Wratten 47) through which the camera flash passes. The resultant blue light continues into the patient's eye, exciting the intraocular free fluorescein to its fluorescing nanometer level. These fundus-reflected lights (blue and fluorescent yellow-green) return out of the eye through an introduced yellow-green filter barrier (such as Kodak Wratten G 15). This filter absorbs the reflected blue light and allows only the emitted fluorescent light to be transmitted and recorded on high-speed black-and-white film in the camera.

Fluorescein's low molecular weight allows it to easily diffuse out of most of the body's capillaries, except for the normal vessels of the central nervous system, including the retinal vascular endothelium. This diffusion leads to the patient's skin becoming jaundiced in appearance for a few hours after testing and the urine becoming brilliant yellow for 24 to 48 hours.

Posterior to the retina, the choroid has fenestrated choriocapillaris endothelial cells that allow intravascular fluorescein to easily leak outward into the extravascular space, creating a relatively uniform fluorescent background during testing referred to as the *choroidal flush*. Fluorescein is incapable of perfusing through a healthy retinal pigment epithelium (RPE). Depending upon the level of melanin pigmentation, the RPE acts as a filter barrier between the retina and choroid, limiting the transmitted and visualized choroidal flush (Fig. 2). This is especially true of the macular areas where melanin is quite dense. Dropout of the RPE will conversely lead to bright areas of visible hyperfluorescence.

There are several tenets behind fluorescein angiography. Normal blood flow time in transit to and through the retina is relatively fixed, normal vascular patterns are well known, and nondiseased retinal vessels are nonpermeable. This allows the patient's fluorescein study to be compared to established standards. In contrast to the choroidal system (Fig. 3), healthy retinal blood vessels have tightly bound endothelial cells that do not allow fluorescein to leak into the extravascular space.

Instrumentation. Angiography camera and appropriate filters, ASA 400 black-and-white film (36 exposures), 35-mm color film, two camera backs (one motor driven with timer), 5 mL of 10% fluorescein dye, 5-cc syringe, 20-gauge (1½-inch) needle, 23-gauge butterfly or scalp-vein needle, normal saline, tourniquet, alcohol swabs, armrest, small bandage, standard emergency room equipment tray, emesis basin, topical ophthalmic mydriatic solutions.

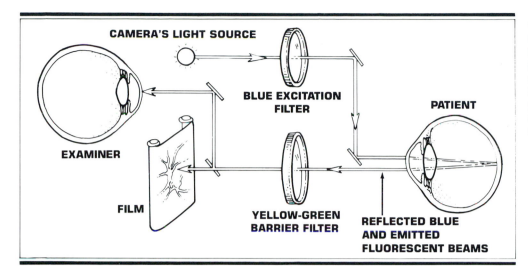

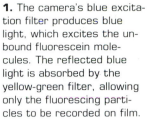

1. The camera's blue excitation filter produces blue light, which excites the unbound fluorescein molecules. The reflected blue light is absorbed by the yellow-green filter, allowing only the fluorescing particles to be recorded on film.

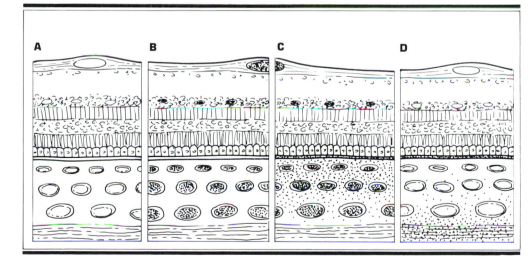

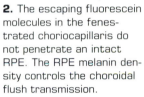

2. The escaping fluorescein molecules in the fenestrated choriocapillaris do not penetrate an intact RPE. The RPE melanin density controls the choroidal flush transmission.

3. A. Pre-fluorescein injection. **B.** Early arteriovenous phase without intravascular fluorescein. **C.** Arteriovenous phase with perfuse choroidal vessel leakage only. **D.** Late phase with extravascular fluorescein only.

Technique. Explain the purpose and procedure of the test to the patient. Mention that this is a photographic test, not an x-ray, and that the injection method is very similar to having blood drawn. Ask the patient to read and sign the fluorescein angiography consent form. Explain that immediately following the injection and up to 30 seconds afterwards, he or she may experience a brief feeling of warmth or transient nausea that will quickly pass. Dilate the patient's pupils fully with topical ophthalmic mydriatic solutions.

Focus the camera eyepiece by turning it counterclockwise to add plus power, relaxing accomodation and blurring the crosshair fixation target. Turn the eyepiece clockwise until the fine crosshairs are in sharp focus. Position the patient comfortably at the camera with a reminder that the forehead must remain against the forehead strap at all times. Focus onto the patient's fundus to ascertain that clear quality photos are possible, and observe the patient's response to the camera's bright light. Take any necessary color photos with the alternate camera back for documentation and comparison with the fluorescein photos. Make sure that the fundus area(s) to be photographed are clearly visible. Change to the motor-driven, timer camera back containing 36-exposure black-and-white ASA 400 film (such as Tri-X film). Use the self-contained high plus camera lens, low strobe power, and red-free filter to photograph a small information card containing the patient's name, date, and other information. Remove the high plus lens, adjust to the proper strobe power, and take photos (2–4) of the involved area(s) using a green (red-free) filter (such as Kodak Wratten 57 or 58). This will increase fundus contrast and identify any areas that appear to fluoresce without dye injection (autofluorescence). Decide which fundus areas will be photographed, which require blood transit studies, and which will need late shots.

Leave the camera focused on the retinal area to be examined, remove the red-free filter, insert the camera's blue excitation and yellow-green blocking filters, and adjust the strobe power to the camera's standard setting. After comfortably positioning the patient's arm on an armrest or table, have the trained or certified person administering the injection insert an intravenous, 23-gauge butterfly needle into the patient's antecubital vein. If this is not possible with these veins, the administrating individual should consider those veins in the back of the hand or the thumb side of the wrist. Inject a small amount of saline and observe to ensure that the fluorescein will not extravasate from the vein due to poor needle placement. A prepared 5-cc syringe of 10% fluorescein is then connected to the butterfly needle using short tubing.

Following a signal from the person injecting, start the camera timer simultaneously with dye injection (Fig. 4). Take a photo upon completion of the injection, which is administered at a rate of 1 cc per second (5 to 7 seconds). Begin taking photos every 1 to 2 seconds for the first 20 to 30 seconds (10 to 12 photos); and then every 10 to 20 seconds for the next minute or two (6 to 10 photos). After the completion of the venous phase, wait 8 to 10 minutes before taking any desired late shots used to reveal late fluorescein leakage, intraretinal dye accumulation, or fluorescein leakage pattern formation. During this 8 to 10-minute waiting period, take any full venous-phase photos of the opposite eye, if indicated. Take late shots of this opposite eye also if desired. If the opposite eye requires a complete fluorescein study on the same day, wait approximately 1 hour before repeating the procedure.

Remind the patient that his or her skin will appear yellow for a few hours and that urine will be yellow for 24 to 48 hours.

Interpretation. Red-free photos showing autofluorescence include retinal pigment granules, myelinated nerve fibers, and certain lipid materials, while pseudofluorescence from imperfect filters is most commonly seen at the optic disc and with drusen.

In the normal fluorescein transit study, antecubital injection of the dye bolus reaches the choroid in approximately 8 to 12 seconds by way of the short posterior ciliary arteries. The choroidal vessel pattern appears in the initial prearterial phase, followed rapidly by the expected fluorescein leakage in the choriocapillaris with its resultant choroidal flush (Fig. 5). Any cilioretinal arteries or optic disc capillaries will also fill at the same time. The intensity of the choroidal flush, being dependent on RPE melanin density, will be noticeably reduced in the darkened macular area where melanin pigment is the most dense and the fluorescent-absorbing retinal xanthophyll pigment is also abundant. The early arteriovenous phase begins immediately afterwards (10 to 15 seconds postinjection). During this phase the arteries quickly fill with fluorescein and early lamellar flow to the veins begins (Fig. 6). Fluorescein characteristically travels along the venous walls to create this lamellar effect. In the late arteriovenous phase complete artery and arteriole filling occurs along with marked venous lamellar flow (Fig. 7). The venous phase at 20 to 30 seconds exhibits maximum venous filling and reduced artery fluorescence (Fig. 8). The choroidal vessels continue to fluoresce but with reduced intensity. The normal fundus is devoid of most of the fluorescein after approximately 10 minutes. Since the entire vessel lumen is seen on angiography versus only the blood column with ophthalmoscopy, vessels will appear larger during angiography.

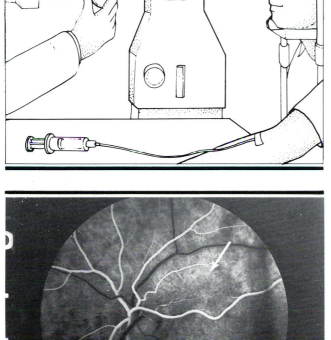

4. Set up for fluorescein angiogram.

5. (below left) In the prearterial phase a uniform choroidal background flush appears (arrows). (Courtesy of Retina Consultants, Providence, RI.)

6. (below right) In the early arteriovenous phase the arteries and arterioles fill with fluorescein (small arrow), while the veins exhibit very early lamellar flow (large arrow). (Courtesy of Retina Consultants, Providence, RI.)

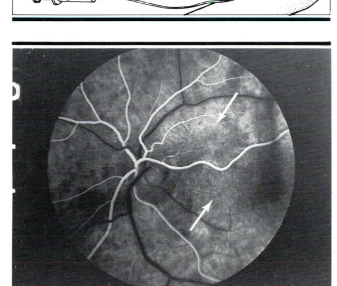

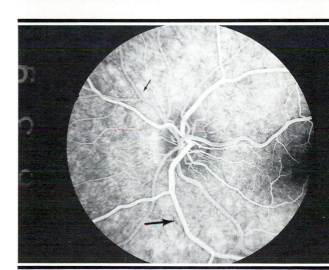

7. In the arteriovenous phase all arterial vessels are filled (small arrow), with marked lamellar flow in the veins (large arrow). (Courtesy of Retina Consultants, Providence, RI.)

8. In the venous phase maximum venous filling (large arrow) is present with reduction in arterial fluorescence (small arrow). (Courtesy of Retina Consultants, Providence, RI.)

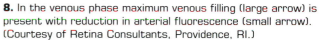

When studying the initial dye transit through the fundus, it is helpful to remember that healthy retinal vessels do not leak fluorescein and that aside from the "black" macular hypofluorescence, the remainder of the choroidal flush is evenly distributed. The examiner looks for areas of hypofluorescence caused by mechanical blockage from hemorrhage, exudates, glial tissue, or pigmentation (Fig. 9), or by vascular compromise from occlusion, nonperfusion, emboli, or arteriosclerosis (Fig. 10). The examiner also looks for areas of hyperfluorescence due to abnormal vasculature or RPE dropout. Abnormal vascular changes include vessel tortuosity, retinal or subretinal neovascularization (Fig. 11) or aneurysm. Vascular leakage may occur due to papilledema, capillary leakage, cystoid macular edema (Fig. 12) or subretinal neovascularization. RPE melanin variations also produce "window defects" with hyperfluorescence from increased choroidal flush transmission due to absence of "filtering" pigment cells.

Complications/Contraindications.   Photophobia from the camera flash, squinting, Bell's reflex, or illness from the injection greatly affect the quality of the photographs. The patient may have to be allowed to briefly close the eyes, blink more frequently when instructed, or sit back for a moment to gain composure in order to obtain at least some angiographic results.

Patients with known hypersensitivity to fluorescein should only be tested when absolutely necessary, following proper medical precautions. Performing FA on pregnant patients should be avoided unless absolutely necessary.

In decreasing order of frequency, the most common side effects reported with FA are nausea, vomiting, urticaria/pruritus, extravasation, dyspnea, and syncope. In addition, there are reported cases of more serious anaphylactic shock and myocardial infarction reactions. For patients whom the test is indicated, the benefits of preservation of vision usually far outweigh the risks involved. In any case, an emergency resuscitation kit should be in the testing room at all times.

Oral fluorescein angiography (see p. 234) may prove of benefit for patients requiring frequent repeated fluorescein studies; those with a fear of injections, inaccessible veins, or cardiovascular problems aggravated by intravenous procedures; pediatric patients; and aphakic patients.

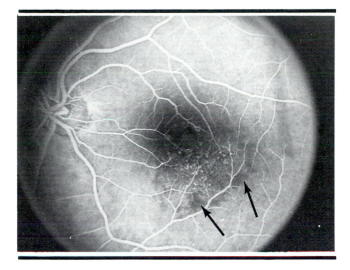

9. Hypofluorescence: diabetic circinate exudative ring blocks normal fluorescence (arrows). (Courtesy of Retina Consultants, Providence, RI.)

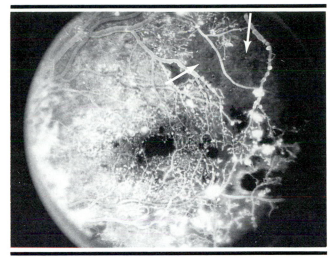

10. Hypofluorescence: diabetic patient exhibiting large areas of non-perfusion (arrows). (Courtesy of Retina Consultants, Providence, RI.)

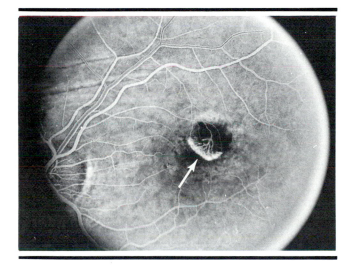

11. Hyperfluorescence: choroidal neovascular membrane (arrow) with feeder vessel. (Courtesy of Retina Consultants, Providence, RI.)

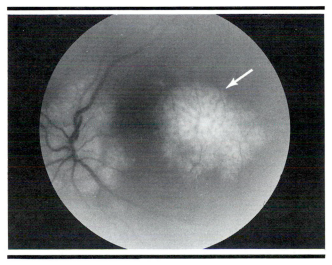

12. Hyperfluorescence: cystoid macular edema (arrow). (Courtesy of Retina Consultants, Providence, RI.)

64   Oral Fluorescein Angiography

Description/Indications. Oral fluorescein angiography is a diagnostic photographic procedure used to examine the eye for certain types of fundus leakage. This noninvasive test is a modification of the intravenous (IV) form and involves the oral administration of ophthalmic fluorescein dye followed by the photographic examination of the fundus. Although it has many similarities to, and a few advantages over, IV fluorescein angiography (FA) (see p. 228), it does not provide as much detailed information as IV angiographic studies. Its greatest value is to examine for late leakage due to conditions such as cystoid macular edema and sensory retinal detachments. When fundus vasculature dynamics or tissue detail are important, the IV method is indicated.

In comparing the different time stages of both procedures, the first visible dye transit with the oral method corresponds approximately to the IV angiographic's mid-arteriovenous phase. It takes at least 15 to 30 minutes for the orally ingested fluorescein to produce this appearance, while its 1-hour mark corresponds to the IV's late venous phase (10 minutes postinjection). Individual gastric absorption rates, recent food consumption, patient's body weight, and the total volume of fluorescein consumed, all affect the photographic results.

Oral fluorescein angiography may be indicated for children, patients with significant fear of needles, poor vein quality and access, cardiovascular risks increased with the use of IV injection, or required frequently repeated late fluorescein studies.

Instrumentation. Fundus camera with appropriate angiography filters, ASA 400 black-and-white film 24 or 36 exposure (Tri-X film), two 5-cc vials of 10% ophthalmic fluorescein, glass, ice, citrus drink, straw, topical ophthalmic mydriatic solutions.

Technique. Instruct the patient to fast for 8 hours prior to testing. Describe the procedure and have the patient sign the consent form. Dilate the patient well with topical mydriatic solution(s). Prepare a liquid citrus drink (such as Tang) over ice and add two 5-cc vials of 10% fluorescein. Increase the fluorescein volume if the patient has not fasted or if he or she has excess body weight. Have the patient remove any stainable dentures. Take any needed pretest color photos. Ask the patient to drink the beverage over several minutes through a straw to prevent lip staining (Fig. 1).

Load the camera back with ASA 400 black-and-white film (Tri-X, 36 exposure). Take red-free photos of the area(s) under investigation. Insert both the required blue excitation filter and the yellow-green filtering lens into the camera. Examine the fundus through the camera every 10 to 15 minutes looking for the first appearance of fluorescein. At this moment begin taking photos at the rate of four photos every 10 to 15 minutes for the next hour (Fig. 2).

Explain to the patient that his or her skin may appear jaundiced for the rest of the day and that the urine will be brilliant yellow for the next 24 to 48 hours.

Interpretation. The primary goal of oral fluorescein is to establish the presence or absence of fluorescein leakage. Conditions such as cystoid macular edema (Fig. 3A), retinal neovascularization (Fig. 3B), and choroidal neovascular membranes, show up quite nicely on the late-phase fluorescein studies. Scheduling the patient for more detailed studies with IV fluorescein may well be the result of this test.

Contraindication/Complications. Oral ingestion of fluorescein dye is not reported to produce any significant side effects as compared with IV fluorescein. Nausea and vomiting are possible. Proper medical precautions must be considered prior to administering this dye to a patient with a reported hypersensitivity. Denture removal will prevent staining. Use of a straw to drink the fluorescein mixture should reduce lip staining.

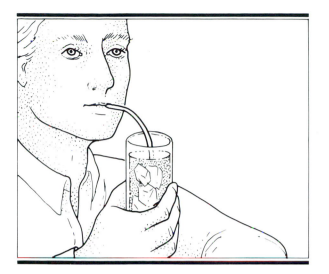

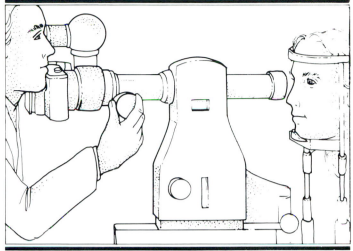

1. The patient drinks the chilled fluorescein mixture with a straw over several minutes.

2. The patient is positioned comfortably in the camera and the proper filters are inserted.

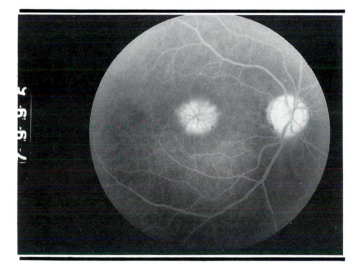

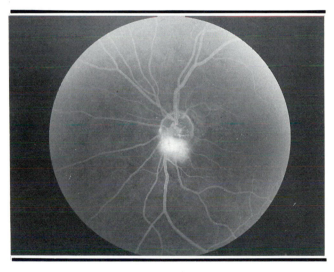

3. A. Cystoid macula edema: late photos reveal residual fluorescein leakage. (Courtesy of James E. Hunter, OD.)

3. B. Optic disc neovascularization: late photos exhibit fluorescein leakage overlying the optic disc. (Courtesy of James E. Hunter, OD.)

65 B-Scan Ultrasound

Description/Indications. B-scan ophthalmic ultrasound (echography) is a diagnostic procedure used for the detection and differentiation of ocular and orbital disorders. Its most common use is in a contact mode for the evaluation of the posterior segment in eyes with media opacification. B-scan ultrasound is also useful in management of identified lesions watching for progression. B-scan instrumentation can be modified to an immersion technique used for anterior segment study.

B-scan ophthalmic ultrasound consists of focused, short-wavelength, acoustic waves with frequencies of approximately 10 MHz. An echographic probe with an internal oval cylinder contains a laterally oscillating piezoelectric crystal near its tip, which converts electrical energy into mechanical energy. This energy is emitted as an advancing acoustic wavefront into the eye (Fig. 1A). This wavefront's intraocular and orbital velocity differs as it passes through various ocular tissues. Distinct tissues reflect, refract, and scatter sound waves in their own characteristic way. The acoustic interface reflections at adjacent tissues create recordable echoes that are affected by the angle of sound wave incidence; different degrees of absorption, scattering, and refraction; and the size and shape of each interface. The emitted sound waves enter the eye, and their reflected components are received by the probe's transducer. These waves are then amplified, filtered, and displayed as a two-dimensional echogram on a video screen (Fig. 1B). The focused beam's reflection or echo is represented as a dot on the screen with its strength indicated by its brightness. The stronger the echo, the brighter the projected dot.

The coalescence of these dots forms the B-scan's two-dimensional screen image. The echogram's horizontal axis represents tissue depth and the vertical axis represents the scanned segment of the globe or orbit. Successive cross-sections are represented on the screen. As the procedure is performed, the examiner tries to summate the two-dimensional sections into a three-dimensional visualization.

The round or oval probe has a line, dot, or logo marker along the shaft near its tip, which corresponds to the lateral-oscillating direction of the crystal. This reference point designates the area represented on the upper portion of the B-scan display or echogram. The probe's surface is represented as the first line on the echogram's left side while the fundus is represented on the right. The best resolution is found centrally on the echographic display.

The value of B-scan is poorly represented by a single echographic polaroid photo. The test is a dynamic kinetic study of the globe and orbit. It is referred to as "real-time" ultrasound because most of the information derived from the procedure is obtained by the examiner during testing. This explains why more practitioners are videotaping the ultrasounds to appreciate the continuous flow of information during testing. Induced tissue mobility during testing for differential diagnosis purposes is an example of the value of dynamic studies.

B-scan ultrasound screening is most commonly indicated in cases of opaque media where information regarding the ocular status posterior to the opacity is desired to determine whether surgical intervention is indicated. For example, B-scan should be performed when a large vitreous hemorrhage (Fig. 2A, B) is present to establish the etiology as vascular leakage, retinal tear or detachment, tumor, or vascular disease with a secondary detachment. Serial B-scans are used to follow this hemorrhage over time until it clears to insure proper diagnosis or to identify complications. B-scan screening is performed both on a high and low-sensitivity or gain setting. The former is more sensitive for gross fundus lesions and vitreal opacities, whereas the latter is capable of resolving subtle fundus elevations.

B-scan yields information about topography—the location and configuration of lesions—along with their gross reflectivity. Positive B-scan screening findings indicate the need for complete B-scan topographic examination (Fig. 3), such as with opaque ocular media, vitreous hemorrhage (previtrectomy), suspected ocular tumors, intraocular foreign bodies, retinal detachment, optic disc anomalies, suspected extraocular muscle disease, and proptosis. A negative B-scan in search of an intraocular or orbital foreign body is followed by a more sensitive CAT scan. When B-scan is used in conjunction with echographic A-scan, it is referred to as *standardized echography*. A-scan provides more information regarding lesion size measurement, internal structure, and intrinsic vasculature.

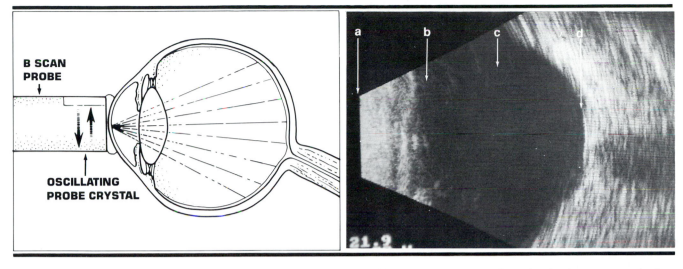

1. A. The echographic probe emits an advancing acoustic wavefront into the eye.

1. B. Normal B-scan. A two-dimensional echogram records tissue specific reflected echoes. The horizontal axis represents tissue depth and the vertical axis the scanned segment of the globe. (a) Probe and corneal surface. (b) Posterior lens surface. (c) Vitreous. (d) Retina. (Courtesy of Retina Consultants, Providence, RI.)

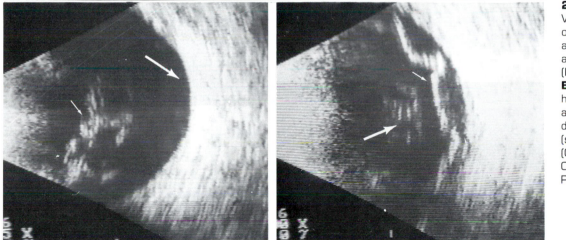

2. A. (far left) Vitreous hemorrhage (small arrow) with attached retina (large arrow).
B. (left) Vitreous hemorrhage (large arrow) with detached retina (small arrow). (Courtesy of Retina Consultants, Providence, RI.)

Section[a]	Probe Marker Orientation
Transverse	
Horizontal: nasal and temporal	Superiorly
Vertical: superior and inferior	Nasally
Vertical: obliques	Superiorly
Axial	
Vertical	Superiorly
Horizontal	Nasally
Longitudinal	
Horizontal, vertical, obliques	Toward center of cornea

[a]The probe's longest diameter is placed parallel to the limbus with transverse sections and perpendicular to the limbus with longitudinal sections.

3. Summary of B-scan sections and probe orientation.

B-scan screening (transverse and axial sections) of eyes with opaque media requires a systematic approach. Transverse or circumferential scans are taken in the eight cardinal meridians beginning at the posterior fundus and progressing anteriorly. These transverse scans (horizontal, vertical, and oblique) assist in determining the presence and lateral extent of a lesion (Fig. 4). The probe is oriented so its longest diameter or the tip marker is parallel to the limbus in all three orientations. Examination therefore occurs circumferentially on both sides of a particular meridian from the posterior to anterior fundus. The meridian lying in the middle of the circumferential scan is referred to as the *designated meridian*. Some practitioners screen only in the four main quadrants.

Axial scans are the next step in B-scan screening. Ultrasound waves are directed straight back through the cornea and lens to assist in documenting certain lesions and membranes relative to the optic nerve. The orientation of axial scans is both horizontal and vertical (Fig. 5).

Complete topographical B-scan includes longitudinal scans in addition to transverse and axial. Longitudinal scans examine the suspected area in an anterior–posterior, radial-like direction (Fig. 6). Here the probe is oriented perpendicular to the limbus with the marker always positioned toward the center of the cornea.

Instrumentation. B-scan ultrasound unit, standard ophthalmic methylcellulose solution, topical ophthalmic anesthetic solution.

Technique. Instill 2 drops of topical ophthalmic anesthetic solution in each eye. Position the ultrasound unit behind the patient to allow you to simultaneously view both the probe and video screen (Fig. 7). Recline the patient and ask him or her to fixate a target on the ceiling, exposing the inferior conjunctiva and sclera. Apply a small amount of ophthalmic methylcellulose to the probe tip to act as a coupling medium.

For initial transverse screening scans, place the probe parallel to the inferior limbus (6 o'clock) directly on the conjunctiva at the limbal border with the marker oriented nasally. Hold the probe steady on the globe and observe the screen. Take three or four overlapping scans as you slide the probe inferiorly from the limbus toward the far inferior fornix area (Fig. 8) at the 6 o'clock position. Continually monitor the echogram for abnormal echoes. Repeat a similar limbal to fornix scanning at every 1½ clock

hour position (6:00, 4:30, 3:00, 1:30, 12:00, 10:30, 9:00, 7:30). Orient the marker superiorly for both nasal and temporal scans, nasally for both superior and inferior scans, and superiorly for any required oblique scans. Perform all scans at both a high and low-gain setting. For example, to evaluate the nasal fundus, ask the patient to fixate nasally while the probe is placed limbally on the temporal conjunctiva with the probe marker oriented superiorly.

To take axial scans, first ensure that there is adequate topical anesthesia. Instruct the patient to look straight up at the ceiling target with the nontesting eye. Place a drop of methylcellulose on the probe tip, then place the probe in direct contact with the cornea. Hold the probe in place as you observe the screen. The first scan is taken with the marker oriented superiorly to perform a vertical axial scan. Rotate the marker to a nasal position for a horizontal axial scan. Perform these at both high and low-gain settings.

For longitudinal scans, orient the probe perpendicular to the limbus by positioning the probe marker toward the center of the cornea for all meridians. Hold the probe on the conjunctiva as you observe the screen. The peripheral fundus will appear superiorly at the top of the echogram, while the optic disc and posterior fundus will be located on the lower portion of the screen.

Although not theoretically correct, many practitioners perform all of the procedures described (see Fig. 3) through the patient's closed lid. They monitor proper eye positioning by observing the opened, nontesting eye and the expected anatomical finding on the screen.

Interpretation. An example of a vitreous hemorrhage with and without retinal detachment is seen in Figure 2. If a lesion is detected with the B-scan screening technique, complete topographical examination (transverse, axial, and longitudinal scans) is indicated in the area of the lesion. The best way to improve interpretation skills is to perform this test on eyes with clear media where the diagnosis is available.

Complications/Contraindications. B-scan should not be performed on an eye that has had recent intraocular surgery or may have a scleral laceration or a perforating injury. When performed properly, B-scan ultrasound presents no danger to the eye or orbit. A minor corneal abrasion or irritation from the probe or testing solution may occur, usually not requiring treatment.

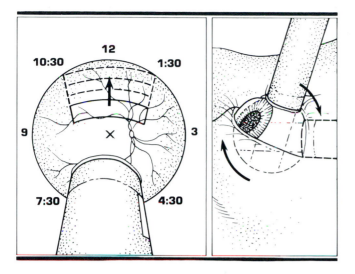

4. Transverse scanning involves moving the "band-like" circumferentially oriented acoustic waves in a posterior-to-anterior globe direction in each of the eight cardinal meridians.

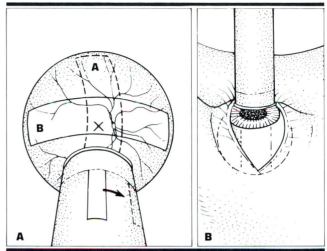

5. Axial scans are performed in two directions. **A.** Vertical, with probe marker superiorly. **B.** Horizontal, with probe marker nasally.

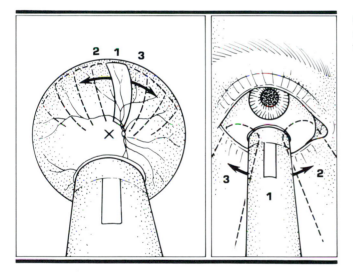

6. Longitudinal scans examine radially in a posterior to anterior direction after a lesion has been identified (probe marker toward central cornea).

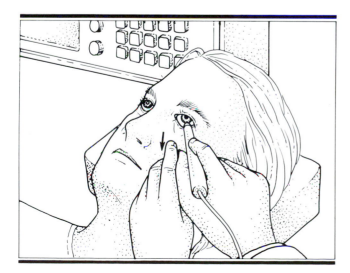

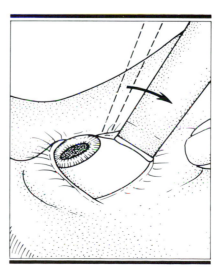

7. (far left) The B-scan screen is positioned behind and close to the patient's head for simultaneous examiner viewing during testing.

8. (left) The probe is slid along the globe in overlapping positions from the limbus toward the furthest extent of the cul-de-sac or fornix.

VIII Suggested Readings

Alexander LJ: *Primary Care of the Posterior Segment.* E. Norwalk, CT, Appleton & Lange, 1989.

Amsler M: *Amsler Grid Book.* London, Hamblin, 1984.

Anderson DR: *Testing of the Visual Field.* St. Louis, Mosby, 1982, pp 240–255.

Barker FM: Vitreoretinal biomicroscopy: A comparison of techniques. *J Am Optom Assoc* 1987;**58**:985–992.

Benson WE: *Retinal Detachment Diagnosis and Management.* Hagerstown, MD, Harper & Row, 1980.

Cavallerano A, Gutner R, Garston M: Indirect biomicroscopy techniques. *J Am Optom Assoc* 1986;**57**:755–758.

Cavallerano A, Semes L, Potter JW: How to perform scleral indentation. *Rev Optom,* Dec 1986, pp 51–59.

Garston M, Cavallerano A: Binocular indirect ophthalmoscopy. *Rev Optom,* Feb 1980, pp 49–57.

Gass JDM: Stereoscopic atlas of macular diseases diagnosis and treatment. St. Louis, Mosby, 1987, pp 12–41.

Glasser JS: Neuro-ophthalmologic examination: General considerations and special techniques, in Duane T (ed): *Clinical Ophthalmology.* Hagerstown, MD, Harper & Row, 1985, vol 2, pp 1–38.

Grala PE: When the patient can't see 20/20. *Rev Optom* 1984;**121**:42–48.

Green RL, Byrne SF: Diagnostic ultrasound, in Ryan SJ, Ogden TE (eds): *Retina.* St. Louis, Mosby, 1989, vol 1, pp 191–271.

Gutner R, Cavallerano A, Wong D: Fundus biomicroscopy: A comparison of four methods. *J Am Optom Assoc* 1988;**59**:388–390.

Havener WH, Gloeckner S: *Atlas of Diagnostic Techniques and Treatment of Retinal Detachment.* St. Louis, Mosby, 1967, pp 1–51.

Oral Fluorescein Study Group: Oral fluorography. *J Am Optom Assoc* 1985;**56**:784–792.

Potter JW, Semes LP, Cavallerano AA, Garston MJ: *Binocular Indirect Ophthalmoscopy.* Boston, Butterworth, 1988.

Schatz H: Fluorescein angiography: Basic principles and interpretation, in Ryan SJ, Schachat AP, Murphy RP, Patz A (eds): *Retina.* St. Louis, Mosby, 1989, vol 2, pp 3–77.

Shammas HJ: *Atlas of Ophthalmic Ultrasonography and Biometry.* St. Louis, Mosby, 1984.

Tolentino FI, Schepens CI, Freeman HM: *Vitreoretinal Disorders: Diagnosis and Management.* Philadelphia, Saunders, 1976, pp 45–108.

Walters GB: The technique of scleral depression. *J Am Optom Assoc* 1982;**53**:569–573.

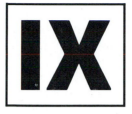

Physical Examination Procedures

66 Preauricular Lymph Node Palpation

Description/Indications. Palpation of the preauricular node area for lymphadenopathy (glandular swelling) is a useful diagnostic procedure, helpful in the differential diagnosis of a "red eye." Adenopathy of these superficial nodes presents as a nodular enlargement and is most prominent in children and young adults, who are most prone to lymphatic hyperplasia.

The preauricular nodes are located immediately anterior to (1 cm), and slightly inferior to, the tragus of the external ear at the temporomandibular joint (Fig. 1). Inflammatory fluid and debris from the superior eyelid and the outer one-third of the inferior eyelid commonly drain into these regional lymph glands. Lymph glands represent a component of the body's defense system. These macrophage-laden nodes act as bloodstream filters by trapping and phagocytizing foreign cells and matter. Anti-inflammatory lymphocytes and plasma cells are also produced in the center of these glands, explaining their characteristic swelling and possible tenderness. Viral conjunctivitis is usually accompanied by preauricular lymphadenopathy, often greater on the side of the more involved eye. Severe bacterial lid conditions such as hordeola, preseptal cellulitis, and impetigo can also produce this lymphatic tissue response.

Instrumentation. None.

Technique. Seat the patient and have him or her turn to face toward you. Place the first digits of your index and middle fingers of each hand in front of the tragus of the external ear (Fig. 2A). With mild pressure feel for the slight bony depression at the temporomandibular joint. Slide the skin with your fingers over the underlying bony structures in a back-and-forth semicircular motion (Fig. 2B) searching for the depression (normal) or an elevated nodular lesion (inflammation). Compare the two sides, noting laterality, asymmetry, size, tenderness, or absence of preauricular nodes.

Interpretation. An enlarged preauricular node can feel just like a small pebble under the skin just in front of the ear. Tender or nontender mobile nodes most often reflect lymphadenitis or hyperplasia in response to acute inflammation. Accompanying ear, nose, and throat symptoms usually suggest a viral conjunctivitis or, less likely, localized bacterial infection. Unilateral, large, visible, tender nodes are commonly found with severe adenovirus infection and with Parinaud's oculoglandular conjunctivitis.

These nodes can be subtle or obvious; therefore, including this technique with every red eye workup will aid the practitioner in making a differential diagnosis. Nodes may stay enlarged for weeks following resolution of ocular infection.

Contraindications/Complications. There are no contraindications or complications in performing this technique, aside from being gentle with those patients who have tenderness associated with preauricular lymphadenopathy.

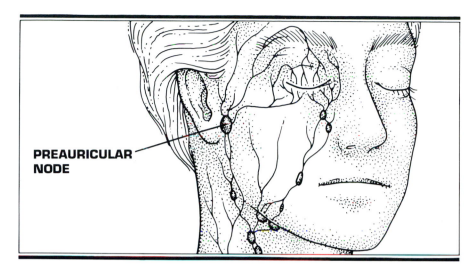

PREAURICULAR NODE

1. The lymphatics of the superior eyelid and the outer one-third of the inferior lid drain into the preauricular nodes, which are located 1 cm in front of the external ear.

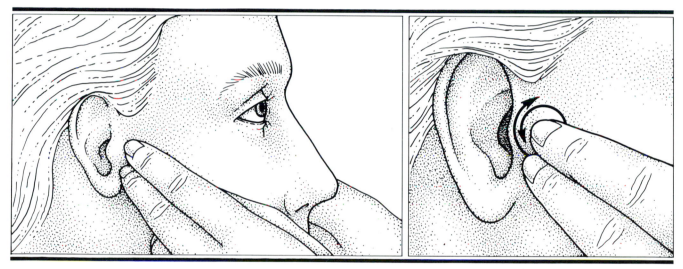

2. A. The first digit of the index and middle finger of each hand are placed in front of the tragus of the external ear.

2. B. Keeping the two fingertips close together, slide the underlying skin back and forth in a semi-circular motion over the node and/or bony depressed area.

67 Digital Intraocular Pressure Assessment

Description/Indications. Measurement of the intraocular pressure (IOP) is an integral component of most ocular evaluations. Goldmann applanation tonometry, either slit lamp mounted or hand-held, is the technique for IOP measurement against which all other techniques are judged (see p. 50). Occasionally, however, the clinician encounters a patient on whom it is impossible to obtain an IOP measurement with standard instrumentation. Patients typically included in this category are very young children, extremely anxious patients, or developmentally delayed individuals. Digital IOP assessment is a technique for grossly evaluating the IOP of these patient types. Digital IOP assessment may be utilized during assessment of a patient with an anterior segment infection when a noncontact tonometer is unavailable.

Using gentle pressure on the globe with the tips of the right and left index fingers, relative assessments of globe softness may be made. The harder the globe the higher the IOP. Incorporating this technique into the routine examination will allow the examiner to gain experience in assessing eyes in which the IOP is known and normal. When a clinical situation arises necessitating digital IOP assessment, the examiner will have already gained confidence in his or her ability to differentiate normal from abnormal globe firmness.

Instrumentation. None.

Technique. Ask the patient to look down. Gently rest the tips of both index fingers on the center of the patient's upper lid (Fig. 1). Push gently on the globe through the lid with the tip of one finger, and the tip of the other finger will rebound slightly (Fig. 2A). Alternately palpate the globe in this fashion two or three times using both fingertips (Fig. 2B). While doing so, subjectively assess the degree of firmness of the globe. Repeat the technique for the opposite eye.

Interpretation. The firmness of the globe is subjectively evaluated as soft, medium, or hard.

Complications/Contraindications. This technique poses no risk to the patient when the globes are intact. Avoid applying excessive pressure to the globe, however, so as not to induce any mild discomfort. Rarely, the patient may object to having the eyes touched and will be unable to cooperate even for this technique. Encourage the patient not to close the eyes, since the normal Bell's reflex will cause the cornea to roll upward beneath the portion of the lid that is palpated, which should be avoided.

Digital IOP assessment is contraindicated for eyes with a recent history of blunt trauma, penetrating ocular injury, or intraocular surgery.

Digital IOP evaluation is a gross assessment that does not substitute for quantifiable IOP measurement when it can be performed. For an acute problem or when glaucoma is suspected, consultation should be obtained for sedation of the patient so that more accurate IOP measurement with instrumentation may be performed.

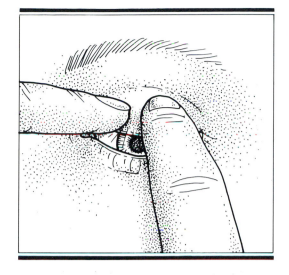

1. Ask the patient to look down and gently rest the tips of both index fingers on the center of the upper lid.

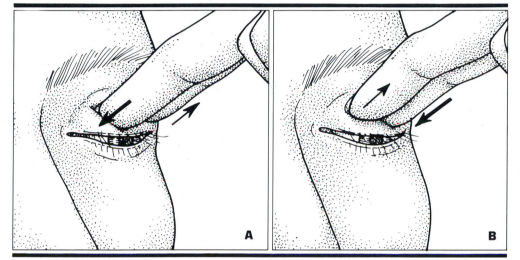

2. A. Indent the globe slightly with one fingertip; the opposite fingertip will rebound slightly. **B.** Alternately palpate the globe two or three times.

68 Globe Reposition

Description/Indications. Orbital congestion, due to a space-occupying lesion, vascular anomaly, or edema, may be evaluated in-office by globe reposition. Both globes are simultaneously reposited manually back into their respective orbits. Any asymmetry in the pressure needed to displace the globe into the orbit is recorded. In addition, patient discomfort during the procedure is noted. Prior to reposit, gentle palpation testing for pulsating exophthalmus can be performed when indicated. A positive pulsation finding is the hallmark of a vascular fistula.

Signs of orbital congestion and indications for globe reposition include: eyelid swelling, conjunctival injection, telangiectasia (pseudoconjunctivitis), chemosis, exophthalmos (unilateral or bilateral), extraocular muscle restriction, diplopia, decreased visual acuity, or ocular discomfort.

As with any less commonly occurring clinical finding, the clinician should perform this technique on many normal patients to become familiar with its normal variants.

Instrumentation. None.

Technique. Seat the patient comfortably at eye level facing you. Instruct the patient to close the eyes. With your hands in the "thumbs up" position, rest the four fingers of each hand perpendicular to the patient's zygomatic arch area or over the preauricular node area (Fig. 1). Place each thumb on the patient's closed lids and attempt to gently push the globes posteriorly into their respective orbital cavities (Fig 2). Compare each side, noting any asymmetry in displacement between the eyes as well as any limitations. Some examiners prefer to reposit each globe individually at first and then simultaneously to aid in their comparison. Also note any discomfort expressed by the patient during testing.

Interpretation. Asymmetry in globe displacement is usually indicative of an orbital problem such as a space-occupying lesion, systemically induced orbital congestion, or a vascular anomaly. Aside from thyroid disease with bilateral exophthalmos, bilateral limited reposition is usually secondary to anatomically shallow orbits. Discomfort upon reposition may accompany inflammation such as retrobulbar optic neuritis.

Contraindications/Complications. Globe reposition should not be performed on anyone with a history of recent blunt ocular trauma, especially if a scleral rupture or laceration is suspected or if a hyphema is present. Other contraindications include any individual who has recently had ocular surgery, is suspected of having a corneal foreign body, or has angle closure glaucoma.

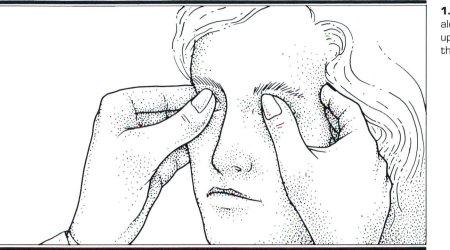

1. Hands and fingers are positioned along the zygomatic arches with upward-directed thumbs resting on the closed eyelids.

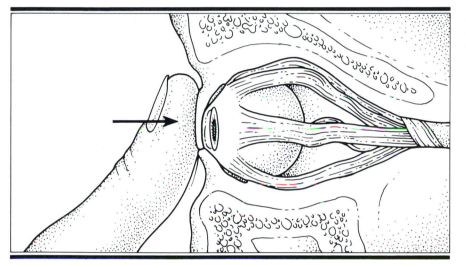

2. Gentle and even pressure is applied to each globe, attempting to displace them posteriorly.

69 Exophthalmometry

Description/Indications. The forward protrusion or backward displacement of the eye(s) may be a sign of a traumatic, infectious, inflammatory, infiltrative, vascular, or neoplastic disorder affecting the orbit or globe. The exophthalmometer measures the anterior projection of the cornea relative to the lateral orbital rim. Each eye is measured in millimeters with the values for each eye compared against the other and against an expected range of "normals." A significant difference between the two eyes or deviations from the norm may be a sign of orbital disease. The progression or resolution of an orbital condition may be monitored by successive comparison of readings over time.

Indications for exophthalmometry include the appearance of proptosis (unilateral or bilateral), enophthalmos (unilateral or bilateral), orbital cellulitis, Grave's disease, or a tumor of the orbit.

The Luedde and Hertel exophthalmometers are two types frequently used. The Luedde exophthalmometer is made of transparent plastic with a millimeter rule on the side. At one end is a notch that conforms to the lateral orbital rim. The Hertel exophthalmometer is composed of two yokes separated by a crossbar with a measuring scale. Each yoke fits over the bony temporal margin of the lateral orbit rim. One yoke is fixed and the other slides to allow their variable separation and measurement of the biocular distance. The biocular distance should be set at the same scale reading each time an individual's measurements are taken. On each yoke is a scale with two mirrors, one above the other. The position of the apex of the cornea, seen on the scale visible in the upper mirror, determines the position of the globe within the orbit.

Instrumentation. Luedde exophthalmometer or Hertel exophthalmometer.

Technique

Luedde Exophthalmometer: Ask the patient to be seated with the head erect, looking straight ahead. With the thumb or index finger, feel for the bony ridge indicating the lateral orbital rim (Fig. 1). Place the notch of the exophthalmometer firmly against the lateral orbit rim (Fig. 2) with the scale facing toward the side. Keep the exophthalmometer perpendicular to the plane of the face. Look from the side view through the transparent exophthalmometer and sight where the corneal apex intersects the mm scale (Fig. 2). If necessary, shine a penlight on the cornea from below to accentuate the corneal image. Take three readings and repeat the procedure for the opposite eye.

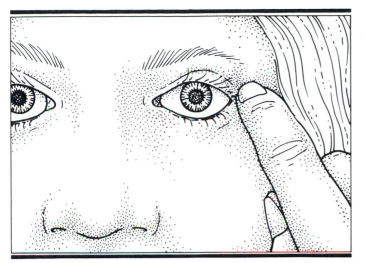

1. Using the index finger, feel for the bony ridge indicating the lateral rim of the orbit. This is where the notch or inner arc of the exophthalmometer is put.

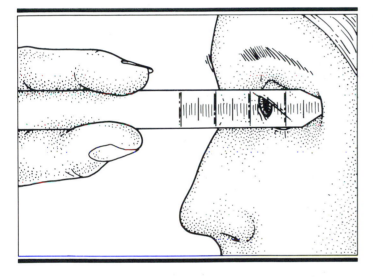

2. The notch of the Luedde exophthalmometer is placed firmly against the lateral orbital rim. View through the clear exophthalmometer, sighting where the corneal apex intersects the scale.

Hertel Exophthalmometer: Prepare the Hertel exophthalmometer (Fig. 3) by loosening the locking screw on the crossbar and ensuring that the numeral scale on the crossbar is erect. Ask the patient to be seated with head erect, looking straight ahead. Sit or stand beside the patient and adjust the patient's chair so that your eyes are both on the same plane. With the thumb or index finger, feel for the bony ridge indicating the lateral rim of the orbit (Fig. 1). Ask the patient to close the eyes and slowly bring the exophthalmometer forward. Keep the exophthalmometer parallel to the floor with the scale on the crossbar visible to the examiner. Place the internal arc of the yoke against the bony temporal orbital rim of the right eye (Fig. 4A). Slide the second yoke along the crossbar until the inner arc wraps around the lateral orbital rim of the left eye. Tighten the locking screw located on the crossbar and note the reading (Fig. 4B).

Ask the patient to open the eyes and to look straight ahead. Look into the two mirrors located above each other. The measurement is taken where the apex of the cornea, seen in the lower mirror, is superimposed on the scale seen in the upper mirror (Fig. 5). Note this point and record. Use the same technique to measure the left eye. Repeat the readings for each eye and compare to previous results. Any discrepancy may indicate poor alignment of the instrument.

Interpretation. An example of a reading is 17/18 @100, indicating a biocular measurement of 100 mm with the right eye measuring 17 mm and the left eye 18 mm. Normal exophthalmometry readings range from 12 to 20 mm for whites and 12 to 24 mm for blacks. Readings greater than this are an indication of possible proptosis and merit further investigation. Measurements between the two eyes are usually within 2 mm of each other. A difference between the two eyes of 3 mm or greater is an indication for further investigation, even if all readings fall within the normal range. A comparison is also made of serial measurements, those taken over time. Any increase in a reading, after using the same biocular base value, must be rechecked and may be an indication for further investigative testing. The deterioration or resolution of an orbital condition can be monitored by comparing successive measurements over a period of time.

The accuracy of the test hinges on the careful alignment of the instrument on the patient's face along with meticulous alignment of the patient's corneal plane in the mirrors and scale of the exophthalmometer. Repeated readings over time require the presetting of the biocular base distance. Poor fixation, convergence, parallax errors, head movement, and blepharospasm may affect the reliability of the results. The Hertel exophthalmometer, being a biocular instrument, is the instrument of choice.

The visual appearance of exophthalmos is not always confirmed with measurements. Factors such as ptosis, lid retraction, and asymmetry of the palpebral fissure may lead to a pseudoexophthalmic appearance. Patient history and old photographs may help in the differential diagnosis.

Contraindication/Complications. This test poses no risk to the patient. Following proper procedure, there are no contraindications to the test. Individuals with facial bone dysformity may not allow for the parallel placement of the instrument on the face, leading to unreliable measurements.

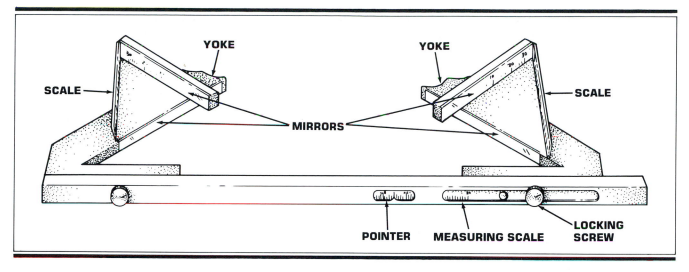

3. The Hertel exophthalmometer.

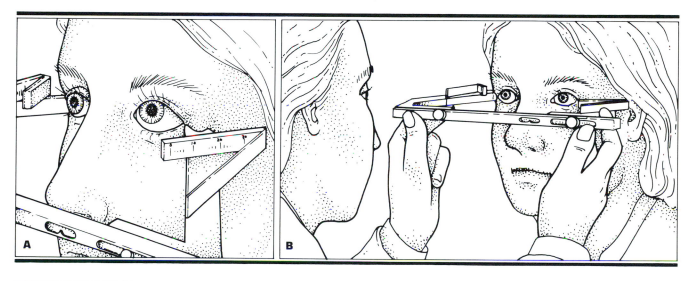

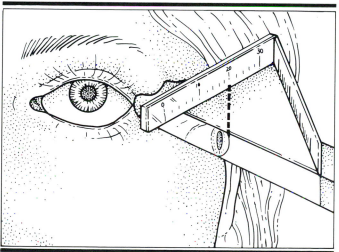

4. A. (above left) The inner arc of the Hertel exophthalmometer is placed on the bony ridge of the lateral wall of the orbit. **B.** (above right) The Hertel exophthalmometer in position on the patient's face.

5. (left) A reading for the Hertel exophthalmometer is obtained where the corneal image, seen on the lower scale, intersects the scale seen in the upper mirror.

70 Infraorbital Nerve Testing

Description/Indications. Direct mechanical injury or indirect edematous compression to the infraorbital branch of the trigeminal nerve (cranial nerve V) can lead to diminished sensation (hypoesthesia) of the skin and subcutaneous tissue along its distribution. In particular, blowout fractures of the orbit are associated with infraorbital nerve damage producing numbness inferior and nasal to the orbit. These areas include the lower lid, the ipsilateral cheek, the lateral aspect of the nose, and the upper lip area.

The maxillary (V2) branch of the trigeminal nerve gives rise to the infraorbital nerve. This nerve travels anteriorly and centrally in the infraorbital sulcus from the lateral posterior aspect of the orbit. Approximately 15 mm posterior to the inferior orbital rim the nerve becomes enclosed in a bony canal, bends inferiorly below the rim, and exits through the infraorbital foramen of the maxillary bone, distributing sensory innervation (Fig. 1).

Direct blunt trauma to the inferior orbital rim may cause various fractures to the bony components with subsequent damage to the surrounding tissue and nerves, leading to hypoesthesia. Blowout fractures involve direct impact to the globe. Globe compression causes compressive, stretching, and rebound expansile damage to the globe itself with a rapid rise in intraorbital pressure. This pressure is frequently released by expulsion of orbital soft tissue through the anatomically thinned orbital floor and medial walls. Any maxillofacial or orbital trauma may affect the integrity of the infraorbital nerve and requires evaluation.

Instrumentation. Cotton-tipped applicator, cotton ball or facial tissue.

Technique. Seat the patient comfortably and remove any spectacles. Instruct the patient to close the eyes and tell you when he or she feels a sensation. Twirl a clean cotton ball, cotton-tipped applicator, or facial tissue to form a wisp. Working first with the noninvolved side, lightly touch the wisp to lateral portion of the lower lid and move nasally along the eyelid (Fig. 2). Pass the cotton wisp downward along the lateral aspect of the nose, temporally across the cheek area, and finally across the upper lip area (Fig. 3). After each area is tested, ask if the patient is able to feel each stimulus. Mentally record the results. Repeat the exact testing sequence to the involved facial side. Ask the patient to compare the sensation on one side of the face to that of the contralateral side. Repeat any area in question, or perform the stimuli simultaneously on each side for direct comparison. Make every attempt to touch the skin with the same amount of pressure with each stroke. Assess the reliability of the patient's responses by at least once not actually touching the patient, but still asking for a response.

Interpretation. History of blunt ocular trauma accompanied by definite or even questionable infraorbital nerve hypoesthesia may indicate the need for motility testing and radiologic examination to rule out a blowout fracture. Infraorbital nerve hypoesthesia is usually temporary. The nerve commonly regenerates within 3 months, with retesting used to follow the restoration of nerve function.

Complications/Contraindications. This test presents no risk to the patient.

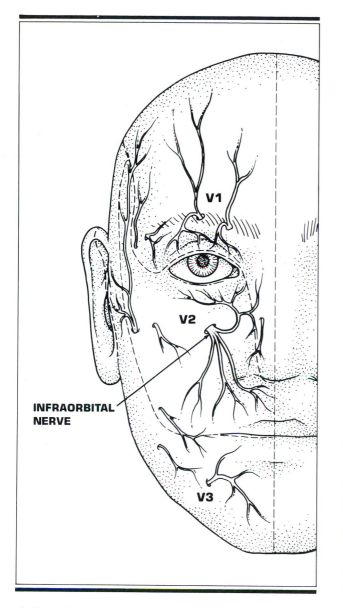

1. The Infraorbital nerve exits its foramen and distributes its sensory fibers to the ipsilateral lower lid, cheek, lateral nasal area, and upper lip.

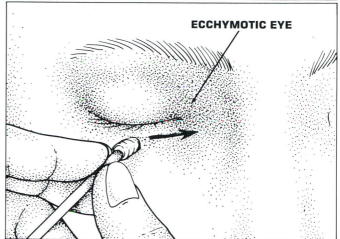

2. Lightly slide a twirled cotton wisp edge along the lower lid asking if the patient feels the stimulus.

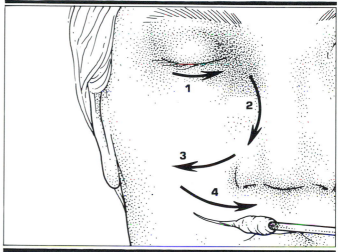

3. After testing the lower lid (1), test the lateral aspect of the nose (2), cheek (3), and upper lip area (4) in a similar manner as Fig. 2.

71 Sphygmomanometry

Description/Indications. Sphygmomanometry is the method of measuring blood pressure (BP) indirectly with a sphygmomanometer (blood pressure cuff) and stethoscope. Measurements are obtained in millimeters of mercury (mm Hg) of the systolic pressure (the arterial pressure at the height of pulsation from cardiac contraction) and the diastolic pressure (the arterial pressure during ventricular relaxation between cardiac contractions) (Table 1). These measurements are obtained by auscultating (listening with a stethoscope) the Korotkoff sounds (Phases I to V) produced by completely compressing the brachial artery with the sphygmomanometer and then releasing cuff pressure until initial refilling occurs.

Primary indications for sphygmomanometry in the optometric office include screening for undiagnosed or uncontrolled hypertension, as well as reinforcing patient compliance with hypertension treatment regimens. In addition, BP measurement may be important in the use of several ophthalmic diagnostic and therapeutic agents, such as topical phenylephrine, hydroxyamphetamine, epinephrine and related compounds, and beta-adrenergic blocking agents; and may aid in or augment the diagnostic process of several ophthalmic conditions such as chronic open-angle glaucoma, low-tension glaucoma, hypertensive retinopathy, retinal embolic phenomena, amaurosis fugax, and papilledema.

The BP cuff is a nonstretchable fabric bag with Velcro cloth strips at the ends for closure and contains an inflatable rubber bladder. An inflating bulb with a pressure release valve and a manometer gauge for measuring pressure in the bladder are connected to the cuff by one or more rubber tubes (Fig. 1). The length of the arterial segment compressed by the inflated cuff influences the accuracy of the BP reading. Sphygmomanometry in the average-sized adult is most accurate when performed with a cuff 12 to 14 cm wide (regular adult cuff). For other patients choose an alternate cuff size having a rubber bladder that encircles at least two-thirds of the arm circumference. The most common cuff sizes utilized in the optometric office are child, adult, and large adult. In the clinical setting the cuff pressure is usually registered by either a mercury or aneroid manometer that is hand-held (combined manometer gauge and inflation bulb), pocket-sized (separate manometer gauge and inflation bulb), wall-mounted, table-mounted, or stand-mounted.

As pressure in the BP cuff is controlled, the Korotkoff sounds are auscultated with a stethoscope. Most stethoscopes have a chestpiece with two components, a bell and a diaphragm (Fig. 2). The diaphragm best transmits high-frequency sounds; the bell best transmits low-frequency sounds such as heart or vascular sounds. Either the bell or diaphragm side of the chestpiece is "clicked" into position to transmit sounds through the stethoscope. Usually the diaphragm side of the chestpiece, or a modification known as a corrugated diaphragm, is used for BP measurement.

Instrumentation. Adult, large adult, or child-sized sphygmomanometer; stethoscope with diaphragm.

TABLE 1. FOLLOW-UP CRITERIA FOR INITIAL BP MEASUREMENT: ADULTS ≥ 18 YEARS

BP Range (mm Hg)	Recommended Follow-Up[a]
Diastolic	
< 85	Recheck within 2 years
85–89	Recheck within 1 year
90–104	Confirm within 2 months
105–114	Refer promptly within 2 weeks
≥ 115	Refer immediately for medical care
Systolic, when diastolic blood pressure is < 90	
< 140	Recheck within 2 years
140–199	Confirm within 2 months
≥ 200	Refer promptly within 2 weeks

Normal BP Readings: Children/Adolescents	
< 142/92	Ages 16–18 years
< 136/86	Ages 13–15 years
< 126/82	Ages 10–12 years
< 122/78	Ages 6–9 years
< 116/76	Ages 3–5 years

[a]If recommendations for follow-up of recorded diastolic and systolic BP are different, the shorter recommended time for recheck and referral should take precedence.
Adapted from the 1988 Report of the Joint National Committee on Detection, Evaluation, and Treatment of High Blood Pressure, U.S. Department of Health and Human Services.

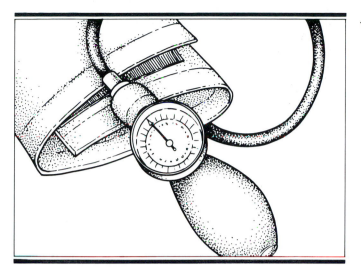

1. A hand-held aneroid sphygmomanometer

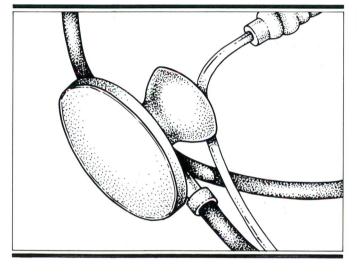

2. This stethoscope chestpiece has both a diaphragm and a bell. Rotating the head will "click" either into position for transmitting sounds.

Technique. It is recommended that BP measurement be taken after 5 minutes of quiet rest and that caffeine consumption, smoking, and exercise be avoided within 30 minutes of measurement. Support the seated patient's arm on the arm of a chair or table just above waist level and slightly bent with the palm turned upward so that the stethoscope head will be positioned at the level of the heart. Free the forearm of clothing and ensure that a rolled-up sleeve does not excessively constrict the upper arm. The BP may be successfully measured through a single layer of thin fabric such as the sleeve of a nylon jacket or lightweight blouse.

Palpate the brachial artery just below the antecubital crease, the bend of the elbow (Fig. 3). Center the bladder of the cuff on the upper arm overlying the brachial artery, aligning the appropriate arrow on the cuff for the arm being used. Wrap the cuff smoothly and secure it snugly so that the lower border of the cuff lies approximately 2.5 cm (1 inch) above the antecubital crease (Fig. 4). Palpate the systolic pressure to avoid an artificially low reading produced by auscultatory gap. Use the forefinger and middle finger of one hand to gently palpate the radial artery at the wrist, and inflate the cuff to approximately 30 mm Hg above the level at which the pulse disappears (Fig. 5). Deflate the cuff smoothly at a rate of approximately 2 to 3 mm Hg per second until the pulse is first palpated, and mentally note the manometer reading. Rapidly and steadily deflate the cuff completely.

Set the earpieces of the stethoscope into your ears so that they angle forward toward your face as the stethoscope is put on. Place the diaphragm of the chestpiece gently but firmly over the brachial artery between the antecubital crease and the lower edge of the cuff, avoiding contact between the chestpiece and the cuff (Fig. 6). Inflate the cuff to approximately 20 to 30 mm Hg above the systolic pressure as determined by palpation. Turn the manometer release valve to slowly and smoothly release air from the bladder at the rate of approximately 2 to 3 mm Hg per second. Mentally note the first audible Korotkoff sound, Phase I (soft tapping sounds), which is the systolic reading. Korotkoff sounds Phases II (swishing murmur), III (crisper sounds, increasing in intensity), and IV (abrupt sound muffling) will be audible with continued deflation of the cuff. Phase V, the disappearance of sounds, is the generally accepted diastolic reading for most patients. Mentally note the manometer reading when Phase V occurred, listen for an additional 10 to 20 mm Hg to confirm sound cessation, and then rapidly and completely deflate the cuff. If repeat measurement is necessary, wait 1 to 2 minutes to permit the release of blood trapped in the forearm venous system. Record the BP reading. If indicated, also take a measurement on the opposite arm.

Interpretation. By convention record both the systolic and diastolic readings to the nearest even-number mm Hg. Indicate the position of the patient and which arm was used for measurement. For example, an entry of "160/100 R.A. Sit" indicates that BP measurement was performed on the right arm with the patient sitting down. If a cuff size other than the regular adult was used, note this information as well. A 5 to 10 mm Hg difference in the readings between the right and left arms is considered normal.

Hypertension is not diagnosed on the basis of a single elevated in-office reading. Usually two or three readings taken in the course of several visits are necessary to diagnose essential hypertension. If two readings are taken during a visit, they are averaged, and if these first two measurements differ by more than 5 mm Hg, additional readings are taken and averaged. However, if you find the BP to be severely elevated (see Table 1), even after a single reading, refer the patient immediately for medical care.

Complications/Contraindications. This procedure poses no risk to the patient; however, patient anxiety will often produce artificially high in-office readings ("white coat" hypertension). If the BP cuff is too small for the patient's arm circumference, falsely high readings will also be obtained. Make certain that the sphygomomanometer is in good working order. It is recommended that aneroid manometers be calibrated against a perfectly working mercury manometer at least annually.

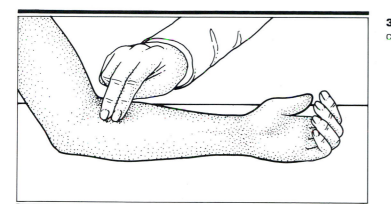

3. Palpate the brachial artery just below the antecubital crease.

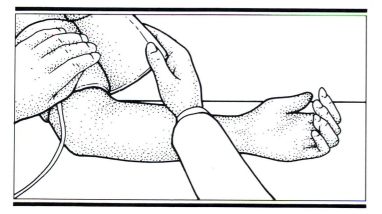

4. Wrap the cuff smoothly and snugly so that the lower border lies approximately 1 inch above the antecubital crease.

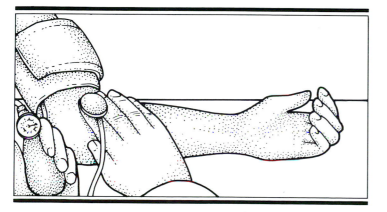

5. To estimate systolic pressure, palpate the radial artery and inflate the cuff until the pulse disappears.

6. Place the diaphragm of the chestpiece gently but firmly over the brachial artery between the antecubital crease and the lower edge of the cuff.

72 Carotid Pulse Palpation and Auscultation

Description/Indications. Bruits ("noises") are rushing sounds heard over medium and large arteries caused by vibrations of the blood vessel walls induced by turbulent blood flow. This blood flow turbulence and vessel wall distortion may be caused by partial vessel lumen occlusion from atherosclerotic plaque formation. Although generally not audible until the vessel is approximately 50% occluded, bruits are detected by auscultating ("listening to") the affected artery with a stethoscope.

The right and left common carotid arteries derive from the right brachiocephalic (innominate) artery and aortic arch, respectively, and course up through the neck between the trachea and sternocleidomastoid muscles. At the angle of the jaw the common carotids bifurcate into the external carotid arteries, which supply the scalp, and the internal carotid arteries, which supply the brain. The first branch of the internal carotid artery is the ophthalmic artery, serving the globe and adnexa (Fig. 1).

Plaque formation within either common carotid artery is more likely to occur at its proximal and distal ends where bifurcation occurs. Auscultation of the carotid arteries for bruits is an in-office procedure that helps to screen for atherosclerotic plaque formation related to certain ocular signs or visual symptoms. The evaluation for common carotid artery bruits will also serve as a barometer for plaque formation elsewhere within the arterial system. A gross assessment of carotid artery integrity may also be made by palpating the pulse of the right and left common carotids.

Indications for carotid auscultation include symptoms or signs of plaque formation within the cerebrovascular arterial system that may occur in the middle-aged to elderly patient. These signs and symptoms may include amaurosis fugax, transient ischemic attacks (TIAs), Hollenhorst plaques, retinal occlusive phenomena, asymmetric diabetic retinopathy, and anterior segment ischemic syndromes; or symptoms of vertebrobasilar artery disease such as equilibrium disorders, bilateral visual disorders, unsteadiness, and auditory symptoms.

Carotid auscultation is performed with a stethoscope. Most stethoscopes have a chestpiece with two components, a bell and a diaphragm (Fig. 2). Either the bell or diaphragm side of the chestpiece is "clicked" into position to transmit sounds through the stethoscope. The diaphragm best transmits high-frequency sounds; the bell best transmits low-frequency sounds such as heart or vascular sounds. As a result, the bell setting is preferred for carotid auscultation; however, the diaphragm may be tried if difficulty in eliciting sounds is encountered.

Instrumentation. Double-head stethoscope.

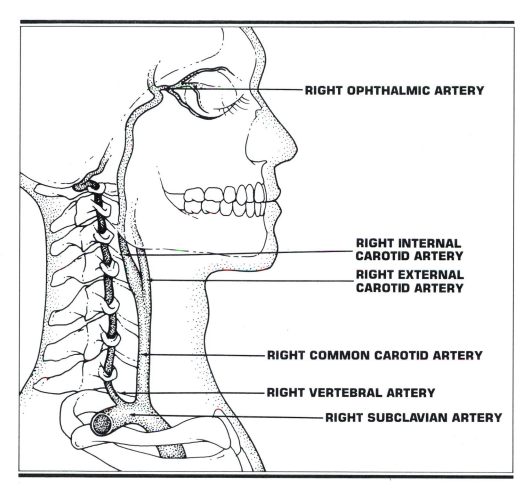

RIGHT OPHTHALMIC ARTERY

RIGHT INTERNAL CAROTID ARTERY

RIGHT EXTERNAL CAROTID ARTERY

RIGHT COMMON CAROTID ARTERY

RIGHT VERTEBRAL ARTERY

RIGHT SUBCLAVIAN ARTERY

1. The common carotid is accessible to auscultation for bruits.

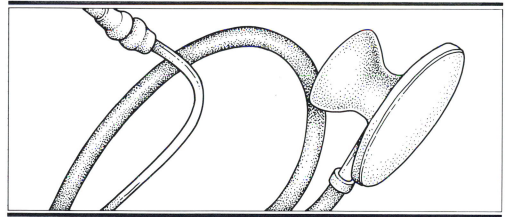

2. This stethoscope chest-piece has both a diaphragm and a bell. Rotating the head will "click" either into position for transmitting sounds.

Technique. Adjust the headrest on the examination chair so that the patient's head is resting back slightly with the chin slightly elevated. Use the tips of the first and second fingers of one hand to gently palpate for the pulse of the right common carotid artery in the fleshy groove lateral to the trachea (Fig. 3). Insert the stethoscope into your ears and turn the chestpiece so that the bell side is transmitting. Once the common carotid is located, gently place the head of the stethoscope over the artery approximately 1 inch above the clavicle (Fig. 4). To minimize the distracting noise of the patient's breathing, ask him or her to stop breathing in mid-expiration. Closely listen for bruits for approximately 10 to 15 seconds, and then ask the patient to resume breathing. Repositioning the stethoscope head further up the common carotid artery, repeat the procedure three or four times along the length of the carotid. Repeat the technique on the left side.

Interpretation. Palpation of the carotid pulse may be graded as follows: Grade 0, no pulse; Grade 1+, detectable but faint pulse; Grade 2+, stronger pulse but decreased in intensity; Grade 3+, normal pulse; Grade 4+, bounding or forceful pulse. Atherosclerotic plaque formation will reduce carotid blood flow, which may be evident as a diminished pulse by palpation.

When a bruit is present, a blowing, whooshing type sound will be heard superimposed on the normal sound of the pulse. If a plaque is present at the distal or proximal end of the common carotid artery, the bruit may become louder as that partially obstructed portion of the artery is auscultated. Bruits may be subjectively graded 1 to 4. Because of normal vessel elasticity, bruits are common but benign in children and young adults. Significant heart murmur may also be transmitted along the vessels and interpreted as a bruit.

Carotid bruits may be indicative of potentially life-threatening cerebrovascular or cardiovascular disease and referral should be made for appropriate medical assessment. The absence of bruit does not necessarily rule out carotid artery plaque formation, however, since the vessel lumen may be occluded to the extent that blood flow turbulence is greatly diminished.

Complications/Contraindications. Care must be exercised so as not to apply excess pressure on the carotid artery when palpating the pulse, or auscultating with the stethoscope. If plaque formation is present, excess pressure may mechanically occlude the vessel, interrupt blood flow, and induce a TIA. During carotid pulse assessment the right and left common carotids should not be palpated simultaneously.

3. Gently palpate to localize the common carotid artery.

4. To auscultate, gently place the bell over the artery approximately an inch above the clavicle. Auscultate at three or four positions along the length of the common carotid.

73   Orbital Auscultation

Description/Indications. Orbital congestion, due to a space-occupying lesion, vascular anomaly, or edema may be further investigated in-office with orbital auscultation. Performing this test on "normal" patients will help the examiner learn the expected orbital sounds.

Signs of orbital congestion and indications for orbital auscultation include eyelid swelling, conjunctival injection and telangiectasia (pseudoconjunctivitis), conjunctival chemosis, exophthalmos, extraocular muscle restriction, diplopia, decreased visual acuity, and ocular discomfort.

Similar in many ways to carotid auscultation (see p. 258), orbital auscultation is performed through the closed eyelid in search of a bruit, diagnostic of a vascular anomaly. Either the patient's subjective awareness of a bruit by reporting head sounds similar to that of "swishing" or running water, or the examiner's detection of a bruit, are both indicators of a positive test. Any detection of an orbital bruit suggests referral to rule out an orbital vascular anomaly, a posteriorly located carotid-cavernous fistula, or, less commonly, an orbital or intracranial tumor.

Instrumentation. Double-headed bell stethoscope.

Technique. Seat the patient comfortably in the examination chair and instruct him or her to close both eyes and hold their breath. Place the bell portion of the stethoscope over the closed eyelid of one eye (Fig. 1A). If a bruit is not heard, slide the bell temporally towards the lateral canthus to enhance the orbital sounds (Fig. 1B). Listen carefully for a "whooshing" bruit sound, which should be synchronous with the heartbeat. It may require listening for 10 to 15 seconds to detect the bruit. Repeat the procedure on the opposite eye for comparison. Multiple attempts may be necessary for subtle bruits.

Interpretation. Any detection of a bruit sound suggests referral to rule out an orbital vascular anomaly, a carotid-cavernous fistula, or less likely, an orbital or intracranial tumor.

Contraindications/Complications. When performed gently, orbital auscultation poses no danger or risk to the patient. Caution should be used when examining an eye that has undergone recent intraocular surgery or has sustained blunt trauma.

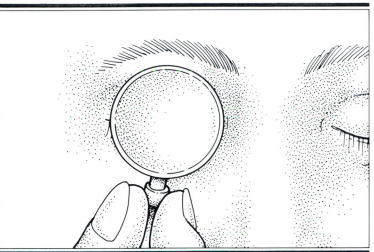

1. A. The bell portion of the stethoscope is placed against the patient's closed eyelid.

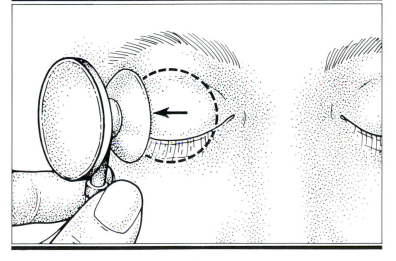

1. B. The bell can be moved temporally toward the outer canthus for enhanced auditory results.

74   Ophthalmodynamometry

Description/Indications.   Ophthalmodynamometry (ODM) is a technique that measures the relative ophthalmic artery pressure. When used in conjunction with other tests and procedures (such as auscultation, angiography, and Doppler studies), a profile of carotid artery insufficiency may be obtained. Carotid artery insufficiency is a vascular condition with both ocular and systemic significance. In this condition the common and/or internal carotid arteries, the major vessels supplying blood to the head and neck, are focally narrowed due to stenosis, artheromatous buildup, or thrombosis, with subsequent decrease in blood flow to the eye and brain. The resultant ischemic condition may cause symptoms that may include transient monocular blindness (amaurosis fugax), headache, aphasia and tingling, paraesthesias, or weakness of a limb. Signs of carotid artery involvement include Hollenhorst plaques, central or branch retinal artery occlusion, venous stasis retinopathy, retinal artery pulsation, asymmetric retinopathy, or unilateral reduced intraocular pressure. There are effective medical and surgical approaches for the treatment of carotid artery occlusive disease if detected; however, if undetected, a great many patients may go on to experience cerebral or ocular stroke.

During ODM, external pressure is applied to the sclera, leading to a rise in intraocular pressure, while the arterial tree at the disc is observed. When the intraocular pressure is greater than the diastolic arterial pressure but less than the systolic pressure, an arterial pulse is observed as the vessel collapses and reopens. The first arterial pulse indicates the diastolic pressure, and loss of this pulse, the systolic pressure. Under normal conditions an arterial pulse is not observed but may be seen in glaucoma, syncope, and aortic valve insufficiency. At least 50% of individuals have a normal spontaneous venous pulse because the intraocular pressure of 15 to 20 mm Hg approximates ophthalmic venous diastolic pressure.

There are two methods of ODM, compression and suction. Compression ODM is most commonly used. The instrument itself has either a linear or dial scale (Fig. 1), which both function by spring tension. The dial type has two indicators, one active and the other passive. The passive indicator will remain at the highest scale reading after pressure is released or the instrument is removed from the eye. The linear type consists of a spring-loaded sliding rod with graduated markings along a cylinder. The movement of the rod, scale, and footplate are controlled by a button that must be depressed for movement to occur. The rod is locked in position when the button is released, holding the last reading on the scale. Any prior measurements must be visually read off the scale by the examiner or an assistant.

A direct or binocular indirect ophthalmoscope (see pp. 186, 192) may be used to observe the retinal arteries during the procedure. Advantages to using the direct ophthalmoscope are that it requires only one person and provides greater magnification. Its disadvantage is the limited field of view such that small ocular movements may cause the examiner to lose sight of the artery during the procedure. Steady, perpendicular globe alignment and compression with the ODM, while simultaneously viewing with the direct ophthalmoscope of the retinal artery, makes this form the most difficult of the ODM procedures to do. The advantages for using a binocular indirect ophthalmoscope (BIO) are the greater field of view, increased working distance allowing for easier access for an assistant to maneuver, greater illumination, and stereopsis. Sufficient magnification is obtained with a condensing lens ranging in power from +14D to +20D. With the increased field of view and reduced magnification, small eye or head movements made during the procedure by the patient may be instantly compensated for by the examiner without losing sight of the artery. The disadvantages of using a BIO are the need for two individuals and discomfort for the patient due to the bright light.

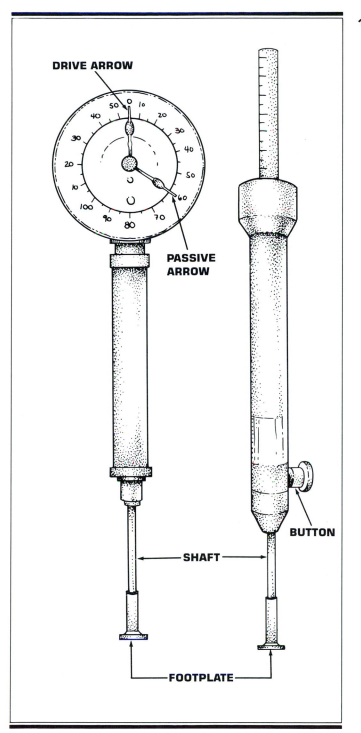

1. A linear and dial ophthalmodynamometer.

Instrumentation. Ophthalmodynamometer, binocular indirect ophthalmoscope, direct ophthalmoscope, mydriatic/cycloplegic solutions, topical ophthalmic anesthetic solution, slit lamp, Goldmann tonometer, sphygmomanometer, stethoscope.

Technique. Explain the purpose of ODM to the patient and how it requires cooperation to obtain reliable results. Measure the intraocular pressure (see p. 50) in each eye and obtain bilateral brachial blood pressure readings (see p. 254). This information is used in the interpretation of ODM results. Dilate each eye. Begin the ODM phase of the procedure once the pupils are adequately dilated. Instill a topical anesthetic solution in each eye. Use moderate room illumination so the scale on the ophthalmodynamometer is visible during the procedure.

Direct Ophthalmoscope: Holding the direct ophthalmoscope in the hand corresponding to the eye being examined, locate a visible major artery on the optic disc near the rim. Hold the ophthalmodynamometer horizontally, like a pencil. Use the thumb, index, and middle fingers to hold the instrument and rest the remaining two or three fingers on the cheek to increase stability of the instrument (Fig. 2). With a linear-scale instrument, the scale and button face the examiner and the thumb or index finger used to depress the button, allowing movement of the rod (Fig. 3). With the patient sitting erect in the examination chair, provide a fixation target at a distance that moves the testing eye up and in. Align the footplate tangentially on the globe, approximately 1 cm behind the limbus at the level of the insertion of the lateral rectus muscle (Fig. 4). Do not angulate the instrument.. Make sure the scale is visible to the individual noting the readings, either examiner or assistant (Fig. 5). Ask the patient to look straight ahead.

Locate the artery to be observed and apply even pressure with the ODM at a rate of approximately 20 grams per second. Have the assistant call the readings off the scale as pressure is increased. Disregard a venous pulse if present, concentrating only on the chosen artery. Stop as soon as the first initial pulse (diastole) is seen, and record the reading directly from the instrument in grams. Return the index pointer to zero or depress the button on the linear scale to reset the rod. Resume applying pressure, going past the initial pulse, and watching the artery until the pulse stops and the vessel collapses (systole). Quickly remove the instrument and record this reading. Take three readings of the diastolic and systolic pressure for each eye, waiting one minute between each. Discard any disparate reading and average the results.

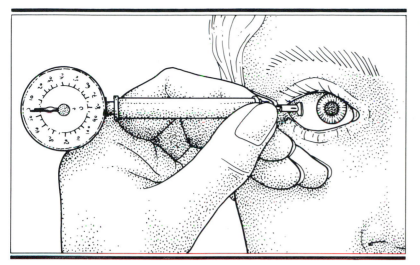

2. The ophthalmodynamometer is held between the thumb and index finger, using the remaining fingers supported on the cheek for stability.

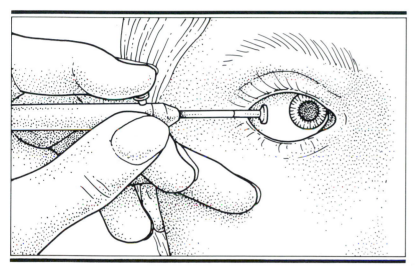

3. The index finger is used to depress the button on the linear ophthalmodynamometer to allow movement of the shaft.

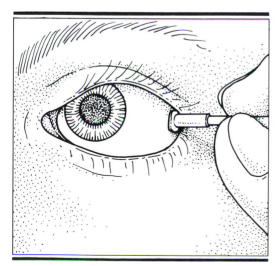

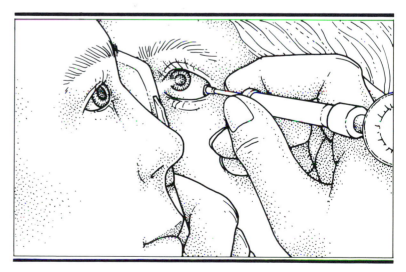

4. The footplate of the ophthalmodynamometer is placed tangentially on the globe with the shaft held horizontally. Allow the shaft to rest in the lateral canthus for stability.

5. ODM being performed with one examiner and the direct ophthalmoscope.

Binocular Indirect Ophthalmoscope: Try both the +14 D and +20 D condensing lens to see which gives you the preferred view of the artery. Locate a large artery on the disc near the rim and have the assistant place the footplate on the globe, 1 cm behind the limbus. Instruct the assistant to begin applying steady pressure when the view of the artery is clear and stable (Fig. 6). Stop as soon as the first pulse (diastole) is seen and record the measurement in grams directly off the scale. Zero the instruments and repeat the procedure. Increase the pressure until the pulse occurs (diastole) then disappears (systole), remove the instrument quickly, and record. Take three separate readings for each eye, waiting 1 minute between each, discard any disparate results, and average the rest.

Interpretation. Readings in grams of pressure approximate but are not equal to those in mm Hg. By using a nomogram the readings in grams are plotted against intraocular pressures to arrive at mm Hg. However, the absolute values in grams are usually used since the relative difference between the eyes is the most important factor.

The diastolic arterial reading is approximately 45 to 60% of the diastolic blood pressure measurement. This gives expected values between 30 and 50 mm Hg. The systolic arterial measure is approximately 54 to 70% of the brachial artery blood pressure, normally between 60 and 85 mm Hg. A greater than 20% decrease from the expected is considered a positive test. For borderline cases, repeat the test at a subsequent visit with the patient standing. For an individual with hypertension, a 20 to 25% reduction is needed before the diagnosis of carotid artery insufficiency can be made. A 20% increase in the diastolic measure as compared to the diastolic blood pressure is suggestive of increased intracranial pressure.

In normal individuals there should be no more than a 10% difference between the eyes. When a 15% difference is seen, the test is considered a positive indicator of carotid artery insufficiency. Any positive test is an indicator for prompt referral to the patient's internist, neurologist, cardiologist, or vascular surgeon.

Contraindications/Complications. Care must be used whenever ODM is performed, especially since the individuals being tested probably have a compromised vascular system. The procedure should not take more than 5 to 6 seconds once pressure to the globe is initiated. If the view of the artery is lost or a pulse not seen after 6 seconds, stop the test and begin again.

Because of a concern for permanently occluding a retinal artery during a systolic phase of the procedure, some authors propose that only diastolic readings be taken. However, it has been shown that without systolic readings some individuals with carotid artery insufficiency will be missed. These individuals may have equal diastolic ODM readings, and any difference between the two eyes may not manifest until systolic ODM measurements are taken. A recommended approach is to take diastolic readings first and if a 20% difference between the two eyes is seen, the test is positive and systolic readings are not indicated. If the test is negative or inconclusive, systolic ODM readings are warranted, especially in symptomatic individuals.

Proper technique and patient cooperation are crucial to obtaining accurate results. Misalignment of the footplate or angulation of the instrument will negatively affect the results. Any of these may also cause the eye to be displaced, losing the ophthalmoscopic view. Cataracts, media opacities, or poor fixation, which affect the examiner's view of the retinal arteries, can affect the results.

Relative contraindications to the test include a recently operated eye, ectopia lentis, recent penetrating or blunt injuries, history of retinal tears or retinal detachment, high myopia with peripheral retinal weakness, or neovascularization of the iris or retina.

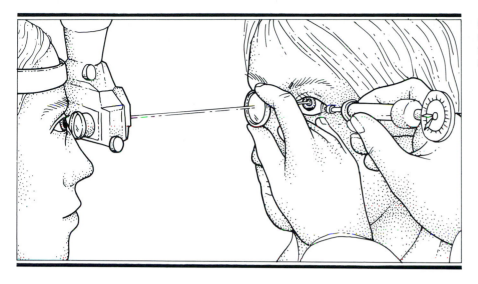

6. ODM using the binocular indirect ophthalmoscope as performed with two people, the examiner and an assistant.

IX Suggested Readings

American Heart Association: *Recommendations for Human Blood Pressure Determination by Sphygmomanometers*. Report of a special task force appointed by the steering committee, 1987.

Berguer R, Weiss H (eds): *The Carotid and the Eye*. New York, Praeger, 1985.

Greenberg DA: Basic evaluation of exophthalmos. *J Am Optom Assoc* 1977;**48:**1431–1433.

Joint National Committee on Detection, Evaluation, and Treatment of High Blood Pressure: 1988 report. *Arch Intern Med* 1988;**148:**1023–1038.

Kaplan NM: *Clinical Hypertension*, 4th ed. Baltimore, Williams & Wilkins, 1986.

Keeney AH: *Ocular Examination: Basis and Technique*, ed 2. St. Louis, Mosby, 1976.

Locke LC: Induced refractive and visual changes, Amos JF (ed): *Diagnosis and Management in Vision Care*. Boston, Butterworths, 1987, pp 313–367.

Miller NR (ed): *Walsh and Hoyt's Neuro-Ophthalmology*. Baltimore, Williams & Wilkins, 1988, pp 994–1017.

Pence NA: Ophthalmodynamometry. *J Am Optom Assoc* 1980;**51:**49–55.

Smith JL, Zeiper IH, Cogan DG: Observations on ophthalmodynamometry. *JAMA* 1959;**170:**1403–1407.

Terry JE (ed): *Ocular Disease: Detection, Diagnosis, and Treatment*. Springfield, IL, CC Thomas, 1984.

Wood, FA, Toole JF: Carotid artery occlusion and its diagnosis by ophthalmodynamometry. *JAMA* 1957;**165:**1264–1270.

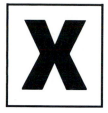

Preoperative and Postoperative Cataract Procedures

75 Interferometry

Description/Indications. The assessment of retinal visual acuity through mild to moderate ocular media opacification can be accomplished in the office with an interferometer. The potential visual acuity expected postoperatively is assessed prior to surgery (for cataract extraction, YAG laser) to prevent disappointment with the postoperative visual results and to avoid unnecessary surgery. This "potential" measurement—along with the patient's overall ophthalmic and medical status, visual needs, and surgical risk(s)—is reviewed prior to surgical intervention.

An interferometer directs two coherent light beams through pinpoint areas of the eye's optical system in Maxwellian view (Fig. 1), creating interference patterns on the retina. The spacing of this moiré fringe pattern (fringe pitch) is a function of the separation of the two pinpoint beam areas (grating angle) within the dilated pupil. Increasing the separation produces a pattern of finer and finer fringe pitch, which requires greater macular resolution (Fig. 2). The last repeatably perceived pitch or grating value, recorded in a decimal system reading, is converted to Snellen potential acuity (Fig. 3). The entire procedure is independent of refractive errors, most media opacities, and spatial orientation of the retinal receptor cells.

Because the production of the interference fringe pattern depends on the amplitude of the electromagnetic wave and not the intensity of light, as little as 2% transmission of each beam is needed to obtain a reading. This characteristic makes the interferometer more valuable for assessing retinal function behind denser cataracts than other types of potential acuity meters.

There are several types of interferometers. The Haig-Streit Lotmar Visometer and Randwal IRAS H-H interferometers use white incandescent light with rotatable gratings to produce the moiré fringes. The Rodenstock Retinometer and Randwal Acuiometer models use neon–helium lasers to produce their coherent light sources. The Retinometer and Visometer are slit lamp mounted, the IRAS hand-held, and the Acuiometer table mounted.

Instrumentation. Interferometer, slit lamp, topical mydriatic solution.

Technique. In this discussion, the Lotmar Visometer is illustrated. Other types of interferometers are similar.

Dilate the patient's pupils with a topical mydriatic solution. Demonstrate the possible fringe pattern responses from the display card (Fig. 4). Explain that partial patterns may be seen and that the patient should look only for band pattern direction, ignoring aberrations or partial scotomas.

Position the well-dilated patient at the slit lamp. Do not perform any prolonged "light" testing (such as binocular indirect ophthalmoscopy or photostress) prior to the test. In a darkened room, examine the red pupillary reflex with slit lamp retroillumination (see p. 62) to locate the less dense or "clearest" area(s) in the cataract or opacity to allow for maximum light transmission. Remove the slit lamp's tonometer apparatus, mount the interferometer on the same post, and plug in its cord to the slit lamp light housing cord.

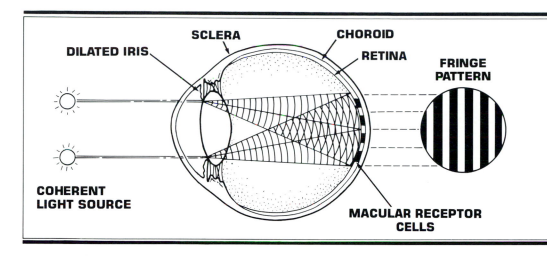

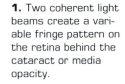

1. Two coherent light beams create a variable fringe pattern on the retina behind the cataract or media opacity.

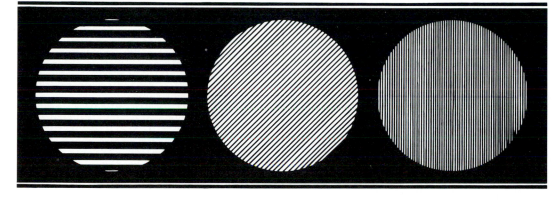

2. As the interferometer's grating angle or beam separation is increased, the fringe pattern becomes finer, requiring greater macular resolution.

DECIMAL SYSTEM	SNELLEN 6 METER TABLE	20 FOOT TABLE
1.0	6/6	20/20
0.8	5/6	20/25
0.7	6/9	20/30
0.6	5/9	15/25
0.5	6/12	20/40
0.4	5/12	20/50
0.3	6/18	20/70
0.1	6/60	20/200

3. Conversion chart: decimal fringe pitch/ pattern to potential Snellen acuity.

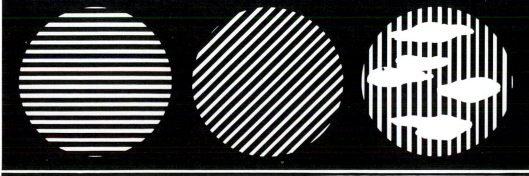

4. A pretest possible response display is demonstrated to the patient.

Set the Visometer instrument initially as follows (Fig. 5):

Lever A (filters)	set in middle position (empty/no filter)
Lever B (entrance pupil)	.5 mm
Knob C (fringe pattern)	.05
Lever D (visual field)	3.5 degrees
Handle E (orientation)	vertical
Voltage switch	5 V

Direct the interferometer light beam into the tested eye. Focus the beam axially to a fine white point on the perilimbal sclera or iris (Fig. 6A). Direct this focused beam into the pupil, remaining at the iris plane (Fig. 6B). Scan horizontally and vertically for the most transparent area in the lens, while keeping the distance to the corneal surface constant. The Maxwellian view is operating at the point where the beam is least visible, indicating greater lens transparency and light penetration. After the patient acknowledges visualization of patterned lines, switch knob B (entrance pupil) to .15 mm and lever A (filter) to green. Begin testing by increasing knob C (fringe pitch) in steps of 0.1, while asking the patient to indicate the azimuthal direction of the fringes (horizontal, vertical, obliques). Press in on handle E (orientation) to obscure the patient's view as band orientations are changed. Bracket the endpoint visual acuity level by presenting one or two fringe orientations at each level, based upon the quickness and accuracy of patient's responses. As the endpoint is approached, usually indicated by slower patient response, four consecutive correct responses are needed for the final VA potential reading. With low media transparency, it is helpful to increase the voltage to 6 or 7.5V and to remove the green filter. To ensure axial stability with only horizontal and vertical adjustment, keep the distance from the back of the slit lamp and the table's rubber cover plate constant during testing after your initial setting is made. For patients with high refractive error, if poor results occur without corrective lenses, repeat the test with the spectacle or contact lens correction.

Interpretation. The instrument's end-point fringe pitch decimal reading (knob C) is converted to Snellen acuity using the supplied conversion table. This acuity reading is the estimated postoperative expected vision result.

The interferometer generally produces more reliable results than the Potential Acuity Meter (see p. 276) in denser cataracts. Its accuracy however, also decreases as cataract density increases, resulting in some false negatives (predicted visual acuity worse than final or actual acuity). Poor dilation, which limits the examiner's ability to bypass denser cataracts, may also lead to false negatives. Tilted retinal receptors generally result in poor Snellen acuity (Stiles-Crawford anomaly); however, if these same receptors are viable, they can result in a normal interferometry reading producing false positive results (predicted visual acuity better than final or actual acuity). False positive results occur in the presence of serous detachment of the macular sensory retina, cystoid macular edema, geographic atrophy of the macular retinal pigment epithelium, visual field defects that involve fixation, macular hole or cyst, recent postoperative retinal detachment, and amblyopia. Viable parafoveal tissue stimulation yielding a test response is believed to be the basis for these false positives. Interferometry, along with the ocular and retinal examination, are all considered in the final visual potential prediction.

Because of poorer oblique visual acuity, it is controversial whether only horizontal and vertical orientations should be used in testing. The PAM (see p. 276) is considered the best instrument to test amblyopic eyes, but theoretically the interferometer can also be utilized by using the 1.5-degree setting on lever D (visual field) to test pure macular integrity.

Contraindications/Complications. This is a noninvasive test that presents no danger to the patient. Eyes that do not dilate well or those in which pupil dilation is contraindicated can test poorly.

CONTROLS	INITIAL SETTINGS	PROCEDURE
A FILTER LEVEL GREY EMPTY GREEN	MIDDLE POSITION (NO FILTER)	Set to green filter; may have to remove with dense opacity.
B ENTRANCE PUPIL .5 .15	.5 MM	Set at .15 mm.
C FRINGE PITCH 0–2.0	.05	Increase in .1 steps.
D VISUAL FIELD 3.5° 2.5° 1.5°	3.5°	Leave at 3.5°.
E ORIENTATION	VERTICAL	Press in on handle when changing orientation.
F SLIT LAMP VOLTAGE	5 V	Increase to 6 or 7.5 V with low media transparency.

5. Interferometer's initial settings and procedure.

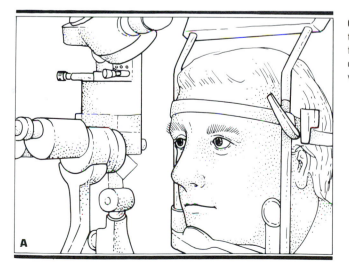

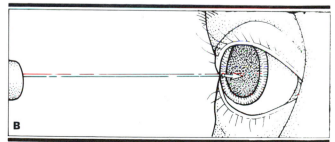

6. A. (left) After the patient is properly positioned in the slit lamp, the light beam is focused at the edge of the iris. **B.** (below) The focused iris beam is then shifted laterally to the pupillary center or toward a less densely opacified area using only horizontal and vertical movements.

76 Potential Acuity Meter

Description/Indications. The assessment of retinal visual acuity through mild to moderate ocular media opacification is performed in the office with a Potential Acuity Meter (PAM). Cataract and other surgical procedures correcting media opacification should be preceded by measurement of the potential visual acuity to prevent unnecessary procedures, surgical risks, and postoperative acuity disappointment.

The PAM uses a Maxwellian view optical system to project a bright miniature Snellen acuity chart through an aerial aperture of 0.1 mm onto the retina (Fig. 1). This single beam can be directed through less dense or "window" areas of mild to moderate opacities to maximize beam transmission. The internally projected eyechart has letters ranging from 20/400 to 20/20 presented simultaneously. An additional number chart is also available. The patient identifies these familiar eyechart letters during testing for the examiner. Since the PAM depends entirely on the intensity of the light reaching the retina for best response, its reliability diminishes with increasing density of the cataract or opacity.

The Guyton-Minkowski PAM (Fig. 2) is slit lamp mounted and portable, utilizing an incandescent light source. The projected Snellen chart is achromatically imaged and "folded" by internal condensing lenses and prisms. A spherical equivalent correction dial with − 10 to + 13 diopter powers is incorporated for best visual performance. This dioptric dial, along with an external examiner's Snellen chart, facilitate testing. The on–off switch and facial illumination knob are also located on this instrument panel.

Instrumentation. PAM, slit lamp, topical mydriatic solution.

Technique. Dilate the pupils with topical mydriatic solution. With slit lamp retroillumination (see p. 62), scan the patient's dilated pupillary red reflex for clear "windows" or less dense opacification. Do not perform any prolonged "light" testing (such as binocular indirect ophthalmoscopy or photostress) before the procedure. Attach the PAM to the slit lamp following the manufacturer's guide. With the Haig-Streit-style slit lamp, this involves placing the mounting pin of the PAM into the focusing post hole, orienting its alignment notch with the slit lamp's alignment tab. Tighten the locking knob and plug the cord into an electrical outlet, then switch the instrument on.

Position the dilated patient in the slit lamp, with his or her refractive spherical equivalent dialed in on the PAM. Direct the patient to close the eyes as the perpendicularly directed light beam is focused on the eyelid (Fig. 3A). Upon opening the lids and with slight downward gaze (approximately 14 degrees), the patient should see the illuminated chart (Fig. 3B). Place the beam in a "window area" using mainly horizontal and vertical movements, with slight inward movement if required (Fig. 4A). Make fine patient subjective alignment adjustments to obtain uniform illumination of the silvered eye chart. Ask the patient to read the chart starting with the largest letters. As the end-point of acuity measurement is approached, attempt a brief subjective vision improvement using the dioptric dial. Two or more letters read correctly at the end-point identifies the final potential acuity reading.

Interpretation. False negative results (predicted visual acuity worse than final acuity) are associated with dense opacification (Fig. 4B) and subsequent poor light penetration with the PAM. Use of the interferometer is then indicated (see p. 272). If this is unsuccessful, entoptic phenomena, electrodiagnostic testing, or ophthalmic ultrasound testing (see p. 236) may be considered.

False positive results (predicted visual acuity better than final acuity) have been found with cystoid macular edema, serous detachments of the macula, and age-related macular degeneration. All allow for the possibility of healthy parafoveal tissue stimulation, yielding an erroneous reading. Maculopathy-related visual acuity loss produces more false positives with the interferometer than the PAM, but still the examiner's fundus impression and patient history are important in preventing false predictions and unnecessary surgery. The brightness level of the PAM chart, greater than a normal Snellen chart, may also contribute to false positive results.

The measurements obtained are intended as "estimates" of the expected acuity. No exact correlation exists.

Contraindications/Complications. This is a noncontact procedure that presents no danger to the patient. Eyes that do not dilate well or those in which dilation is contraindicated can test poorly. Overaccommodation due to closeness of the instrument to the eye, especially with younger patients, may require adjustment of the dioptric dial.

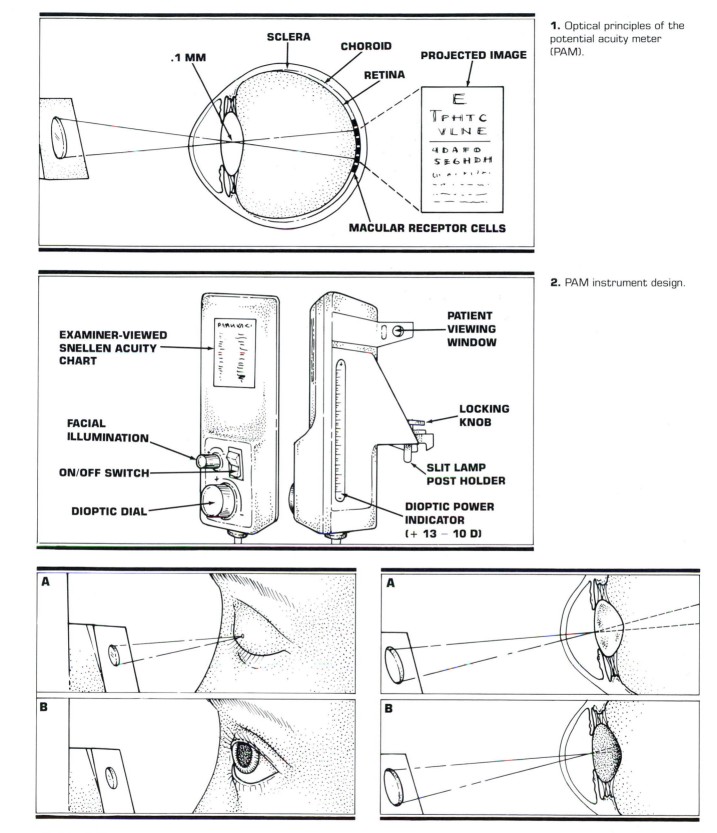

1. Optical principles of the potential acuity meter (PAM).

2. PAM instrument design.

3. A.(top) After proper patient positioning, the light beam is focused on the patient's eyelid. **B.** (bottom) The patient is asked to open the eyes and look into the illuminated opening.

4. A. (top) The beam is directed through the least dense window area of the cataract or media opacity. **B.** (bottom) A dense cataract will not allow light transmission to the retina. This is an example of a possible false negative result.

77 A-Scan Ultrasound: Biometry

Description/Indications. The axial length of the eye can be measured with quantitative A-scan ultrasound. An ultrasonic transducer crystal, placed in front of the eye, emits and receives sound waves along the patient's optical axis. This probe crystal's rapid emission of sound waves, alternating with emission suppression and subsequent retinal-rebound wave reception, yields a time–amplitude recording. This is then converted into an electrical distance measurement and displayed on an oscilloscope screen along with other pertinent patient information (Fig. 1). Each spike on the graph represents a specific ocular tissue area (Fig. 2). The deflected lines represent the measured time intervals between echoes recorded along the optical axis.

To arrive at the proper intraocular lens (IOL) dioptic power used for implantation, the examiner combines the linear value of axial length as determined by A-scan with the two major corneal meridian curvature measurements, an anterior or posterior IOL "constant" adjustment value (surgeon-selective), and the desired final spectacle lens power.

A hand-held or slit lamp mounted probe/transducer is connected by a cable to a microprocessor with a display screen (Fig. 3) which gathers, stores, and calculates all necessary IOL implantation data. The transducer tip has a small light emitting diode (LED) to assist patient fixation. An attached printer for one-dimensional linear tracing is interconnected for permanent recording and interoffice communication.

Instrumentation. A-scan ultrasound unit with printer, keratometer, topical ophthalmic anesthetic solution, alcohol swabs, slit lamp.

Technique. Take multiple, accurate keratometry readings on a calibrated, focused instrument prior to ultrasound measurements. Record the average of each of the two major corneal meridians without noting the axis.

Turn the ultrasound unit on and enter the day's date and patient's name (if desired). If not recently done, calibrate the instrument following the manufacturer's instructions. The probe should be aseptized with a sterile alcohol swab, allowing sufficient time to air dry (2 to 3 minutes). Anesthetize both corneas with a topical ophthalmic anesthetic agent (such as proparacaine hydrochloride). Set the instrument in the automatic mode if available, or in the manual mode. Use the manual mode if no readings are obtainable in the automatic mode or if closer analysis of the "in vivo" reading is needed. Place the unit's pedal on the floor by your foot. Select the proper crystalline lens status entry (cataract, aphakic, or normal) for the tested eye. An improper lens status selection (phakic versus aphakic) in the automatic mode will cause the instrument to continue to search for the presence or absence of a lens structure, never selecting an "acceptable" reading. Ask the patient to fixate a target straight ahead with the nontested eye or directly at the probe's LED with the tested eye if better fixation is needed.

Two techniques for probe positioning are described.

Hand-Held: Secure the patient's upper lid gently against the superior orbital rim with the thumb of the nontesting hand, and secure the lower lid against the inferior rim with the ring finger of the opposite hand. Using the thumb, index finger, and side of the middle finger to hold the probe, stabilize your hand on the inferior orbital rim and place the tip of the probe perpendicular to and in light contact with the corneal apex. Attempt to align the probe tip with the optical axis, avoiding pressure that could create corneal compression (Fig. 4).

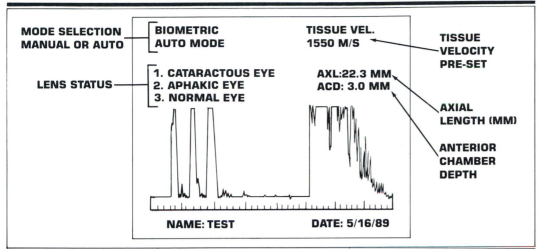

1. A-scan's oscilloscope screen with a diagram of an acceptable reading.

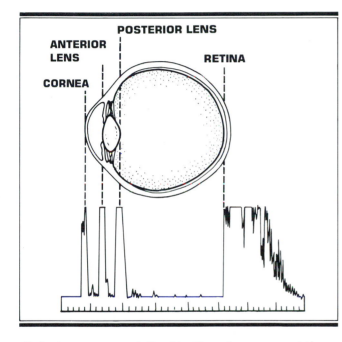

2. Anatomy—screen relationship. These lines represent the measured time intervals between tissue echoes along the patient's optical axis.

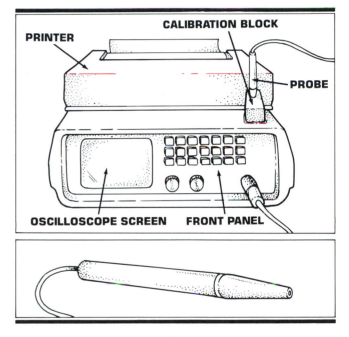

3. A-scan/biometry unit.

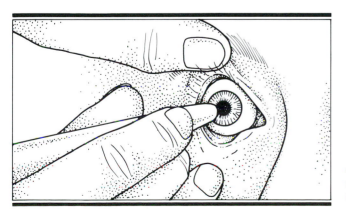

4. Hand-held probe technique. With the hand securely positioned on the lower orbital rim, the transducer probe is placed in light contact with the cornea.

Slit Lamp Mounted Probe: Place the probe in the applanation tonometer biprism holder and position the patient in the slit lamp. Ask the patient to fixate straight ahead with the opposite eye. Move the probe forward, similar to the technique of applanation tonometry (see p. 50), using the joystick to perpendicularly align and lightly touch the corneal apex (Fig. 5). Make every effort to avoid corneal compression.

Corneal contact will cause a continuous emission of ultrasonic waves, signified by repeated "beeping" sounds. With proper corneal alignment the screen, positioned for simultaneous viewing, should display approximately equal spike heights for the cornea, anterior and posterior lens surfaces, and retina (Fig. 2). Subtle probe realignment may be needed at times to produce this result.

The automatic mode accessory makes the judgment of spike equality and reading acceptability and signals this by emitting a high-pitched sound. This is followed by cessation of the beeping sounds and a freezing of the screen recording (variations exist between units). In the manual mode, the examiner views the screen simultaneously and freezes an acceptable frame with depression of the foot pedal. After a poor reading, the anterior chamber depth (ACD) reading location is replaced by a message indicating where the first problem occurred (Fig. 6A, B). Multiple readings are obtained and averaged to ensure accuracy; a minimum of six readings per eye is suggested. After each reading, regardless of mode, depress the foot pedal to clear the graph before taking the next reading. Make sure that the anterior chamber depth measurements (ACD) are consistent between readings to ensure against corneal compression.

Most A-scan units utilize a microprocessor to calculate IOL power. A printed readout of the best scan diagram is made, accompanied by the IOL calculations. Perform biometry on both eyes to allow for comparison. The average expected axial length difference is 0.2 to 0.3 mm between eyes. If inconsis-

tencies exist recheck for corneal compression.

Interpretation. Three of the more common methods used for IOL power calculations are linear regression, Binkhorst, and Colenbrander. To perform the calculations, select the method used by the surgeon (Fig. 7). The average of each major keratometry meridian (K1 and K2), the average ultrasound axial length (AXL), the surgeon's anterior and posterior IOL constants (A1 and A2), and the desired final postoperative spectacle lens power (7 and 9), are entered into the microprocessor in their respective screen spaces. Multiple IOL dioptric powers are automatically calibrated for spectacle powers at the desired Rx and for powers above and below the specified Rx value. Both anterior and posterior chamber lens values are calibrated. Two IOLs (anterior and posterior chamber) with the appropriate powers are brought to surgery, since a surgical plan calling for posterior chamber implantation may have to be changed to an anterior chamber design during surgery. When the final desired spectacle Rx is greater than +2.00 diopters from Plano power, additional methods of calculation need to be considered and compared.

Contraindications/Complications. This procedure is noninvasive and safe. It requires that the examiner be accurate and precise with all readings and calculations. Repetition with consistent readings is the key to success. Caution should be exercised to prevent corneal compression with the probe, creating an artificially shallowed anterior chamber depth and subsequent underestimation of actual axial length. Poor patient fixation, which may be reduced by using the probe's fixation light, can lead to poor results. Small pupils with significant lenticular opacification may require pupil dilation if initial testing is poor. An induced corneal abrasion or anesthetic reaction are possible but rare. Infrequent or incorrect calibration of any instrument, or incorrect data entry, can yield poor postsurgical acuity results

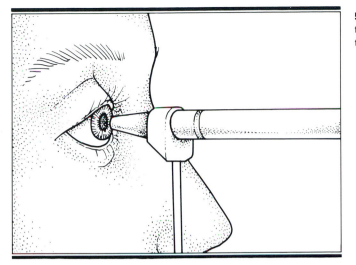

5. Slit lamp mounted probe technique. With the probe positioned in the tonometer holder, its tip is placed in light contact with the cornea using the joystick.

→ **1. CATARACTOUS EYE**
 2. APHAKIC EYE
 3. NORMAL EYE

→ **1. CATARACTOUS EYE**
 2. APHAKIC EYE
 3. NORMAL EYE

6. A. Unacceptable biometry reading showing poor retinal echo.

6. B. Unacceptable biometry reading showing poor lens echoes.

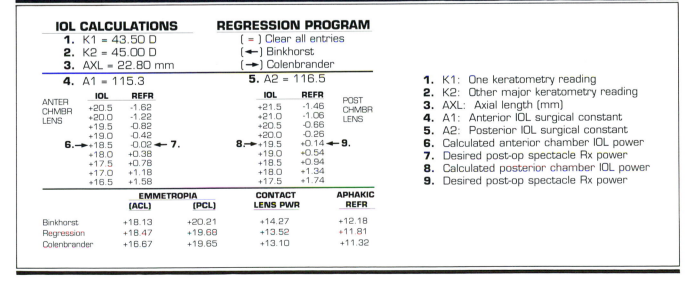

IOL CALCULATIONS

1. K1 = 43.50 D
2. K2 = 45.00 D
3. AXL = 22.80 mm
4. A1 = 115.3

REGRESSION PROGRAM

[=] Clear all entries
[←] Binkhorst
[→] Colenbrander

5. A2 = 116.5

ANTER CHMBR LENS	IOL	REFR
	+20.5	-1.62
	+20.0	-1.22
	+19.5	-0.82
	+19.0	-0.42
6.→	+18.5	-0.02 ← 7.
	+18.0	+0.38
	+17.5	+0.78
	+17.0	+1.18
	+16.5	+1.58

	IOL	REFR	POST CHMBR LENS
	+21.5	-1.46	
	+21.0	-1.06	
	+20.5	-0.66	
	+20.0	-0.26	
8.→	+19.5	+0.14 ←9.	
	+19.0	+0.54	
	+18.5	+0.94	
	+18.0	+1.34	
	+17.5	+1.74	

	EMMETROPIA		CONTACT LENS PWR	APHAKIC REFR
	(ACL)	(PCL)		
Binkhorst	+18.13	+20.21	+14.27	+12.18
Regression	+18.47	+19.68	+13.52	+11.81
Colenbrander	+16.67	+19.65	+13.10	+11.32

1. K1: One keratometry reading
2. K2: Other major keratometry reading
3. AXL: Axial length (mm)
4. A1: Anterior IOL surgical constant
5. A2: Posterior IOL surgical constant
6. Calculated anterior chamber IOL power
7. Desired post-op spectacle Rx power
8. Calculated posterior chamber IOL power
9. Desired post-op spectacle Rx power

7. Example of IOL calculations.

78 Suture Cutting

Description/Indications. Current cataract surgery suturing techniques consist of the more common interrupted pattern (Fig. 1A) and the running or continuous design (Fig. 1B). The interrupted suture technique consists of six to eight radially placed sutures located between the 10 and 2 o'clock position above the superior limbus closing the corneal/scleral surgical incision. After tying each suture (Fig. 2A), the knot is rotated superiorly abutting the scleral suture opening (Fig. 2B). The knot's loose ends are trimmed (Fig. 2C) and then covered with the surgical conjunctival flap (peritomy) (Fig. 2D).

Running or continuous sutures connect the cornea and sclera using a single interlacing/shoestring-like suture. Nondissolvable 10/0 nylon suture material is the most commonly used material for both techniques.

Suturing techniques can affect the final shape of the cornea (Fig. 3A). Ideal suturing technique places the sutures equidistant, at the same tissue depth, with equal tissue involvement on each side of the incision, positioned as radially as possible and tied with equal tension. Tight wound closure will steepen the central cornea in the meridian of the tight suture(s) since the circumference of the globe is decreased, resulting in a shortened radius of curvature. Indicators of tight sutures are induced postoperative corneal astigmatism, corneal wrinkling, perisutural tissue necrosis, and posterior gaping of the wound. With the interrupted suturing technique, wound compression results in a shortening (steepening) of the vertical corneal meridian, yielding with-the-rule astigmatism (Fig. 3B), in contrast to the running/continuous suturing technique, which usually results in against-the-rule astigmatism. Loose interrupted suture(s) can create wound gap with subsequent against-the-rule astigmatism (Fig. 3C). Cutting tight suture(s) in the meridian 90 degrees from the correcting minus cylinder axis reduces the astigmatic value. Therefore, a patient with 3 diopters of induced postoperative refractive cylinder at axis 180 will require cutting of the interrupted suture at the 12-o'clock (axis 90) position.

The appropriate time for cutting sutures is variable. It is dependent upon the closure technique, suture material, the amount of topical steroid used postoperatively, and the quality of healing. Good wound healing exhibits closed incision edges, the absence of an overlying conjunctival bleb, and a negative Seidel test (see p. 290). Thus, both the sutures and wound need to be examined before sutures are cut. If the wound appears healed, removal can be attempted. It is rare to cut sutures before 6 weeks postoperatively. This removal of sutures to adjust induced astigmatism is usually accomplished within 3 months.

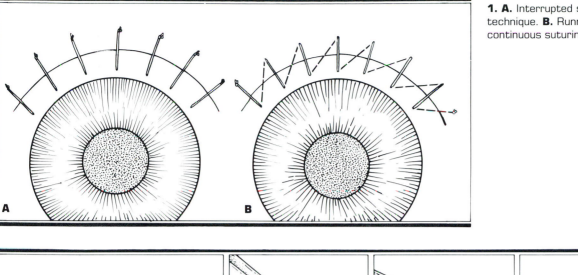

1. A. Interrupted suturing technique. **B.** Running/ continuous suturing technique.

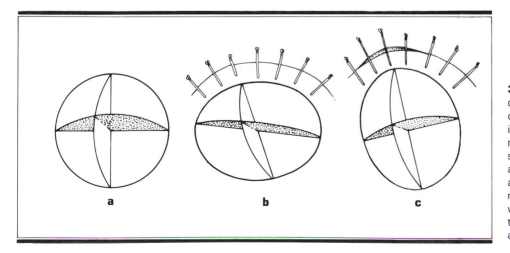

2. A. Sutures are tied to close the surgical incision **B.** The suture knot is grasped and rotated superiorly abutting the scleral suture opening. **C.** The knot's loose ends are trimmed. **D.** The suture lies flat as the surgical conjunctival flap is repositioned over the incision.

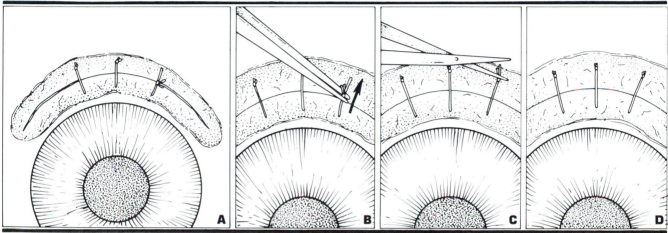

3. (a) The design and tightness of the sutures affects the final corneal curvature. This cornea is spherical. (b) Tight interrupted sutures will shorten and steepen the vertical meridian(s), inducing with-the-rule astigmatism. (c) Loose interrupted sutures can create wound gap and a flattened vertical meridian, with resultant against-the-rule-astigmatism.

Instrumentation:. Keratometer, slit lamp, blade breaker and blade or scalpel, topical ophthalmic anesthetic, broad-spectrum antibiotic ophthalmic drops, jeweler's forceps, sterile fluorescein strip, sterile saline solution.

Technique. Obtain keratometry readings and the present refractive status. With this information, use the slit lamp to identify the surgical suturing technique and the probable tight suture(s). This suture(s) should be located approximately 90 degrees from the correcting minus cylinder. Topically anesthesize the globe by instilling 2 drops of topical tetracaine solution, or place a cotton-tipped applicator saturated with topical proparacaine hydrochloride at the suture site for 15 to 30 seconds. Place 2 drops of a broad-spectrum antibiotic solution in the eye prophylactically before cutting any suture. Position the patient in the slit lamp with instructions to keep his forehead firmly against the headstrap. Have the patient look slightly downward, securing the upper lid with the thumb of your noncutting hand (Fig. 4A). Hold the cutting instrument in your opposite hand. Brace the instrument hand on the patient's bridge of the nose or inferior orbital rim. From a perpendicular direction move the blade forward, lightly contacting the inferior edge of the suture (corneal side) through the conjunctiva with the blade tip (Fig. 4B). The taut suture should "snap" upward when cut. The superior area will show the residual subconjunctival radial suture above the surgical incision (Fig. 4C) while the inferior suture end should disappear into the sclera. The suture usually remains subconjunctival and is removed only if it penetrates the conjunctival surface. Perform a Seidel test to ensure that no wound leakage has been induced. Instill 2 additional antibiotic drops into the eye following the procedure for further prophylaxis.

Running suture cutting can have greater tension-releasing effect and increased variability than the interrupted type. Usually, a longer waiting period is used prior to cutting these sutures. Since running sutures techniques vary, more knowledge of the specific surgical technique used and the expected healing process is necessary prior to intervention.

Interpretation. A patient presenting 6 weeks postoperatively with induced corneal astigmatism may require one or more sutures cut. For example, if the keratometry readings are 44.50 D at 180 and 48.00 D at 90, and the refractive correction is $+2.00 - 3.00 \times 180$, the tight suture(s) at the same axis (90) as the steepest k-reading (90 degrees away from the minus cylinder axis) should be cut (Fig. 5). Usually the refractive cylinder axis and the keratometry axis are approximately the same. If not, single suture cutting is done based on the keratometry reading.

Sutures are rarely cut before 6 weeks postoperatively, unless one wishes to correct a very high induced cylinder at the fourth or fifth week. Expect a 1.50 to 2.00 D cylinder change with each suture cut. A maximum of two sutures are cut at one session, and this is only done in cases of very high induced astigmatism (6 to 8 D). Cutting more than two sutures at one time reduces refractive predictability and increases the chance of wound gap. A small to moderate amount of residual with-the-rule astigmatism remaining after surgery will reduce over the years as healing continues.

Contraindications/Complications. Premature suture cutting prior to proper healing can lead to poor wound closure (wound gap), subsequent aqueous leakage, and possible endophthalmitis. Improper sterile or surgical technique may lead to secondary external and/or internal infection. Incorrect suture cutting calculations and selection can yield a less than desirable astigmatic result. A subconjunctival hemorrhage may result from this procedure and the patient should be so advised.

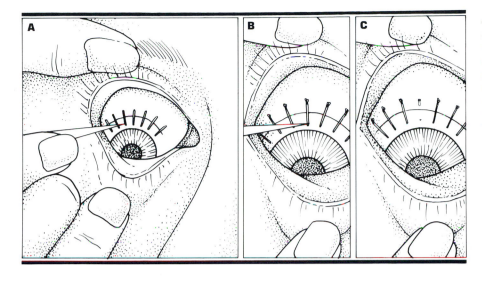

4. A. The patient's lids are secured and the blade-holding hand is stabilized. **B.** The blade tip is gently passed through the conjunctiva to nick the inferior edge of the tight suture. **C.** The loosened residual suture is seen above the incision line, while the inferior end retracts back into the scleral suture opening.

5. An example of interrupted suture's induced astigmatism correction.

Post-Op K Reading 44.50×180/48.00×90
Post-Op Refraction +2.00−3.00×180 20/20

Cut Suture at Axis 90°
(90° from correcting minus cylinder axis)

Post-Suture Cut K-Reading 44.50×180/46.25×90

Post-Suture Cut Refraction +0.75−1.00×180 20/20

79   Suture Barb Removal

Description/Indications. Sutures used to close cataract surgery incisions can later become elevated to produce symptomatic irritation. The frequently used nondissolvable 10/0 nylon sutures have the potential to weaken, stretch, break, or rotate with time. During surgery, interrupted suture knots are rotated superiorly abutting the scleral suture openings, and then covered with the surgical conjunctival flap. The suture knot or broken suture end can rotate, elevate, and perforate the bulbar conjunctiva as a barb; to cause foreign body sensation, marked discomfort, or a secondary papillary reaction of the superior palpebral conjunctiva. A loose protruding suture with good wound closure should be removed. Two to three months postoperatively is the desired waiting period for relatively safe, uncomplicated suture barb removal. In some instances, a bandage soft contact lens is fit over the sutures to maintain patient comfort, allowing more time for further wound healing prior to suture removal. Symptomatic elevated sutures frequently have a small area of surrounding conjunctival edema, elevation, and injection accompanied by a fine mucous tag on the barb itself (Fig. 1A,B,C). Three types of sutures are usually responsible for this irritation. It can be an elevated knot of an intact suture, an elevated knot of a broken suture, or the knotless end of a broken suture.

Instrumentation. Topical anesthetic, broad-spectrum topical ophthalmic antibiotic solution, slit lamp, lid speculum, sterile jeweler's forceps, scalpel or blade-breaker with razor blade, sterile cotton-tipped applicator.

Technique. Locate the involved suture with the slit lamp and identify the suturing pattern as interrupted or running (see p. 282). Attempt to determine whether the barb is the result of a broken suture (knot or loose end) or a rotated, protruding but intact suture. Make sure the wound is well healed and the globe is otherwise not infected or inflamed. Instill 1 or 2 drops of a broad-spectrum antibiotic solution prior to beginning barb removal. Topically anesthetize the globe using either the more potent tetracaine ophthalmic drops or a sterile cotton-tipped applicator saturated with proparacaine hydrochloride applied directly to the barb area for 15 to 30 seconds.

Align the patient properly at the slit lamp with instructions to keep the forehead firmly against the headstrap rest. Depending upon the degree of difficulty of the suture removal as well as patient cooperation, either a sterile lid speculum (see p. 90) or the examiner's or assistant's fingers can be used to secure the eyelids. Without a speculum, ask the patient to look downward and secure the upper lid against the superior orbital rim with the thumb of the noncutting hand. Stabilize the opposite hand, which is holding the instrument, on the patient's bridge of the nose or inferior orbital rim, depressing the lower lid with your ring finger simultaneously. Ask the patient to continue looking downward throughout the procedure.

In the case of a broken interrupted suture, working with the slit lamp, grasp the knot with the jeweler's forceps and gently pull the entire suture out (Fig. 2). If only the knotless end is visible (Fig. 3A), have an assistant hold the eyelids or use a lid speculum. Hold the jeweler's forceps with the noncutting hand and stabilize the other hand on the patient's nose or inferior orbital rim, holding a bladed instrument. Gently grasp the loose suture end with the forceps and pull upward, exposing as much of neck of the suture as possible (Fig. 3B). Trim the suture by passing the sharp edge of the blade under the forceps as close as possible to the conjunctival surface in a direction away from the cornea. The cut end should snap back into the scleral opening (Fig. 3C). Instill additional antibiotic drops after this procedure. A careful Seidel test (see p. 290) should be performed before dismissing the patient. Do not attempt to pull the entire suture out by the knotless end, as the internal knot will be forced to travel through the narrow scleral suture canal, possibly widening it and creating potential aqueous leakage.

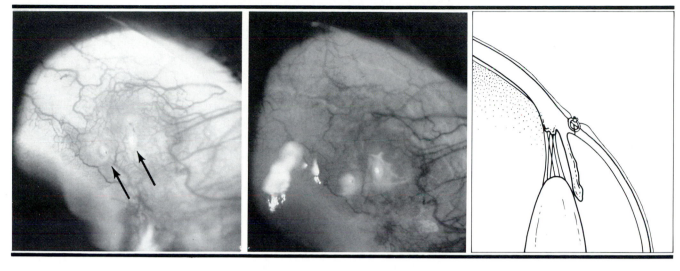

1. A. Protruding suture barbs (*see also* Color Plate 79—1.A.) (Courtesy of David E. Magnus, OD.)

1. B. Same protruding suture barbs seen with fluorescein and the cobalt filter. (*See also* Color Plate 79—1.B.) (Courtesy of David E. Magnus, OD.)

1. C. Cross-section of barb showing protrusion through the conjunctival surface.

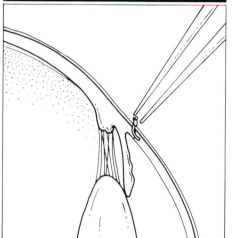

2. The broken suture barb is grasped by the knot with jeweler's forceps and gently pulled out.

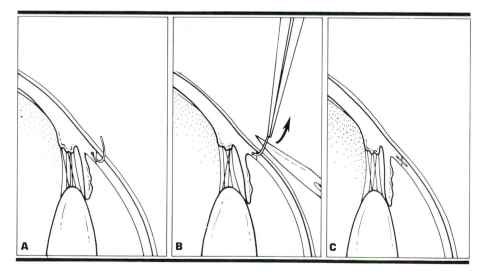

3. A. Protruding knotless suture end. **B.** Grasp the suture end with forceps, pull upward to extend and expose it, and then cut with a blade at its base. **C.** After the suture is cut, it snaps back inward, becoming subconjunctival.

In the case of an unbroken interrupted suture that has eroded through the conjunctiva (Fig. 4A), first gently pull on it with the sterile jeweler's forceps to determine if it is fragile enough to break. If not, gently grasp it with the forceps and lift it upward away from the conjunctival surface sufficiently to allow the sharp-bladed instrument tip to be passed under it (Fig. 4B). With an away-from-cornea motion, cut the suture on either side of the knot using the sterile blade breaker or scalpel. Grasp the knotted end of the cut suture with the forceps and pull gently for removal (Fig. 4C). Instill additional antibiotic drops. Perform the Seidel test.

Running suture barb repair is similar, except that the suture has to be cut at two points on either side of the protruding barb. Once the suture is cut twice, use the forceps to remove the free segment. Familiarize yourself with the specific running suture pattern before making any cuts.

Contraindications/Complications. Wound leakage caused by wound gap or dehiscence is possible if sutures are removed prior to adequate postoperative healing. Leakage is also possible from the suture opening where the knot or knotless end of the suture is pulled out. Some practitioners advocate pulling the exposed knotless end of a broken suture, when no knot is visible, back through the scleral suture canal, anterior chamber, corneal-scleral junction, and out, followed by several days of topical antibiotic drops. These patients require close follow-up for aqueous leakage. Tissue "openings" or technique injury may both cause secondary bacterial infection. The Seidel test and topical broad-spectrum antibiotics must be utilized to safeguard against these sequellae.

Since different running suture techniques exist and since the cutting of a running suture can have more tension-releasing effect on an eye than an interrupted suture, extra care must be taken. Be sure that the area has had more than adequate time to heal and that the specific running suture technique and its repair technique are known to the examiner. When in doubt concerning suture removal, consult the surgeon whenever possible.

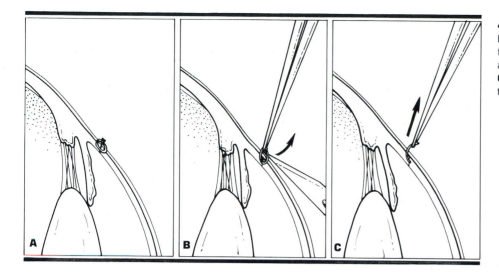

4. A. Intact suture as protruding barb. **B.** The suture is grasped with forceps, elevated, and then cut with a blade passed inside the loop. **C.** The cut suture is grasped with the jeweler's forceps and removed.

80   Seidel Test

Description/Indications. The Seidel test is used in evaluating for possible wound/aqueous leakage through an external fistula following ophthalmic surgery (such as cataract extraction), suture removal, or suspected penetrating injury to the globe. A common sign of wound/aqueous leakage is a diffuse conjunctival filtering bleb-like appearance overlying the involved area, which can frequently be difficult to distinguish from typical postoperative conjunctival chemosis. Microcystic subepithelium changes to the overlying conjunctiva may also occur. Other more obvious indicators of wound gap or a penetrating injury are peaking of the pupil with iris plugging at the wound opening, a large shift to against-the-rule astigmatism, a shallow anterior chamber, hypotony as measured by tonometry, decreased visual acuity, corneal laceration, and prolapsed intraocular contents. Wound leakage creates an unequal pressure gradient between the anterior and posterior chambers. The higher pressure in the posterior chamber may push the iris toward the gap in the surgical wound. This can lead to iris prolapse and/or pupillary block secondary to a forwardly displaced vitreous.

If the Seidel test is positive, the aqueous is best observed leaking externally using a slit lamp with a fluorescein-saturated tear film. With close observation, wound leakage is identified by clear aqueous streaming into the fluorescein, a localized brilliant green fluorescein appearance at the leakage site, or dots or bubbles forming on the involved surface (Fig. 1A and B).

Instrumentation. Slit lamp with cobalt filter, sterile fluorescein strips, sterile ophthalmic saline solution.

Technique. Three ways to perform the Seidel test are as follows:

1. Instill fluorescein from a saturated sterile strip into the eye. Carefully search the wound or sutured area with the slit lamp and cobalt blue filter for indicators of wound/aqueous leakage (clear aqueous leakage, localized brilliant hyperfluorescence, bleb-like formation, or surface bubbles (Fig. 2A). If the IOP is extremely low and no positive Seidel test is apparent, gently press the eyelid against the globe and observe the suspicious area very closely again for leakage.

2. Ask the patient to look in the opposite direction of the area to be examined. After instilling a saturated fluorescein strip, pool the fluorescein tear lake over the suspicious area using the lower lid. Examine for signs of wound/aqueous leakage (Fig. 2B).

3. Hold a sterile dry fluorescein strip in apposition to the area of concern while viewing through the slit lamp. Look for a trickle of aqueous moistening the strip (Fig. 2C). This is a less preferred technique.

Interpretation. A positive Seidel test necessitates an immediate surgical referral to prevent endophthalmitis or other postsurgical complications such as hypotony or poor visual acuity. When wound leakage is suspected, but Seidel testing is negative, intermittant leakage following intraocular pressure changes may be occurring. Referral in this case is also indicated.

Contraindications/Complications. Instillation of contaminated fluorescein or saline can lead to serious infection. Failure to instill an adequate amount of fluorescein can yield a false negative result. All manipulation of a postoperative eye or an eye with a suspected penetrating injury must be performed with extreme care.

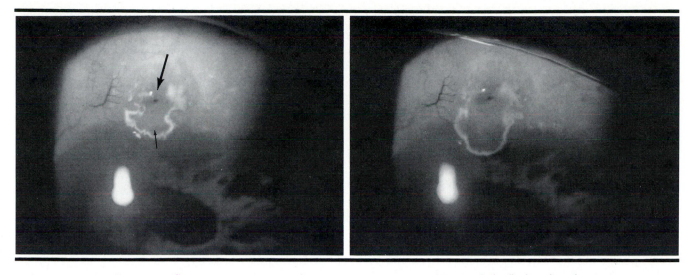

1. A. A localized brilliant green fluorescence occurs at the wound site (large arrow), with clear aqueous leaking into the fluorescein (small arrow). (*See also* Color Plate 80—1.A.) (Courtesy of David E. Magnus, OD.)

1. B. The bright fluorescein is displaced as the aqueous continues to leak. (*See also* Color Plate 80-1.B.) (Courtesy of David E. Magnus, OD.)

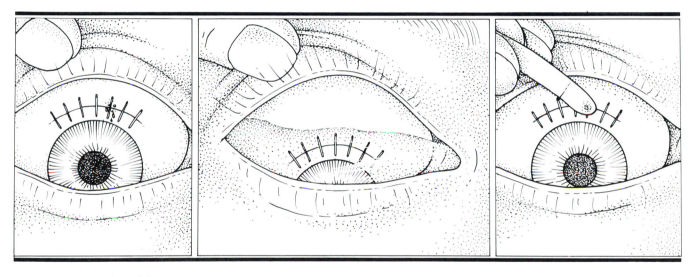

2. A. After saturation of the tear film with fluorescein dye, the wound area is closely examined for hyperfluorescence, bleb-like changes, and possible surface bubbles.

2. B. The fluorescein dye is pooled over the suspected area of leakage by using the lower eyelid, while slit lamp and cobalt filter examination is performed.

2. C. A dry sterile fluorescein dye strip is held against the suspected wound leakage area while the examiner watches for wetting of this strip from externally leaking aqueous.

X Suggested Readings

Faulkner W: Macular function testing through opacities, in Milder B (ed): Focal points 1986: Clinical modules for ophthalmologists. *Am Acad Ophthalmol* 1986;**4**:1–10.

Guyton DL: Preoperative visual acuity evaluation, in Smolin G, Friedlaender M (eds): *Int Ophthalmol Clin* 1987;**27**:140–147.

Jaffe NS: *Cataract Surgery and Its Complications.* St Louis, Mosby, 1984,

Melore GG, Accettura J: Suture barb syndrome. *South J Optom* 1987;**5**:70–73.

Minkowski JS, Guyton DL: New methods for predicting visual acuity after cataract surgery. *Ann Ophthalmol* 1984;**16**:511–516.

Pederson JE: Hypotony, in Duane T (ed): *Clinical Ophthalmology.* Hagerstown, MD, Harper & Row, 1985, vol 3, pp 1–2.

Ritch R, Shields MB, Krupin T: *The Glaucomas.* St. Louis, Mosby, 1989, pp 282–283.

Index